# Barrel Cortex

The barrel cortex contains the somatosensory representation of the whiskers on the face of the rodent and forms an early stage of cortical processing for tactile information. It is an area of great importance for understanding how the cerebral cortex works because the cortical columns that form the basic building blocks of the cerebral cortex can be seen within the barrel cortex. In this advanced graduate- and research-level text, Kevin Fox explores three main aspects of the barrel cortex: development, sensory processing, and plasticity. Initial chapters introduce the topic, describing those animals that have barrels, the functional anatomy of the system, and the cellular and synaptic physiology of the cortical microcircuit. The book concludes with a chapter covering the numerous fields where the barrel cortex is used as a model system for solving problems in other areas of research, including stroke, angiogenesis, and understanding active touch.

KEVIN FOX is currently Professor and Head of Neuroscience, and Head of Research in Biosciences at Cardiff University, as well as Director of the Experimental MRI Centre. He gained his Ph.D. in Neuroscience at the University of London and has worked in the USA at Washington University St. Louis as a McDonnell Fellow, Brown University Rhode Island, and University of Minnesota Medical School Minneapolis as an Assistant Professor.

It is almost 40 years since THOMAS WOOLSEY discoverd the barrel field in studies carried out in his father's laboratory in Wisconsin. His pioneering work with Henrick Van der Loos, Dan Simons and others has given rise to a large and growing community of scientists who find the barrel cortex an ideal system in which to study numerous questions about the brain. He continues to innovate with the barrel cortex, most recently using in-vivo imaging methods such as hyperspectral interferometry, MRI, and microPET. Tom Woolsey is currently the Director of the James L. O'Leary Division of Experimental Neurology and Neurological Surgery at Washington University St. Louis.

# Barrel Cortex

KEVIN FOX

Cardiff University, Cardiff, UK

*Foreword by*
THOMAS WOOLSEY

Washington University School of Medicine, St. Louis, MO, USA

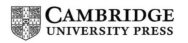

CAMBRIDGE
UNIVERSITY PRESS

CAMBRIDGE UNIVERSITY PRESS
Cambridge, New York, Melbourne, Madrid, Cape Town, Singapore, São Paulo

Cambridge University Press
The Edinburgh Building, Cambridge CB2 8RU, UK

Published in the United States of America by Cambridge University Press, New York

www.cambridge.org

First published 2008

Printed in the United Kingdom at the University Press, Cambridge

*A catalog record for this publication is available from the British Library*

ISBN 978-0-521-85217-3 hardback

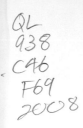

This book is dedicated to Richard, William and Anwen

# Contents

The Plates are between pages 48 and 49.

# Foreword

Understanding the brain – its structure, connections, functions and the genetic bases of these properties – remains the central riddle in biology if not science. A number of different strategies to attack this issue have focused on many aspects of the nervous system and have, at an ever-increasing pace, begun to home in on the core questions. In neuroscience, the details of the underlying mechanisms have become tractable in the past decade and a half. But, similar to understanding the relationship of atomic interactions to the weather that they must cause, taking detailed neural mechanisms back to the level of the functioning nervous system has been arduous. Nevertheless, there is great promise that in the not too distant future the problem will be solved. Seemingly complicated behaviors and strategies could be explained entirely from understanding the components, their connectivity, their functions and their cohorts.

This quest could be made easier by focus on a part of the brain that is both easily accessible and straightforward to study and that provides a "standard" context to position data of different sorts from different studies by different laboratories. Further, it would offer greater promise if it could be manipulated genetically, developmentally and behaviorally and was reasonably similar to many other brain regions so as to permit ready translation to them. In this volume, Kevin Fox (whom I have had the good fortune to know since he worked in St. Louis in the late 1980s and early 1990s) has elegantly and concisely summarized the major findings on a region of cortex that we have both studied.

The barrel cortex, the whiskers that activate it and the intervening neural pathways have been increasingly the subject of focus by a growing number of groups for some time. At the time I first described barrels in the context of somatosensory function related to the whiskers, they seemed a kind of curiosity. In 1970, with the late Hendrik Van der Loos, we advanced the hypothesis that they may be a visible form of the functional columnar organization detailed by Mountcastle and subsequently rapidly confirmed this in many cortices of many species, including humans. It is of interest that Mountcastle cited Lorente de Nó's summary based in part on original histological studies in Madrid in the 1920s as the anatomical correlate of functional columns. The barrels were quickly proven to be visible parts of columns in the rodent somatosensory cortex.

It has been personally gratifying to me to see the explosion of information that relates in many ways to the barrels and, likely, the cortex in general. However, it has also become more challenging to keep pace with new findings and to place them in a reasonable context. Fortunately, Kevin Fox has picked up this gauntlet and has produced this insightful, succinct and readable volume. It is an excellent summary of a large body of work that will be of use to those familiar with this "field" as well as to those contemplating entering it. It is with considerable personal satisfaction and admiration that I have been asked to write this Foreword. It is a privilege that I did not imagine 40 years ago, much less now.

THOMAS A. WOOLSEY
Washington University in St. Louis

# Preface

The field of barrel cortex research has grown rapidly over the past few years. Today, studies are directed not only at understanding the barrel cortex itself but also at understanding issues in related fields using the barrel cortex as a model system. In the three years it has taken to write this book, over 300 papers have been published on barrel cortex. While this rising tide of information has made writing a challenge, the fundamental studies of the preceding 34 years have provided a solid foundation and context in which to place the new work. Fortunately for me, the story has been enhanced by research in recent years and not entirely rewritten by it.

One of the reasons for writing this book has been the realization that barrel cortex research has matured to a point where a survey and a summary has become possible. The field has been characterized by classic studies that illuminate this and other areas of neuroscience and by a constant innovation in techniques and ideas. In fact, the barrel cortex has served as a test-bed system for several new methodologies, partly because of its unique and instantly identifiable form, and partly because the species that have barrels, the rodents, are the most commonly used laboratory mammal. The classic studies on the basic anatomy and physiology of this cortical area have certainly facilitated subsequent studies on barrel cortex. Two fundamental innovations have driven the field further. One is the invention of the thalamocortical slice, which has enabled detailed synaptic and cellular studies of barrel cortex. The other is the development of genetic manipulation in the mouse, which has enabled a host of new questions to be addressed, either about the function of the molecules involved in cortical processes or, by using the expression of fluorescent proteins, about the life of dendrites, spines and cellular subtypes.

As the innovation continues, many new laboratories are using barrel cortex as a system in which to explore their own particular questions without necessarily having access to, or time to research, the literature on the area being used in their experiment. A further reason for writing this book now is to provide an easy way of learning about the barrel cortex for those new to the field and to provide an easy route into the literature on which it is based. I hope that the book will be of benefit not only for those embarking for the first time on studies on barrel cortex but also for those who are already experts but need a rapid reference to direct them toward the numerous seminal discoveries that have been made in this field over the past 37 years.

KEVIN FOX
Cardiff, UK

# Acknowledgements

I am most grateful to my colleagues and friends for help with this book at various stages of its gestation. I would like to thank Asaf Keller and Egbert Welker for early discussions on the genesis of the book and for reading some of the first chapters produced. I should also like to thank Randy Bruno, Barry Connors, Peter Kind, Neil Hardingham and John Isaac for detailed comments on individual chapters. A number of people have either wittingly or unwittingly contributed to the book by discussing scientific issues with me over the years, or by carefully answering what must have seemed like bizarre emails on esoteric points of barrel cortex research. Thanks then also to Tom Woolsey, Reha Erzurumlu, Ehud Ahissar, Dirk Feldmeyer, David Kleinfeld and Mark Jacquin. Last but not least I would also like to thank Gavin Swanson for asking me to write the book, Martin Griffiths for helpful discussion and patience during its genesis and Karen Ingham for her beautiful front cover.

# *Abbreviations*

| | |
|---|---|
| 2-DG | 2-deoxyglucose |
| 5-HT | 5-hydroxytryptamine (serotonin) |
| ACI | adenylyl cyclase type 1 |
| AMPA | alpha-amino-3-hydroxy-5-methyl-4-isoxazolepropionic acid |
| APV | 2-amino-5-phosphonovaleric acid |
| BDNF | brain-derived neurotrophic factor |
| CaMKII | calcium-calmodulin kinase type II |
| CO | cytochrome oxidase |
| DiI | 1,1′-dioctadecyl-3,3,3′,3′-tetramethylindocarbocyanine perchlorate |
| DSI | depolarization-induced suppression of inhibition |
| EPSP | excitatory postsynaptic potential |
| FS | fast spiking |
| FSU | fast-spike units |
| GABA | gamma aminobutyric acid |
| GluR | glutamate receptor |
| HRP | horseradish peroxidase |
| $I_{Kca}$ | calcium-activated potassium channel current |
| $I_t$ | low-threshold calcium channel current |
| IB | intrinsic bursting |
| IPSP | inhibitory postsynaptic potential |
| LTD | long-term depression |
| LTP | long-term potentiation |
| LTS | low-threshold spiking |
| mGluR | metabotropic glutamate receptors |
| MI | motor cortical area I |
| NMDA | $N$-methyl-D-aspartate |
| PHA-L | *Phaseolus vulgaris* phytohemagglutinin |
| PKA | protein kinase A |

| | |
|---|---|
| PKC | protein kinase C |
| PLC | phospholipase C |
| POm | posterior medial thalamic nucleus |
| RA | rapidly adapting |
| RS | regular spiking |
| RSU | regular spike units |
| SA | slowly adapting |
| SI | somatosensory cortical area I |
| SII | somatosensory cortical area II |
| VPm | ventroposterior medial thalamic nucleus |

# 1

## Introduction to the barrel cortex

### 1.1    Introduction

The barrel cortex is a remarkable structure. Its form has captured the imagination of researchers for decades and its versatility has ensured that it finds a place in each new wave of neuroscience research. Since its discovery by Woolscy and Van der Loos in the early 1970s, researchers have used barrel cortex to study some of the most pressing questions in neuroscience. How does the cortex develop? How does active touch work? What makes neurons plastic? In each case, the value of the barrel cortex has been to help neuroscientists to relate structure with function through its unique and easily defined form.

In order to understand how these questions are being addressed currently, it is useful to understand some of the basic structural and functional features of the barrel cortex. The first three chapters of this book address some of the fundamental anatomy and physiology of the barrel cortex. For the expert in the field, most of what is written in these chapters will probably be quite familiar but will hopefully still serve as a useful reference to the original studies. While most of the original anatomical studies span the 1970s and 1980s, new neuroanatomical findings are still being described into the current century. Curiously, a review of this anatomical literature has not previously been written. For those less familiar with barrel cortex, the anatomical pathways linking the periphery to barrel cortex are described in Chapter 2 along with the intracortical connections, the study of which, at the time of writing, is still an active area of research. Chapter 3 deals with the cellular and synaptic physiology of the cortex. Many of these features of cortex are presumably common to all cortical areas but have been studied most completely in barrel cortex to date. We begin here by looking at three questions: What animals have barrels? What are barrels? Why are barrels important for neuroscience research?

## 1.2    System overview

### 1.2.1    *What animals have barrels?*

The barrel cortex is part of the somatosensory cortex. It receives and processes tactile information derived from the whiskers on the contralateral face of the animal. In cross-section, the cortex is a six-layered structure where the main input layer is layer IV (see Figure 1.1C, D; color version in the plate section). The barrels that give the barrel cortex its name are located in layer IV. If a horizontal section is taken through layer IV, the distinctive pattern of the barrels can be seen. The barrel pattern replicates the pattern of whiskers on the face of the animal such that each whisker corresponds to a single barrel. The topological position of the barrel within the barrel cortex is identical to the topological position of its corresponding whisker. Figure 1.1 (Plate 1 in color section) shows a picture of the whiskers on the face of a young rat together with a section through barrel cortex layer IV showing the same pattern in barrels. A pathway comprising just three synapses connects the primary afferents carrying information from the whisker follicle receptors to the cortex and the final link in this pathway is made into layer IV of the cortex to produce the characteristic barrel pattern.

The whiskers are an important tactile sense organ for rodents in the same way as the hands are an important sense organ for humans and other primates. The sensory innervation of each whisker follicle is quite high, reflecting the importance of the information they transmit. In rats, each of the larger follicles receives terminations from approximately 200 trigeminal ganglion cells and the smaller follicles closer to 50. Each muzzle contains about 36 large whiskers, which can be whisked back and forth by muscles in and around the whisker pad, and numerous smaller vibrissae, which do not move and are located around the lip and front of the snout. In total, the muzzle on each side of the face contains approximately 165–210 whiskers depending on the species and strain of animal, which corresponds to the same number of barrels in each hemisphere of the cortex. The area of cortex devoted to the whiskers reflects the high innervation levels of the whisker follicles. In the mouse, the barrel cortex represents approximately 13% of the cortical surface area in total and 69% of the somatosensory cortex (Lee and Erzurumlu, 2005). Figure 1.2 shows a picture of the relative proportions of the body representations for a human and a rodent. The vibrissae are as over-represented in rodents as the hands and lips are in humans. In absolute terms, the barrel field comprises 4.7 to 6.4 mm$^2$ in the rat and 2.1 to

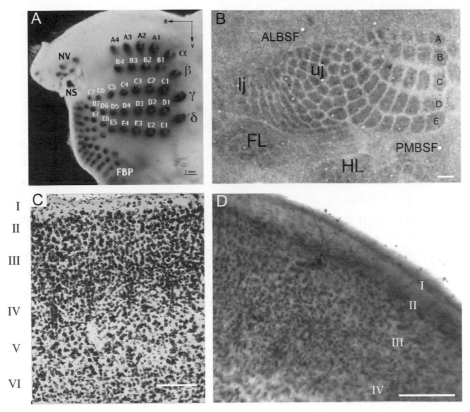

**Figure 1.1.** Somatotopic organization of the barrel cortex. A. A section through the muzzle of the rat reveals the pattern of vibrissae follicles arranged in five rows labeled A to E. The vibrissae are conventionally numbered from 1 at the back and increasingly higher numbers toward the nose (left). (Reproduced with kind permission of S. Hairdarlui and E. Ahissar.) B. The same pattern is replicated in barrel cortex. This cytochrome oxidase-labeled section through layer IV of the somatosensory cortex reveals barrels organized in five rows. The posterior medial barrel subfield (PMBSF) is on the right and corresponds to the large vibrissae that are actively whisked. The anterior lateral barrel subfield (ALBSF) is to the left and represents the smaller vibrissae around the upper jaw (uj) and nose region and lower jaw (lj). Other components of the body can also be seen such as the forelimb (FL) and hindlimb (HL). (A, B reproduced from http://www. neuro-bio.pitt.edu/barrels/pics.htm.) C. A cross-section through the cortex reveals the six-layer structure and the barrels in layer IV, which appear like staves of a barrel. (Nissl stain adapted from Woolsey and Van der Loos [1970] with kind permission of Elsevier and the authors.) D. Nissl stain through barrel cortex showing the barrels and a pyramidal neuron labeled with biocytin located at the top of layer III. (See color plate section.)

2.8 mm$^2$ in the mouse (Woolsey and Van der Loos, 1970; Welker and Woolsey, 1974). If the lower jaw, buccal pad and lip areas are included, the rat barrel field is closer to 10 mm$^2$ (Riddle and Purves, 1995). The absolute dimensions of the barrel cortex can vary from animal to animal (Riddle and Purves, 1995).

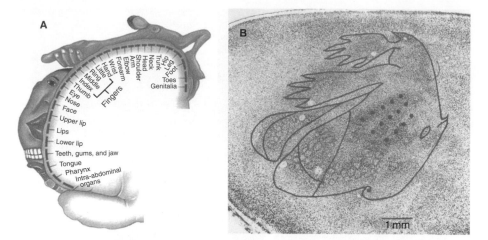

**Figure 1.2.** Relative magnification of the body surface representation in somato-sensory cortex. A. In humans, a large area of cortex is devoted to the face, lips and hand representation compared with the back, even though the surface area of the back is larger than these. This diagram shows a cross-section through the human cortex at the level of the somatosensory representation. The location of areas responding to touch on particular locations of the skin on the contralateral side of the body are labeled and the corresponding distorted map of the body drawn above the cortical surface to depict the homunculus. B. A Nissl-stained section through rat somatosensory cortex shows the location of the barrels. Electrode recordings show that the areas of the body responding to touch correspond to the drawing of the body surface superimposed on the Nissl stain. The rat cortex has an even larger proportion of its cortex devoted to the face than in humans. (Reproduced from Welker [1976], with kind permission of Wiley and the author.)

All animals that have barrels have whiskers of some sort. The whiskers themselves are located in specialized hair follicles that have a follicle sinus, and in this respect they are unlike the hair follicles that give rise to the common fur. When the sinus is pressurized with blood, the individual vibrissa is held more rigidly within the follicle and the receptors are pressed closer to the whisker, thereby increasing the receptor's sensitivity to any mechanical stimuli transmitted via the whisker (see Section 2.1).

A large number of species have whiskers, from rodents through carnivores, insectivores, bats, shrews and marsupials to primates (Table 1.1). Perhaps surprisingly, only a subset of animals with whiskers (or sinus follicles) actually has barrels.

Almost all the rodents that have been studied to date do have barrels (Table 1.1). The beaver is an exception to this rule, and it has been suggested that barrels may be less easy to distinguish the larger the brain (Woolsey *et al.*, 1975a). Squirrels have barrels that are notably less distinct than in rats and mice but none the less present.

Table 1.1. *Comparative analyses of different species that have whiskers; not all have barrels, notably the carnivores, and not all whisk*[a]

| Order/suborder or superfamily | Species common name | Barrels | Whisking | Reference |
|---|---|---|---|---|
| Rodent/Myomorpha | Mouse | Y | Y | Van der Loos and Woolsey, 1973 |
| | Rat | Y | Y | Killackey, 1973 |
| | Hamster | Y | Y | Rice *et al.*, 1985 |
| | Gerbil | Y | Y | Woolsey *et al.*, 1975a |
| | Muskrat | Y | N | Woolsey *et al.*, 1975a |
| Rodent/Sciuromorpha | Chipmunk | Y indistinct | N | Woolsey *et al.*, 1975a |
| | Grey squirrel | Y indistinct | N | Woolsey *et al.*, 1975a |
| | Prairie dog | Y indistinct | N | Woolsey *et al.*, 1975a |
| Rodent/Castorimorpha | Beaver | N | N | Woolsey *et al.*, 1975a |
| Rodent/Cavimorpha | Guinea pig | Y | N | Woolsey *et al.*, 1975a |
| | Chinchilla | Y | Y | Woolsey *et al.*, 1975a |
| Rodent/ Hystricomorpha | Porcupine | Y | Y | Woolsey *et al.*, 1975a |
| Insectivora/Talpidae | Tree shrew | N | N | Woolsey *et al.*, 1975a |
| Insectivora/Lipotyphla | Mole | Y | N | Catania and Kaas, 1997 |
| Lagomorpha | Rabbit | Y indistinct | N | Rice *et al.*, 1985 |
| Carnivora/Feloidea | Cat | N | N | Rice *et al.*, 1985 |
| Carnivora/Canoidea | Dog | N | N | Woolsey *et al.*, 1975a |
| | Raccoon | N | N | Woolsey *et al.*, 1975a |
| Carnivora/Pinipedia | Seal | ? | N | |
| | Walrus | ? | N | |
| | Sea lion | ? | N | |
| Mustelids | Ferret | Y | N | Mosconi and Rice, 1991 |
| Marsupials/ Phalangeroidea | Wallaby | Y | N | Waite *et al.*, 1991 |
| | Australian opossum | Y | N | Weller, 1972 |
| Marsupials/ Didelphoidea | American opossum | N | N | Woolsey *et al.*, 1975a |
| Primates | Squirrel monkey | N | N | Woolsey *et al.*, 1975a |
| | Rhesus monkey | N | N | Woolsey *et al.*, 1975a |

N, no; Y; yes

[a] Not all species with whiskers are included.

Barrels can also be seen in animals as diverse as rabbits and marsupials, but not in the common carnivores that have been studied so far. Curiously, the cat has whiskers and barrel-like structures in the brainstem nuclei (barrelettes) but, along with other carnivores, has no detectable barrels in the cortex (Nomura *et al.*, 1986). One of the most spectacular sets of whiskers to be found in the animal kingdom is possessed by another carnivore, the walrus (Figure 1.3; color version in plate section). However, it is not known whether this animal, nor indeed whether pinnipeds in general, has barrels within its somatosensory cortex (Table 1.1).

Most of the suborder of rodents known as myomorphs (which includes rats and mice) both have barrels and "whisk" their whiskers, that is they move their whiskers back and forth rhythmically to sample the space around them. This active tactile behavior is analogous to palpating a surface with the fingers, where the tips of the fingers are rhythmically brought into contact with and retracted from the surface being explored. Animals whisk at very different frequencies; for example, the chinchilla whisks at about 1 Hz while the rat whisks at 7 Hz (Woolsey *et al.*, 1975a). Unfortunately, once again, a simple rule cannot be made between animals that whisk and animals that have barrels, because several animals with barrels do not whisk, including myomophs such as the muskrat (Woolsey *et al.*, 1975a), several other rodents, rabbits, moles, and various marsupials (Table 1.1).

The marsupials are an interesting set of animals with regard to the evolution of the barrels because they represent a primitive mammalian form. Many Australian marsupials have barrels, including the wallaby and opossum. Curiously, the American opossum does not have barrels despite being very closely related to the Australian opossum. It seems likely that they had a common ancestor that had barrels, which were then lost in the American opossum during their separate evolution once the continents drifted apart.

### 1.2.2    *What are barrels?*

What exactly is a barrel and what makes it so visible? Whereas the thalamic afferents innervating cortical layer IV usually form a relatively continuous distribution of terminations in primary sensory cortex, in barrel cortex the thalamic afferents form discrete clumps separated on all sides by gaps with sparse thalamocortical afferent branches. The gaps that surround the barrels are known as the septae. The dense clumping of thalamocortical afferents form the center, or core, of each barrel, as can be seen in Figure 1.4. Cells tend to be sparse within the centers of the barrels and denser in the barrel wall, though the difference is greater in mice than rats. The cells in the wall of the barrel tend to project their dendrites in toward the center of the barrel (Simons and

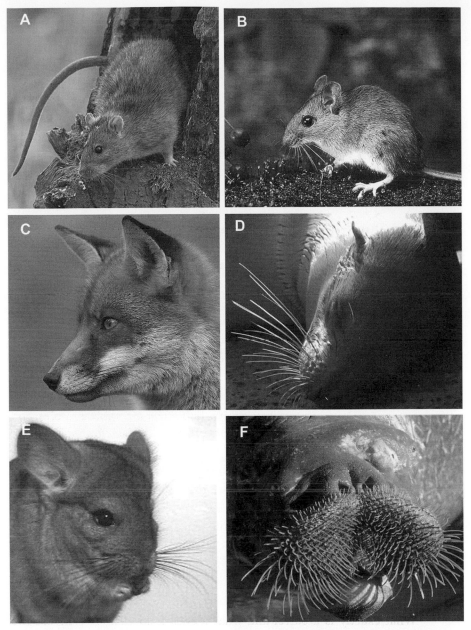

**Figure 1.3.** Many species of animals have whiskers. A. The rat is a common laboratory species for studying barrel cortex (*Ratus norvegicus*). (Courtesy of Stephen Round, reproduced with kind permission.) B. The mouse is a valuable laboratory species that can be genetically manipulated and is frequently used to study barrel cortex (pictured is the common wood or field mouse *Apodemus sylvaticus* a cousin of the laboratory mouse, which is derived from the house mouse *Mus musculus*). C,D. Foxes (C) along with other carnivores such as sea lions (D) have whiskers but are unlikely to have barrels because other carnivores such as cats do not. E. The chinchilla has whiskers and barrels. F. The walrus has an impressive set of whiskers but it is not known whether this species has barrels. (See color plate section.)

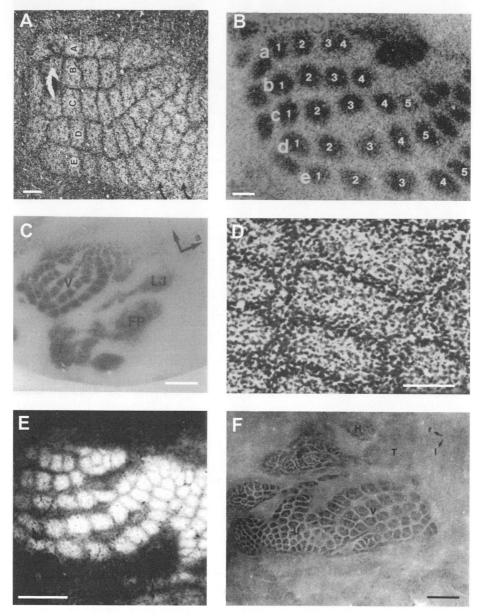

**Figure 1.4.** Barrels can be seen by a variety of methods. A. A stain for tenascin, which is an extracellular matrix molecule, labels the areas outside the mouse barrel cortex in a fenestrated pattern. (Reproduced from Cooper and Steindler [1986] with kind permission of the authors and Wiley.) B. Acetylcholinesterase is located on presynaptic terminals of the thalamocortical afferents at young ages and so labels barrel field in rats. (Reproduced from Schlaggar et al. [1993] with kind permission of the authors and Macmillan Publishing.) C. Similarly, the 5-hydroxytryptamine 1b receptor labels thalamocortical afferents at young ages in rats. (Reproduced from

Woolsey, 1984), again sparing the surrounding septal area between the barrels, where they pick up synaptic contacts from the thalamocortical afferents (Figure 1.4). The simple spatial separation of cells in the walls and thalamic afferents in the center of the barrel is sufficient to see barrels under a micro-scope in an unstained slice, presumably owing to the small difference in refrac-tive index between the myelinated axons and the (unmyelinated) cells.

The barrel itself is most often visualized using cytochome oxidase (CO). This enzyme is present in mitochondria, which are particularly dense at synapses. Since the synapses are far denser in the barrel centers than either the walls of the barrel or the septal areas, so too is the CO. Staining for CO, therefore, shows up the barrels rather well, but only shows the inside of the barrel up to the inside edge of the barrel wall (Land and Simons, 1985). Other mitochondrial enzymes can also be used to the same effect, for example succinate dehydrogenase (Belford and Killackey, 1979).

The other major method for visualizing barrels is a Nissl stain. The Nissl stain shows where the barrels are located by showing up the differences in cell density. Differences in cell density across barrels are greater in mice than rats and, on a practical note, it can be difficult to see barrels using Nissl stains in rats older than about one week of age. Since the major cell density difference occurs between the edge and the center of the barrel, Nissl stains most readily show the barrels if a horizontal section is taken through the barrel field. However, it is possible to see the walls of the barrels in a coronal or transverse section through the layers of the cortex, where they form curved structures reminiscent of barrel staves (Figure 1.4). This is the resemblance that prompted Woolsey and Van der Loos to name this part of the somatosensory cortex "barrel" cortex.

Other methods can be used to see the barrel pattern, most notably staining for various receptors and enzymes such as nicotinic receptors, serotonin

---

**Caption for Figure 1.4 (cont.)**

Bennett-Clarke *et al.* [1993] with kind permission of the authors and the National Academy of Science.) D. A Nissl stain shows up the variation in cell density across the barrels, which appears relatively cell sparse in the middle and denser at the cell wall surrounding the barrel in the mouse. (Reproduced from Woolsey and Van der Loos [1970], with kind permission of the authors and Elsevier.) E. 1,1′-Dioctadecyl-3,3,3′,3′-tetramethylindocarbocyanine perchlorate (DiI) is a lipophilic dye that can be used to label fixed tissue. Here the thalamocortical afferents have been labeled in layer IV of the rat barrel cortex in this fluorescent micrograph. (Reproduced from Boylan *et al.* [2000], with kind permission of the authors and Wiley.) F. One of the earliest stains to be used for studying barrel cortex was succinic dehydrogenase, a mitochondrial enzyme, present at synapses and hence particularly dense in the barrels. (Reproduced from Koralek *et al.* [1990], with kind permission of the authors and Wiley.)

(5-hydroxytryptamine [5HT] receptors, such as $5HT_{1B}$ and acetylcholinesterase (Bennett-Clark *et al.*, 1993; Schlaggar *et al.*, 1993; Bina *et al.*, 1995). These methods rely on the differential distribution of the molecule involved on the thalamo-cortical afferents rather than the neurons. However, the general usefulness of these receptors for viewing barrels is limited to the first couple of weeks of postnatal life because their expression is developmentally downregulated (see Chapter 4). Finally, elements of the extracellular matrix such as tenascin are particularly dense in the septal areas surrounding the barrel and can, therefore, be used to see a negative or fenestrated picture of the barrels by marking where the barrels are not (Cooper and Steindler, 1986).

The essential elements of a barrel are, therefore, a core of thalamic axons and a barrel wall of two to three cell layers in thickness. The middle of the barrel has a lower cell density than the outer wall but nevertheless does contain cells. In the mouse and rat, the larger barrels are located at the posterior medial part of the barrel field (Figure 1.1), which is, therefore, known as the posterior medial barrel subfield, and the smaller barrels are at the anterior lateral part. In both species, the barrels are arranged in five rows conventionally labeled from A to E (Figure 1.1). Rows A and B contain just four barrels while the other three rows contain approximately 8–10 barrels within the posterior medial subfield. The pattern accurately reflects the pattern of whiskers on the face of the animal; for example the gerbil, which has seven rather than five rows of whiskers, also has seven rather than five rows of barrels in the cortex (Woolsey *et al.*, 1975a).

The barrels in the mouse tend to be narrower in the dimension along the rows than in the orthogonal direction along the arcs. The larger barrels are about 200 μm in width and about 100 μm along the axis of the row. Each large barrel contains approximately 2000 neurons (Pasternak and Woolsey, 1975). Of the neurons present, about 75% are excitatory and 25% inhibitory (Ren *et al.*, 1992). The cells within layer IV principally project to layers above and below them. A strong projection is sent vertically to layers II/III and a smaller but important projection to layer Va directly below. Both these projections tend to preserve the topography of the barrels because they do not spread appreciably into surrounding barrels. In addition, layer IV projects to cells in layer VI.

The cells in the septal regions surrounding the barrels have a different set of major inputs and outputs, which make it probable that they form a partly separated interdigitated circuit within the barrel cortex. Whereas cells located within a barrel tend to connect with other cells within that barrel, cells in the septal regions form a wide mesh of connections with septal regions several barrels apart. They tend not to receive as great a thalamic input from the ventroposterior medial thalamic nucleus (VPm) as the barrel cells but do receive callosal input from the barrel field in the other hemisphere unlike the barrel cells and in addition receive an innervation from the posterior medial thalamic nucleus (POm; Koralek *et al.*, 1988). The vertical connections of septal cells within layer IV tend to run radially and not to diverge greatly into neighboring barrels. The septal and barrel projections from layer IV are, therefore, separate to some extent and so a level of parallel processing exists at this stage within the barrel field. The detailed connectivity of the system is explored more in Chapter 2.

### 1.2.3    *Why are barrels important?*

Why should anyone study barrels? They are after all specializations in primary sensory cortex of a subset of mammalian species and no one would expect them to be present in humans. There are many answers to this question; probably as many answers are there are people working in the field. But the two main reasons why barrels have become important in neuroscience is a combination of practical experimental advantage and the theoretical connection between barrels and the basic functional unit underlying the structure of the cerebral cortex – the cortical column.

The cortical column and the columnar hypothesis is described in more detail in Chapter 5, but briefly, the idea is that the cortex is composed of a vertical array of cells running orthogonal to the six-layered structure of the cortex (Figure 1.1). Each column measures about 300 µm across, on average, and runs through the depth of the cortex, which would be about 1.5 mm for a mouse and 2 mm for a rat. Each column of cells would be composed of an archetypical circuit that would be repeated in each column. The difference between neighboring columns is that they receive different functional input from the thalamus. For example, within the visual system, neighboring columns might represent neighboring areas on the retina, and in the barrel cortex, neighboring columns represent neighboring whiskers on the face. Each column is thought of as performing the same basic transformation on the input from the thalamus, and an extreme form of this theory would hold that one could transplant columns from one place to another in the cortex and they would perform the same job. In practice, this can only really be done during early development because the connections from the thalamic and intracortical connections will not otherwise form properly. Where cells have been transplanted or inputs rerouted to different cortical areas, a good deal of function has been replicated by the transplanted cells, as discussed in Chapter 4.

Therefore, one rationale for studying barrel cortex is that the barrels identify the location of cortical columns and cortical columns are an important fundamental element of cortical structure. The similarity between columns in the barrel cortex and columns elsewhere in the brain means that one can understand a great deal about the cortex in general by understanding the columns in the barrel cortex in particular. This not only includes understanding connections within the column itself, but also understanding the connections the column makes with other columns and with subcortical structures. These connections are described in Chapter 2.

Of course, there are many differences and peculiarities of individual cortical areas that obscure the underlying pattern of columnar architecture, chief of which are the differences between the proportions of layers between different cortical areas. Indeed, these are among the features that allowed the different cortical areas to be defined in the first place (Brodmann, 1909). For example, barrel cortex has a well-developed layer IV in common with other primary sensory cortical areas such as primary visual cortex and primary auditory cortex. In contrast, primary motor cortex (MI) has a poorly defined layer IV.

Despite these differences, many would argue that there are sufficient similarities between cortical areas to warrant studying barrel cortex in order to understand cortex in general. Indeed, even if barrel cortex is only a good model for sensory cortical areas, one would imagine studying it would still be worthwhile. The practical advantages inherent in studying the barrel cortex have made it one of the most studied cortical areas in recent years. The fact that the analogue of the column can be seen (at least in layer IV) allows anatomical and physiological results to be aligned against a common reference, which is important for detecting patterns of connectivity and functional similarities across multiple experiments (Feldman and Brecht, 2005). The fact that the barrels can be seen in slices has allowed cellular recordings to be made in cortex while stimulating identified thalamocortical and intracortical pathways (Agmon and Connors, 1991). The distinctive pattern of the barrels has been of great benefit in studying both pattern formation and development of a cortical area in general.

The diversity of scientists studying the barrel cortex is remarkable. Geneticists look to see if the barrel cortex is present following a mutation as a standard test of normal forebrain development; developmental neuroscientists use barrel cortex to understand the principles of pattern formation; behaviorists and systems neuroscientists use barrel cortex to understand the process of active touch. Neurologists study the barrel cortex to better understand stroke and cerebral blood flow, and computational neuroscientists model barrel cortex in order to understand cortical processing in general. All these studies occur in addition to numerous others focused on the function of the barrel cortex itself.

Before exploring the different fields of barrel cortex study, we begin first by describing the basic components of the barrel system starting with the basic anatomical pathways in Chapter 2 and their physiological properties in Chapter 3. The fruits of the diverse studies mentioned above are then covered in Chapter 4 with regard to development, Chapter 5 for sensory processing, Chapter 6 for synaptic plasticity and Chapter 7 for systems plasticity. The final chapter considers some of the more recent, but none the less flourishing, new fields that have found practical advantage from studying particular questions in the barrel cortex (Chapter 8).

# 2

---

# Anatomical pathways

Since the 1970s, a detailed description of the anatomical pathways of the vibrissae system has evolved in the literature. The process has been facilitated by the ability to discern topographical arrangements at each stage of the somatosensory pathway by virtue of the barrel pattern itself and by the careful application of dye-tracing techniques by a number of laboratories. The connectivity of the barrel cortex still remains a challenge because of its intricate complexity, and it has only recently become ammenable to description as a result of dual intracellular recording and glutamate uncaging methodologies. In this chapter, we describe the pathways leading from the whisker follicles (Section 2.1) through the brainstem (Section 2.2) and thalamus (Section 2.3) to the barrel cortex (Section 2.4). Where appropriate, the physiology of subcortical pathways are discussed but a more detailed consideration of barrel cortex physiology is reserved for subsequent chapters. We begin here at the periphery by considering the anatomy of the vibrissa follicle.

## 2.1    Whisker follicle innervation

The follicle itself is composed of a series of concentrically arranged membranes. Closest to the vibrissa itself lies a thick basement membrane, often referred to as the glassy membrane, which ensheaths the vibrissa hair (Figure 2.1). Outside the glassy membrane is a mesenchymal sheath that forms the inner surface of the follicle sinus. Outside this lies the vascular sinus itself, which is bounded on the outside by another thick highly collagenous membrane that forms the outside of the follicle sinus. The bottom of the sinus is bounded by the dermal papilla, where the hair grows at the top at the point where the collagenous membrane constricts and merges with the dermis. Most

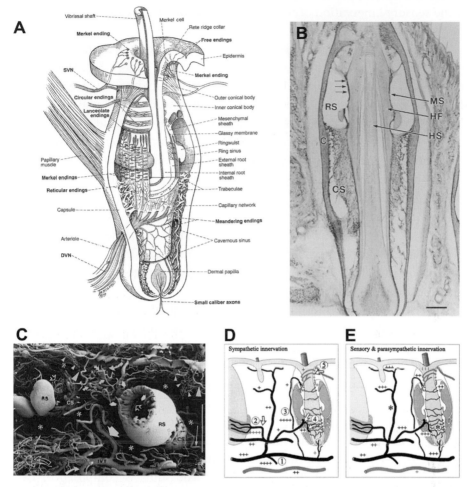

**Figure 2.1.** The structure of the vibrissa follicle. A. Diagram showing the structure and innervation of a rat follicle (SVN, superficial vibrissae nerve; DVN, deep vibrissae nerve). (From Rice *et al.* [1993], reproduced with kind permission of Wiley and the author.) B. Cross-section through a follicle sinus complex (scale bar = 200 μm; abbreviations as in C). C. Vasularization of the follicle imaged by scanning electron microscopy of a vascular cast showing the ring sinus (RS), cavernous sinus (CS), a vein (V) and the intervibrissal trunk artery (IVT). (MS, mesenchymal sheath; HF, hair follicle; HS, hair shaft; C, capsule; scale bar, 500 μm). D,E. Diagram of sympathetic (D) and parasympathetic (E) innervation of the vasculature associated with the follicle. (Innervation density: +, weak; ++, moderate; +++, dense; ++++, very dense. Blood supply: 1, arterioles suppling the facial muscles; 2, arterioles supplying papilliary muscles (see A); 3, proximal portion of the superficial vibrissal artery; 4, arterioles and precapilliaries in the cavernous sinus; 5, circumferential venous channels in the outer connical body in E, asterix the intervibrissal artery, which shows dense parasympathetic innervation. (Parts C–E reproduced from Fundin *et al.* [1997], with kind permission of the authors and Wiley.)

of the sensory innervation of the follicle lies between the sinus and the glassy membrane.

Two sensory nerves innervate the follicle; these are known as the superficial vibrissa nerve (SVN) and the deep vibrissal nerve (DVN) (Figure 2.1). Most of the innervation is carried by the DVN. In the rat, approximately five-sixths of the axons from a single follicle are derived from the DVN and one-sixth from the SVN (Waite and Jacquin, 1992). The SVN innervates an area at the top of the follicle known as the inner conical body and comprises circumferentially oriented nerve endings wrapped around the follicle. In addition, the SVN supplies a number of Merkel's discs located in the epidermis at the rete ridge at the top of the follicle (Figure 2.1A).

Each whisker follicle has its own unique DVN and SVN. In other words, axons within these nerves do not branch to innervate more than one follicle (Zucker and Welker, 1969). Approximately 1–200 axons innervate each large follicle in the whisker pad (70–170 myelinated and 25–60 unmyelinated) in the mouse (Lee and Woolsey, 1975) and rat (Li et al., 1995).

The primary afferents terminating in the trigeminal nuclei make contact at their peripheral end in a variety of receptor specializations (Figure 2.1). Receptor endings in the vibrissae follicles can be classified into two broad types; slowly adapting (SA) such as Merkel's discs, and rapidly adapting (RA) such as lanceolate endings. The lanceolate endings are either arranged vertically and exit via the DVN or are wrapped around the follicle circumferentially and exit via the SVN (Figure 2.1). In addition, a number of free nerve endings surround the vibrissae follicle, including reticular endings.

Apart from its shear size, the vibrissae follicle is distinct from the follicle of a normal hair because of the follicle sinus. The sinus is composed of two main chambers, the ring sinus and the cavernous sinus at the base of the follicle (Figure 2.1C). The autonomic innervation of the arterioles controls inflation of the sinuses and hence the rigidity of the follicle. The main locations of action of the autonomic innervation are indicated in Figure 2.1D, E (Fundin et al., 1997).

The infraorbital nerve carries axons from the vibrissae follicle receptors to the brainstem. At its peripheral extent, it divides into fascicles each supplying one row of vibrissae (Dorfl, 1985). The infraorbital nerve then courses out of the back of the vibrissa pad before running dorsally and caudally beneath the ventral surface of the eye orbit at the infraorbital foramen. The nerve merges with the motor and mandibular branches of the fifth cranial nerve at the level of the trigeminal ganglion. The trigeminal ganglia containing the cell bodies of the infraorbital nerve axons lie on the base of the skull. The axons then exit the ganglion within the fifth nerve to innvervate the brainstem nuclei.

## 2.2    Brainstem nuclei and their projections

### 2.2.1    *General organization of the trigeminal nuclei*

There are four primary termination zones in the brainstem for trigeminal ganglion cells that relay information from the follicles; these are known
collectively as the trigeminal nuclei. The trigeminal nuclei form four groups,
which are known by various synonyms: the principal nucleus of the V nerve
(Vp), the oral nucleus (Vo), the interpolar nucleus (Vi) and the caudal nucleus
(Vc). There are various synonyms for these nuclei, with the Latin names often
being preferred to the English names; hence the principal nucleus is often
referred to as principalis and the others as oralis, interpolaris and caudalis. In
addition, because oralis, interpolaris and caudalis are in the spinal part of the
brainstem they are often designated as the spinal 5 nuclei, hence SP5o, SP5i and
SP5c (Figure 2.2).

Figure 2.3 shows a coronal section through the brainstem at the level of the
trigeminal nuclei. All four nuclei have a complete representation of the whiskers
in the rat and mouse because the whisker pattern is present in the trigeminal
afferents. The pattern is clear in CO-stained tissue but is less distinct in oralis for
both the rat (Chiaia *et al.*, 1992; Jacquin *et al.*, 1993a) and mouse (Ma, 1991).

In the trigeminal nuclei, the structures equivalent to cortical barrels are called
barrelettes. The barrelettes run rostrocaudal as individual cylinders in the rostral
nuclei, and the topgraphic pattern can, therefore, be seen in transverse section

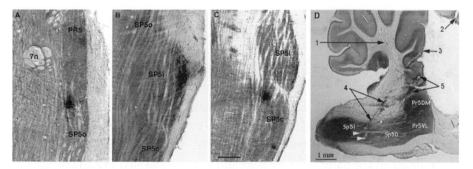

**Figure 2.2.** Location and structure of the brainstem trigeminal nuclei. A. Horizontal
section through the brainstem showing principalis (PR5) and oralis (SP5o) nuclei.
B. Horizontal section showing a more caudal section with SP5o, interpolaris (SP5i)
and caudalis (SP5c) nuclei indicated from rostral (top) to caudal (bottom).
C. Horizontal section through (SP5c). Scale bar 500 μm. (Reproduced from Veinante
*et al.* [2000], with kind permission of the authors and Wiley.) D. Saggital section
through the brainstem nuclei showing the location with respect to the cerebellum (1)
and visual cortex (2). The arrows mark two electrode tracks. (Reproduced from
Haidarliu *et al.* [1999], with kind permission of the authors and Elsevier.)

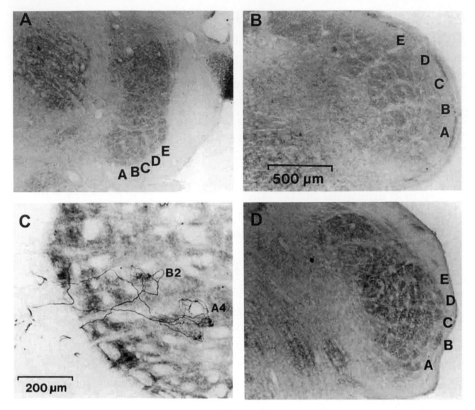

**Figure 2.3.** Cross-sections through the brainstem trigeminal nuclei showing the barrel pattern of the barrelettes using cytochrome oxidase staining. A,B. Cross-sections through principalis (A) and interpolaris (B) nuclei. C. Interpolaris nucleus showing innervation of the B2 and A4 barrelette by primary afferents. D. The caudalis nucleus. The 500 μm scale bar in B also applies to A and D. (Reproduced from Jacquin *et al.* [1995], with kind permission of the authors and Wiley.)

through the brainstem (Figure 2.3). The barrelette rows run dorsal to ventral within principalis but rotate slightly clockwise by 90 degrees as they move caudal through oralis and interpolaris. In caudalis, the representation is reversed as a mirror image of the pattern in the other nuclei (Jacquin *et al.*, 1993a).

The interconnections of the vibrissal nerves with the trigeminal nuclei and the outputs of the nuclei with other brain areas have mainly been studied in the rat. Therefore, the overview given here relates to the rat rather than the mouse. The primary afferents enter the brainstem and branch to send an ascending axon to the principalis and a descending axon to the spinal portions of the trigeminal nuclei, namely oralis, interpolaris and caudalis. The majority of axons do not bifurcate, but those that do so make contact with all four trigeminal nuclei. In principalis, the terminations of the primary afferents are dense ellipsoid sprays with terminal swellings (boutons) that are largely confined to the CO-labeling patches that exhibit the topographic pattern (see Figure 2.3C), whereas in oralis the terminations lack the complex terminal arborization and have fewer boutons (Jacquin *et al.*, 1993a).

The primary afferent termination patterns tend to be localized and distinct in interpolaris and caudalis, where the pattern is as clear as it is in principalis. Oralis, therefore, appears different from the other three trigeminal nuclei in several respects: it has a less distinct CO-labeled barrelette pattern; it does not have discrete and tightly arborized primary afferent terminations; and the primary afferents it receives do not have a high density of terminal boutons. The difference is further demonstrated by measurements of 2-deoxyglucose (2-DG) uptake, which gives an index of the level of activity in a particular neuronal population. In animals acutely deprived of all but one or two whiskers, 2-DG uptake is high in the topologically related barrelette for principalis, interpolaris and caudalis, while in oralis uptake is difficult to see (Jacquin *et al.*, 1993b).

One further point is worth noting regarding inputs to the trigeminal nuclei; the fur innervation that lies between the vibrissae must project somewhere. It appears that the comparatively sparse projection from the fur sends afferents to all the main brainstem nuclei, without obvious organization; for example, it does not project to areas between the vibrissae representation (Arvidsson and Rice, 1991). However, a difference can be seen in caudalis where the DVNs from the vibrissae follicles tend to project to deeper layers of caudalis (IV and V) while the fur inputs terminate more superficially in layers I–III (Arvidsson and Rice, 1991).

### 2.2.2 *Projection patterns of the trigeminal nuclei*

Principalis and interpolaris are the two main trigeminal nuclei that project to the somatosensory thalamus (Figure 2.4A). Retrograde tracer injected into the VPm mainly labels principalis (Figure 2.4B). Anterograde tracer injected into principalis mainly labels VPm (Chiaia *et al.*, 1991) and POm only sparsely (Figure 2.5). Principalis and VPm form the main lemniscal pathway for tactile information from the face to the cortex and this pathway is analogous to the dorsal column to ventroposterior nucleus (VPn) lateral component (VPl) pathway for the hand and foot representations of the somatosensory system. Interpolaris also projects to the thalamus but has a slightly different termination pattern from principalis. The main projection from interpolaris is to the ventrolateral part of VPm (see Figures 2.4 and 2.5), where it contacts the ventrolateral part of the nucleus and does not overlap extensively with the termination pattern of principalis (Section 2.3).

The three spinal trigeminal nuclei all have projections to the superior colliculus and to the cerebellum although not from the same sets of cells

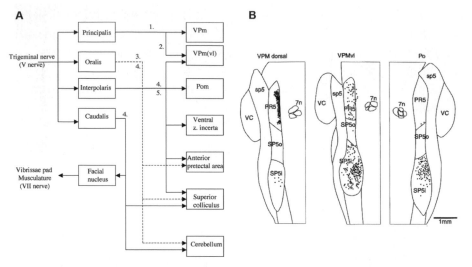

**Figure 2.4.** Brainstem projections to thalamus and other midbrain targets.
A. Connections from the four brainstem trigeminal nuclei (top left) to the ventro-posterior medial nucleus (VPm), its ventrolateral component (VPM(vl)), the posterior nucleus of the thalamus (Pom), zona incerta (z. incerta) and other locations as indicated. Data orginate from the following sources: 1, Chiaia *et al.* (1991); 2, Pierret *et al.* (2000); 3, Hallas and Jacquin (1990); 4, Veinante *et al.* (2000); 5, Jacquin *et al.* (1989). B. Diagram of horizontal sections throught the brainstem showing the number of cells labeled following retrograde transport of fluro gold from VPm, VPm(vl) and the posterior thalamic nucleus (Po). VC, ventral cochlear nucleus; other abbreviations as in Figure 2.2. (Reproduced from Pierret *et al.* [2000], with kind permission of the authors and the Society for Neuroscience.)

(Figure 2.4A). Caudalis also has a projection from deep laminae to the facial nucleus ipsilaterally and thereby provides a route for direct sensory feedback to the vibrissae musculature, presumably to provide some level of sensory control over movement. Feedback is particularly important because the whisker pad muscles do not contain spindle organs, which usually form part of a sensory–motor servo-control of muscle contraction elsewhere in the body.

The trigeminal nuclei also project to one another. In general, each nucleus connects with each other nucleus with the exception of oralis, which appears not to project to interpolaris (Jacquin *et al.*, 1990). The connections from principalis back to the spinal trigeminal nuclei are notably weaker than the connections running from the spinal trigeminal nuclei to principalis.

### 2.2.3　Receptive field properties of trigeminal nuclei cells

The receptive fields of trigeminal nuclei cells are strongly influenced by the properties of their primary afferents. Vibrissae follicle primary afferents can

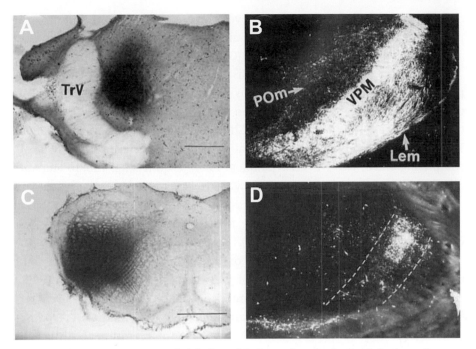

**Figure 2.5.** Anterograde labeling of thalamus from brainstem injections of WGA-HRP (wheatgerm agglutinin–horseradish peroxidase). A,B. Injection in principalis labels the ventroposterior medial thalamic nucleus (VPM) and the posterior medial thalamic nucleus (POm), shown as bright (A) and dark (B) field image (Lem, lemniscus). C,D. Injection in interpolaris labels a subsection of VPM and gives lighter labeling in POm, as shown in bright (C) and dark (D) field images (dashed line indicating the boundary between VPM and POm). (Adapted from Chiaia *et al.* [1991], with kind permission of the authors and Wiley.)

be classified into two broad classes, SA fibers associated with Merkel's discs, and RA fibers such as those associated with Ruffini and lanceolate endings. The SA fibers produce tonic firing in response to a constant whisker displacement whereas the RA fibers will fire briefly during a displacement of the vibrissa but remain silent while it is held steady in its new position. Primary afferents tend not to show spontaneous activity (in agreement with the majority being RA) and can respond to deflections as small as 0.1 degrees (Gibson and Welker, 1983a, b).

Both SA and RA fibers increase their firing rate for an increases in the velocity of a vibrissa deflection, but only the SA fibers code linearly for deflection amplitude (Shoykhet *et al.*, 2000). The velocity thresholds of many fibers are less than 3 degrees/second, but in general a variety of thresholds can be observed. Velocity thresholds range over three orders of magnitude for the population of primary afferents, which means that different stimulus velocities are coded by different subsets of fibers (Gibson and Welker, 1983b).

Many of the properties of principalis cells are very similar to those of the primary afferents. However, one obvious difference is that the primary afferents only respond to one whisker, whereas trigeminal neurons often respond to more than one (Jacquin et al., 1988a; Chiaia et al., 2000; Minnery et al., 2003). There is some agreement that principalis receptive fields are relatively small, comprising one or two whiskers (Shipley, 1974; Jacquin et al., 1988b; Veinante and Deschenes, 1999). However, multiwhisker input is observed in principalis and depends in part on the much larger receptive fields in interpolaris. Ablation of interpolaris input causes receptive fields to decrease in size from three whiskers to one (Timofeeva et al., 2004).

Principalis neurons exhibit phasic on and off responses as well as tonic responses to sustained displacement of the whisker, corresponding to the SA and RA properties of the fibers that innervate them. Most neurons are directionally selective, but the SA responses are more selective than the RA responses (Minnery et al., 2003). There is some variability in the literature regarding the proportion of SA cells present in principalis and estimates range from approximately half the cells (Jacquin et al., 1988b; Veinante and Deschenes, 1999) to as many as 90% (Minnery et al., 2003). A possible reason for the discrepancy is that cells with SA responses are more direction selective than RA cells, requiring all directions to be tested to identify an SA response.

Interpolaris neurons tend to behave similarly to principalis cells except that their receptive fields are larger, often comprising as many as 16 whiskers (Woolston et al., 1982). The receptive fields of interpolaris neurons vary depending on where they project. Local circuit neurons projecting within the brainstem nuclei have single whisker receptive fields on average, while those projecting to VPm have an average of eight whiskers (range 3–16; Woolston et al., 1982). Neurons projecting to the cerebellum are intermediate in nature and have receptive fields of three whiskers on average, with a range of 1–10 (Woolston et al., 1982; Jacquin et al., 1995). Interpolaris neurons projecting to VPm have large receptive fields partly owing to convergence of the primary afferents on to the dendrites of interpolaris neurons. Although the terminal clusters of the primary afferents are quite localized, the VPm projecting cells have large dendritic trees extending across several barrelettes (Jacquin et al., 1986, 1989). The barrel cortex is capable of controlling the size of the receptive field in interpolaris to some extent because acute or chronic ablation of the contralateral cortex increases the receptive field size of local circuit neurons in interpolaris (Jacquin et al., 1990).

## 2.3    Thalamic circuits

### 2.3.1    General organization of the somatosensory thalamus

The somatosensory thalamus lies in the ventral and posterior aspect of the thalamus. It is bounded on its medial side by the ventrolateral nucleus, at the front by the anterior thalamic nucleus, by the posterior nucleus at at its caudal extent and on the lateral side by the reticular nucleus (Figure 2.6). The VPn is the main nucleus for rapid transmission of somatosensory information and comprises two areas: the lateral VPl is concerned with hand, body and foot representations, and the medial component (VPm) is concerned with the face representation (Figure 2.6).

The posterior group of nuclei are located toward the caudal end of the ventrobasal complex, and flank VPm on the medial side before wrapping around the back of it at its caudal extremity. The POm receives a projection

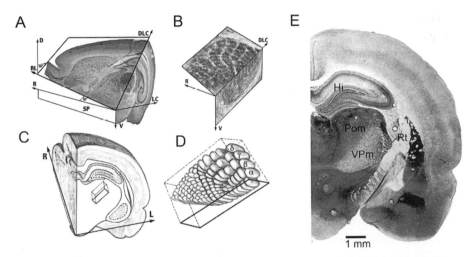

**Figure 2.6.** Three-dimensional organization of the barreloids within the thalamus. A. Section through a hemisphere in a plane designed to run orthoganal to the barrel pattern (D, dorsal; DLC, dorsolaterocaudal; L, lateral; LC, laterocaudal; R, rostral; RL, rostrolateral; SP, saggital plane; V, ventral.). B. The barrel pattern stained with cytochrome oxidase. C,D. Complete set of barreloids showing their location and orientation within a normal coronal section through the hemisphere (caudal aspect). Note that one plane of the box has been marked with heavier line for registration between C and D. (Reproduced from Haidarliu and Ahissar [2001]. E. Coronal section through the rat brain 3.6 mm caudal to bregma stained using acetylcholinesterase immunohistochemistry. Note the location of the ventroposteriomedial nucleus (VPm), the posterior medial nucleus (POm) and the reticular nucleus of the thalamus (Rt). (Adapted from Paxinos and Watson [1986], with kind permission of the authors and Academic Press.)

from the spinal component of the brainstem trigeminal nuclei (Figures 2.4B and 2.5) and together with VPm contains a second complete representation of the whiskers in the thalamus (Diamond *et al.*, 1992a). In the rat and mouse, POm is the main posterior nucleus and is not as complex or differentiated as in the primate, for example (Jones, 1985). However, it is important to distinguish it from the very caudal part of the posterior thalamic nucleus known as the caudal division (POc), which projects mainly to the second somatosensory area (SII) rather than barrel cortex and appears to have multimodal receptive fields (Diamond, 1995).

### 2.3.2   *The ventroposterior medial thalamic nucleus*

As mentioned above, VPm is the main relay for vibrissae information from the trigeminal nuclei to the cortex. The barrel pattern can be discerned in CO-stained transverse sections through the thalamus (Van der Loos, 1976). The barrel-like forms in the thalamus are only 1–200 µm in diameter and form banana-shaped tubes of cells called barreloids. Frustratingly, the banana-shaped barreloids run at an angle to every stereotaxic coordinate axis starting anterior dorsal and medial and ending up in a posterior ventral and lateral location. The E-row of whiskers lie most anterior and the A-row most posterior (see Figure 2.6).

If a retrograde tracer is placed in VPm, it heavily back-labels cells located in principalis and interpolaris in the brainstem (Figure 2.4). A similar injection located in POm will chiefly label cells in interpolaris (Figure 2.4). It has been estimated that about 90% of the cells in principalis project to VPm alone, 7% to POm and 2% to both (Chiaia *et al.*, 1991). Far fewer cells project from interpolaris, but again the main projection is to VPm alone (75%) followed by 17% that project solely to POm and 7% to both. Although interpolaris and principalis both project to VPm, their projections are not overlapped to any great extent. While the interpolaris projection innervates the caudal tails of the barreloids – the ventrolateral component of the VPm (VPm(vl)) – the principalis projection innervates the main body or core of the barreloids (Pierret *et al.*, 2000). If each barreloid is thought of as a banana-shaped structure running from the anterior medial part of the nucleus and curving to reach the ventrolateral aspect, then the ventrolateral ends of the banana preferentially receive input from interpolaris.

The dichotomy between the VPm(vl) pathway from interpolaris and the VPm core pathway from principalis is maintained further in the different projection patterns emanating from the two components of VPm. While the core of the barreloids forms the main projection into layer IV of the cortex and in turn innervates the core of the barrels, the VPm(vl) projection is more elaborate and varied. Some cells project to SII, while others project to the dysgranular zone.

Some VPm(vl) cells send a collateral to the dysgranular zone as well as a projection to the barrels. However, whereas the VPm core projection is focused quite strongly on layer IV, with a collateral projection to the border of layer Vb and layer VI, the VPm(vl) projection is not as strongly confined and projects to layer V and supragranular layers in addition (Pierret *et al.*, 2000).

### 2.3.3    The thalamic reticular nucleus

The rat and mouse somatosensory thalamus is somewhat atypical among the phylogeny in that it does not contain inhibitory interneurons within the VPm nucleus itself. Instead, the inhibitory cells are displaced in a shell surrounding the VPm nucleus at its outer edge in the reticular nucleus. The reticular nucleus is only two or three cells thick and is bounded on its outer edge by the internal capsule. As its name suggests, it is a reticulated structure and this is because many fibers pass through it in order to travel to and from the thalamus. Cortical projections descending from layer VI pass through the reticular nucleus and into VPm, issuing a collateral as they do so. Similarly, VPm axons pass through the reticular nucleus in the other direction on their way to the cortex and also produce a collateral. In this way, excitation from thalamocortical and corticothalamic cells both activate the reticular nucleus. The reticular nucleus cells themselves project back into the thalamus, providing a recurrent feedback inhibition to the VPm neurons. There is evidence that the inhibitory feedback projection is more diffuse than the precise somatotopy of the excitatory input the reticular nucleus receives from VPm and therefore the reticular nucleus creates an element of lateral inhibition to the VPm neurons (Lavallee and Deschenes, 2004). This mechanism can serve to sharpen the receptive fields of the excitatory thalamic neurons. In addition, it provides a limit to the duration of the excitatory drive to the cortex (Section 5.2.4) and tends to reduce sustained responses.

Neurons in VPm can form an oscillatory circuit in combination with the reticular nucleus, which lead to the characteristic thalamic spindle-firing characteristic of slow wave sleep and anesthesia. The VPm cells fire in a repetitive burst of spikes at a frequency of approximately 8–12 Hz. This is largely caused by the intrinsic currents present in the VPm and reticular neurons such as the T-type calcium channel ($I_t$) and the calcium-sensitive potassium channel ($I_{KCa}$). There is some evidence that the reticular nucleus can act as a pacemaker for spindle generation (Steriade *et al.*, 1985). Hyperpolarization is necessary for thalamic spindle generation because it allows the T-type calcium channels to be de-inactivated and thereby contribute to a depolarization that leads to a burst of spikes. The hyperpolarization can either derive from the reticular nucleus activating gamma-aminobutyric acid (GABA) receptors or, once the spindle wave has started, by $I_{KCa}$ (Figure 2.7).

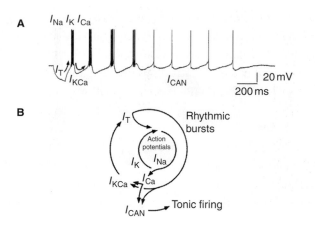

**Figure 2.7.** Oscillatory behavior of thalamic reticular neurons. A. Intracellular recording from reticular neurons showing the characteristic oscillating membrane potential where each depolarizing phase is crowned with a burst of spikes. The occurrence of the main currents involved in this "spindle-like" oscillation are indicated on the trace. B. The cycle of currents is shown for the slower rhythm (outer circle) and spike production (inner circle). Exit to tonic firing mode occurs when the calcium-activated non-selective cation current $I_{CAN}$ is activated (see text for current nomenclature). (Adapted from McCormick and Bal [1997] and reproduced with kind permission of the authors and Annual Reviews Inc.)

The reticular nucleus also serves as a means of communication between thalamic nuclei. The VPm does not send excitatory connections to the other somatosensory thalamic nuclei such as POm (see below). However, reticular neurons receive excitatory drive from VPm and, in turn, project to other thalamic nuclei including POm (Crabtree *et al.*, 1998).

### 2.3.4   *The posterior medial thalamic nucleus*

The medial part of the POm sends a projection to the cortex in a manner that complements the projections of VPm (Figure 2.8). An anterograde injection of tracer in POm will produce a fenestrated pattern of connections in layer IV of the barrel cortex and outline the septal areas (Koralek *et al.*, 1988). Traces of individual axons from POm show that they spread far more laterally within barrel cortex than the clustered connections from VPm that form the centers of the barrels. The POm projection to cortex terminates in layers I–V and not just in layer IV (Figure 2.8C), whereas the VPm projection is concentrated on layer IV with collaterals to Vb/upper VI. The projection from POm is particularly dense in layer V whereas the VPm projection is particularly dense in layer IV. However, the fact that much of the POm projection surrounds the barrels has led to the idea that it may serve a function in integrating information within the barrel

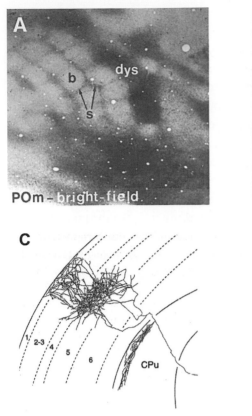
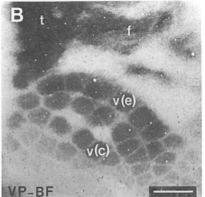
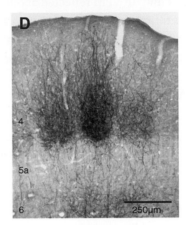

**Figure 2.8.** Two types of thalamic input to the cortex with complemetary innervation patterns. A. An injection of horseradish peroxidase (HRP) into the posterior medial thalamic nucleus (POm) labels the septal areas at the level of layer IV and not the barrels, which appear white in this horizontal section bright field image (b, barrel; s, septum; dys, dysgranular zone; CPu, caudate putamen). B. In contrast, injection of HRP into ventroposterior thalamic nucleus (VP) labels the barrels themselves and not the septal areas, which appear as white (v(c), C-row barrels; v(e), E-row barrels). Scale bar = 600 μm. (Adapted from Koralek *et al.* [1988], with kind permission of the authors and Elsevier.) C. Coronal section of reconstructed single axon fills from the POm-innervating barrel cortex. Note how layers V and I/II receive a large arborizing termination pattern. (Reproduced from Deschenes *et al.* [1998], with kind permission of the authors and Elsevier.) D. Coronal section of barrel cortex following HRP injection in VPm labels the centers of the barrels rather than the septae. (Reproduced from Pierret *et al.* [2000] with kind permission of the authors and the Society for Neuroscience.)

cortex by allowing transmission of information between neighboring barrel-columns (Diamond, 1995).

The main brainstem input to POm is derived mainly from interpolaris rather than principalis, as mentioned above (Figure 2.4). A further source of input derives from the deep layers of the superior colliculus (Roger and Cadusseau, 1984). The third major input is derived from the cortex itself. However, whereas the cortical input to VPm is derived from layer VI neurons, the cortical input to POm is derived from layer V (Hoogland *et al.*, 1987). The cortical projection to POm terminates in large glomerular synapses, which can form as many as eight asymmetric synapses enclosed in glial wrapping (Hoogland *et al.*, 1991). This has led to the idea that the corticothalamic projection to POm may be a feedforward rather than feedback connection.

The three sources of projection achieve some level of topography within POm because a rough map of the whiskers can be discerned in electrophysiological mapping studies (Diamond *et al.*, 1992b). The map in POm is like a mirror image of the map in VPm reflected about the border of the two. For example, the face representation is closest to VPm and the forelimb and hindlimb representation more medial. However, the mapping in POm is highly diffuse compared with that in VPm, which is probably because two of its main inputs, namely interpolaris and cortical layer V cells, have large receptive fields.

It has been suggested that one of the roles of the "secondary nuclei" in the thalamus is to serve as a modulatory relay of information from one cortical area to another (Sherman and Guillery, 2002). Transcortical relay is achieved by cortical cells projecting from primary sensory areas back to secondary thalamic nuclei, which, in turn, project to secondary cortical areas. In the case of the barrel system, the first somatosensory area (SI) barrel cortex projects to POm, which then projects to SII. Support for this idea comes from the finding that cells in POm require cortical input to express responses to the whiskers. Inactivating the cortex by applying a local anesthetic suppresses responses in POm while leaving responses in VPm unaffected (Diamond *et al.*, 1992b). The strong synaptic effect of cortex on POm is a consequence of the nature of the synapses, which tend to be large appositions encapsulated in a glial cell, and their location relatively close to the soma, which gives them a strong depolarizing effect (Hoogland *et al.*, 1991).

The dependence of POm on cortical drive would suggest that the inputs from interpolaris and the superior colliculus are the minor party in controlling the responses of POm neurons. However, one further aspect of POm connectivity needs description in this regard. Neurons in the zona incerta also project to POm and they provide an inhibitory input to the nucleus. When zona incerta cells are themselves inhibited, POm neurons become far more responsive (Trageser and Keller, 2004). It is likely that the unmasked whisker responses are derived from the ascending inputs from interpolaris rather than cortex, judging by their short latency. However, at the time of writing, it has not been explicitly tested whether the cortical inputs are enhanced instead of, or as well as, those from the brainstem, or for that matter from the superior colliculus. These findings raise the possibility that modulation of zona incerta can alter the balance of ascending versus descending influences on POm.

## 2.4    Barrel cortex

### 2.4.1    *Thalamic inputs to barrels and septal areas*

The main thalamic projection into the barrels is derived from VPm. Axons course in an anterior direction from VPm before turning dorsally and reflexing caudally through the white matter underneath the barrel cortex. In doing so, the axons twist the map pattern so that it ends up being reflected about the mediolateral axis. This is achieved by the individual axons twisting about one another similar to strands twisting in a rope (Bernardo and Woolsey, 1987), causing the axons from the higher numbered barreloids to swap position with those from the lower number barreloids within a row. The axons do not travel in a strict topographic map however, suggesting that a trophic factor must reorganize the axons once they reach the cortex.

Within the cortex, thalamic axons project collaterals horizontally at the border of layer V and VI and branch profusely within layer IV in clumps separated from one another by the septal zones (Figure 2.8D). Early studies using axon degeneration methods had shown that VPm neurons terminate in barrels (Killackey and Ebner, 1973). Even earlier studies with Golgi stain-impregnated axons also revealed terminal clusters in layer IV (Lorente de Nó, 1922) though their source was not clear at that time. Tracers such as horseradish peroxidase (HRP) and 1,1'-dioctadecyl-3,3,3',3'-tetramethylindolocarbocyanine perchlorate (DiI) allowed detailed mapping of thalamic axons within the barrels in the rat (Killackey and Belford, 1979) and mouse (Bernardo and Woolsey, 1987). It was noted that axons can branch within layer IV and send an axon out of the barrel hollow before looping back in, again suggesting that trophic factors organize the final position of the axons (Bernardo and Woolsey, 1987). Within the barrel hollow, thalamic afferents form numerous boutons and synapse with stellate, pyramidal and aspiny stellate cells within layer IV, forming approximately 19% of the synapses there (Benshalom and White, 1986; Keller and White, 1987).

In the mouse, approximately 10–23% of all asymmetric (presumed excitatory) synapses on spines of spiny stellate cells are formed by thalamic axons (Benshalom and White, 1986). Different types of GABAergic cell (utilizing GABA as transmitter) receive different proportions of their input from thalamic axons, with bipolar cells receiving somewhat more input than multipolar cells (17% versus 10%) (Keller and White, 1987). The parvalbumin-positive subtype of GABAergic cells are most prevalent in layer IV and include both basket cells and chandelier cells (Section 3.2) and receive multiple contacts from single thalamic axons (Staiger *et al.*, 1996). As a class, inhibitory cells receive approximately 8% of their connections from thalamic inputs. Similarly, the extent of thalamic innervation can differ between classes of excitatory pyramidal cells. Layer V and VI pyramidal cells can pick up thalamic connections on their apical dendrites as they course through layer IV. Tufted pyramidal cells, for example, which can also be characterized by their spike firing patterns as intrinsic bursting cells (Section 3.1.3), show little or no direct thalamic input (Agmon and Connors, 1992) while pyramidal cells projecting back to the thalamus receive 13% of their input from thalamocortical synapses (White and Hersch, 1982), which is a similar percentage to the spiny stellate cells.

The great majority of cells in mouse barrels have dendrites that are oriented in toward the centers of the barrels, and only about 15% have dendrites that project to surrounding barrels (Woolsey *et al.*, 1975b). Cells in the barrel wall have highly asymmetric spread of dendrites, which only project from one side of the cell body into the barrel, while the other side of the cell body appears bald (Figure 2.10D, below). A similar asymmetric disposition of dendrites also occurs in the rat barrel cortex (Feldmeyer *et al.*, 1999). In the mouse, cells within the barrel hollow have a more symmetrical distribution of dendrites, but the dendrites are still confined within the barrel (Woolsey *et al.*, 1975b). This arrangement allows the cells in each barrel to collect synaptic drive principally from thalamic axons within an individual barrel.

In the rat, smaller subdivisions of the barrels can be identified by the occurrence of thin veins, which run through and divide the main corpus of the barrel into two to three compartments or sub-barrels (Louderback *et al.*, 2006). The veins can be seen because they stain less well for CO than the synapse-rich areas between. Just like the walls of the barrels, the internal veins are the location of synapse sparse cell bodies. The thalamocortical terminals are sparse in the clefts dividing the barrels (Louderback *et al.*, 2006). The function of the sub-barrels may be related to directional selectivity of cells in the barrel cortex and the directional subdomains (Bruno *et al.*, 2003; Andermann and Moore, 2006).

The synapses contacting septal cells have not been studied as closely as those located within barrels. Nevertheless, using electron microscopy, it has been found that the POm projection, which preferentially innervates the septal areas, forms boutons in cortex that can be identified as making synaptic contacts (Lu and Lin, 1993). The termination zones of POm axons are layers I to V of the barrel cortex. This might suggests a wider distribution of layers are affected by POm than by VPm and there may be a quantitative argument for this view.

However, as noted above, VPm neurons make contact with cells in all layers of the cortex because the dendrites of cortical cells reach into layer IV and the VPm axons do reach into layer I and III (White, 1978; Pierret *et al.*, 2000).

Barrel cortex also receives other thalamic inputs with characteristic termination patterns. The intralaminar nuclei terminate in layers V and VI and are part of a widespread and diffuse thalamic projection to the cortex in general that crosses boundaries between different functional areas (Herkenham, 1980). The intralaminar nuclei are thought to play a role in general arousal levels (Steriade *et al.*, 1981) and preferentially activate N-methyl-D-aspartate (NMDA) receptor-driven responses in layer V of the somatosensory cortex (Fox and Armstrong-James 1986). One further thalamic projection occurs from the ventromedial thalamic nucleus to layer I of the cortex. While this projection is densest in frontal cortex, it does project to a lesser extent to occipital and parietal cortex including the somatosensory areas (Herkenham, 1979). This nucleus conveys nociceptive information to cortex (Monconduit *et al.*, 1999) and is important for a variety of cortically dependent behavioral tasks including spatial working memory (Bailey and Mair, 2005).

### 2.4.2    *Excitatory intracortical pathways*

The small percentage of synapses formed on cortical cells by thalamic projections from the thalamus highlights the fact that some 70% of cortical synapses result from intracortical connections between cortical cells. This high level of self-connectivity is almost certainly responsible for the high level of sensory processing and plasticity possible in the cortex.

The intracortical connectivity of the barrel cortex has principally been studied using two main methods; by injections of tracers such as HRP and DiI and by paired intracellular recording. Tracer injections give an overall picture of density of the projection, but sparse information about the connectivity of particular cell types. Paired intracellular recordings give good information about the connectivity of the cells involved but none about how common the connection might be. Recently, a third method of gauging the number and strength of input from a particular intracortical pathway has been used. This utilizes uncaging of caged glutamate in a systematic pattern in slices of barrel cortex while recording from an individual neuron. The cell can be labeled with intracellular dye and characterized electrophysiologically in addition to obtaining a good survey of its intracortical inputs using this method.

In this section, a detailed description of intracortical connections is given with an emphasis on axonal trajectories of individual cell types and layers. Cortical circuitry is discussed further in Chapter 3 from the standpoint of function. Before describing particular intracortical pathways, it may be

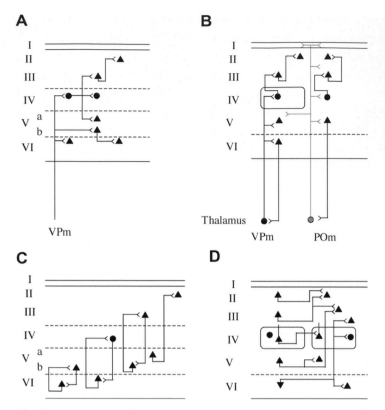

**Figure 2.9.** Features of intracortical excitatory pathways. A. Serial feedforward pathways allow columnar transmission of information from the ventral posterior medial thalamic nucleus (VPm) through layer IV to layers III and II and layer Va. Direct input from VPm also activates cells at the layer Vb/VI border and transmission to VI from V also occurs. B. VPm and the posterior medial thalamic nucleus (POm) projections target different layers and different barrel/septal subdivisions. C. Recurrent excitatory circuitry between different layers. NB: a distinction is not made in the diagram between excitatory connections on to inhibitory and excitatory cells, but it should be noted that the VI to IV pathway includes connections on to inhibitory cells. D. Horizontal pathways between barrels occur in all layers and between some layers (notably V and VI). The interbarrel layer IV to IV pathway is far sparser than the others indicated here and reserved for star pyramid interconnections.

worthwhile first to give the general picture of excitatory intracortical barrel cortex connectivity (see Figure 2.9).

1.  Columnar projections are made by layer IV barrel cells to supra- and infragranular layers (Figure 2.9A, B).
2.  Layer II/III and V cells reciprocally connect within columns (Figure 2.9C).

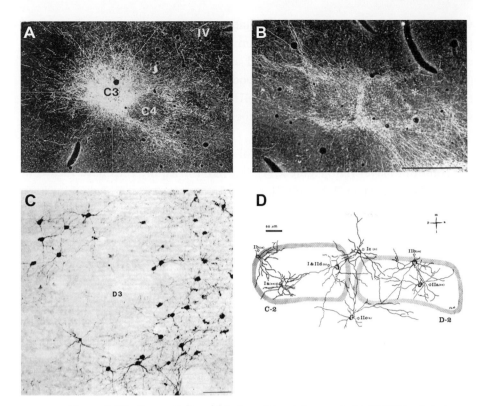

**Figure 2.10.** Connectivity within layer IV septal areas. A. An injection of phyto-hemagglutinin-L (PHA-L) from *Phaseolus vulgaris* in the C3 barrel labels some radially projecting axons but the pattern is biased to trajectories along the septae. B. An injection of PHA-L outside the field of view labels septae along three barrels within layer IV. Scale bar = 500 μm (A,B). C. Retrograde labeling of cells from intracortical injections preferentially labels septal neurons. Scale bar = 100 μm. (Reproduced from Hoeflinger *et al.* [1995], with kind permission of the authors and Wiley.) D. Cells located in barrels have asymmetric dendrites that project into the barrel center and avoid the septal area. (Reproduced from Woolsey *et al.* [1975a] with kind permisson of the authors and the US National Academy of Science.)

3. Layer IV and VI cells reciprocally connect within columns (Figure 2.9C).
4. Radial connections are sparse in layer IV barrels but spread consider-able distances in extragranular layers (Figure 2.9D).
5. Septal connections differ from barrel connections within layer IV in that they connect over larger radial distances (Figure 2.10).

### 2.4.2.1  *Layer IV connections*

Layer IV contains three main types of neuron: the aspiny or sparsely spinous GABAergic inhibitory cell; the spiny stellate cell; and the star pyramid, which is an intermediate form of excitatory cell half way in form between a pyramidal cell and a stellate cell (Simons and Woolsey, 1984). The inhibitory cells tend to have their dendrites and axons confined within single barrels (Harris and Woolsey, 1983). Their cell bodies tend to be located in the walls of the barrels in common with the other cell types. Their axons are usually directed superficially but send recurrent branches back into the same barrels within layer IV (Porter et al., 2001).

The spiny stellate cells and pyramidal cells chiefly project vertically within the column to layer II/III (Figure 2.11), but like the aspiny cells have recurrent collaterals to the layer IV barrels (Harris and Woolsey, 1983). The dual intracellular recording method demonstates that some layer IV cells connect with layer Va cells (Feldmeyer et al., 2005). It is not yet known whether the connection is made on to the basal dendrites or as a result of the apical dendrite passing through layer IV and contacting a local arborization of the layer IV cell axon.

In general, the horizontal connections from layer IV barrels are fewer and of shorter range than those in other cortical layers, as can be seen from HRP injections (Bernardo et al., 1990a; Hoeflinger et al., 1995). This finding is also supported by the observation that the probability of paired recordings between layer IV cells decreases rapidly outside the barrel wall (Feldmeyer and Sakmann, 2000). One exception to this rule is that septal areas are interconnected within layer IV over several barrel widths (Figure 2.10). An injection of PHA-L into D1 back-labels cell bodies around the D3 barrel (Figure 2.10C) and individal axons appear to travel within layer IV and have synaptic swellings within the septum (Hoeflinger et al., 1995). The other exception is to this pattern of connectivity is made by the star pyramid cells in layer IV. Although layer IV is characterized by the small granular stellate cells, nevertheless approximately one third of cells actually have a clear apical dendrite and a pyramidal somatic appearance. It has been shown that pyramidal cells can connect between barrel-columns (Schubert et al., 2001, 2003), suggesting that they form a subcircuit within the barrel system. Theoretically then, the stellate cells may be concerned with columnar connectivity and the pyramidal cells with columnar and intercolumnar connectivity. In support of this idea, spiny stellates and star pyramids also form local connections within layer IV, but preferentially with the same cell type: that is, spiny stellate to spiny stellate and star pyramid to star pyramid (Cowan and Stricker, 2004). It has been estimated that an individual spiny stellate cell connects to approximately 20–30% of the other layer IV cells within reach of its axon, which considering that the axonal projection covers most of the barrel indicates that layer IV cells are highly interconnected within the barrel (Feldmeyer et al., 1999).

Projections from layer IV to layer II/III cells in barrels have been studied in rat barrel cortex and comprise extensive complex arbors that largely stay confined

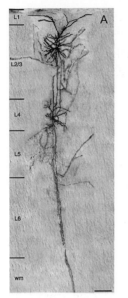

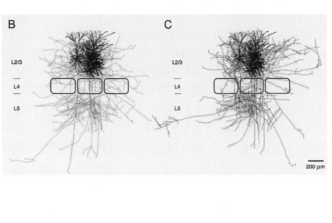

**Figure 2.11.** Axonal projection patterns within barrel cortex. A. An example of a layer IV cell projecting superficially to a surpagranular layer cell. The axons of both the pyramidal cell and the layer IV spiny cell project through layers V and VI toward the white matter (wm). Scale bar = 100 μm. (Reproduced from Lubke *et al.* [2003], with kind permission of the authors and Oxford University Press.) B,C. Examples of projection patterns of two pairs of synaptically coupled layer III pyramidal cells showing their vertical connections to layer V and interbarrel connections within all layers but reaching their greatest lateral extent in layer V. (Reproduced from Feldmeyer *et al.* [2006], with kind permission of the authors and Cambridge University Press.)

within the barrel-column and partly send diagonal axons into the near side of the neighboring columns (Feldmeyer *et al.*, 2002). Most, if not all, of the layer IV axons ascend as well as descend within the column (Figure 2.11). However, more than 90% of the connections of stellate and star pyramidal cells are made within layer IV and layers II/III (Lubke *et al.*, 2000). The connections with layers II/III cells are relatively reliable but evoke small excitatory postsynaptic potentials (EPSPs). This implies that convergence of input is required for layer IV to activate layers II/III pyramidal cells. Layer III pyramidal cells that lie on the boundaries of layer IV and III also send their basal dendrites into layer IV where they can make direct contact with the thalamocortical arbors. Both features conspire to preserve the same principal whisker identity in transmission from layer IV to III.

Studies using caged glutamate photolytically released in slices of rat barrel cortex have shown that layer III cells receive a strong functional connection from layer IV, within the barrel-column (Shepherd *et al.*, 2005). Similarly, where the layer III cell lies directly above a septum, inputs are directed preferentially from the septal layer IV cells beneath it rather than from the nearest layer IV barrel cells (Kim and Ebner, 1999). However, the layer IV to layers II/III connection is weaker from the septum than from the barrels, perhaps partly because of the difference in cell density in the two areas. A stronger connection to superficial layers, particularly layer II, comes from layer Va in the septal column (Shepherd *et al.*, 2005). Therefore, in so far as the septal and barrel cells receive POm and VPm inputs, respectively, the streams remain separate at this particular locus in the cortex (see Figure 2.9). However, the same cannot be said for the layer IV input to layer Va, because the layer Va cells receive direct POm input immediately beneath the barrel as well as VPm-derived input from layer IV (Feldmeyer *et al.*, 2005).

### 2.4.2.2  *Layer II and III connections*

Layer II cells form a distinct stratum within mouse cortex close to the white matter. The transition between II and III can be seen in Nissl stains and from filled cells. The transition between layer II and III is less distinct in the rat barrel cortex, which often leads authors to refer to the upper and lower halves of layers II/III. In mouse barrel cortex, layer II pyramidal cells often lie sideways with a horizontally directed apical dendrite, or the apical dendrite bifurcates almost immediately after leaving the cell body in a diagonal or horizontal direction. The dendrites of layer II cells often branch extensively within layer I (Feldmeyer *et al.*, 2006). Layer II cells can send axons down into layer III and V and recurrent collaterals course up into the layer I white matter above them. The lateral extent of the layer II axons can be extensive, spanning several barrels. In general, at the time of writing, far less is known about layer II connectivity than generic supragranular layer connectivity.

Layer III pyramidal cells have axons that both descend to infragranular layers and send lateral branches out to neighboring columns and other layer II/III cells within the same column (Lorente de Nó, 1922; Bernardo *et al.*, 1990a; Gottlieb and Keller, 1997). Pairs of synaptically coupled layer III cells have been recorded within the span of a barrel-column and are estimated to interconnect with as many as 270 other local pyramidal cells (Feldmeyer *et al.*, 2006). Some layer III cells are projection neurons, sending axons into the white matter to SII. In doing so, many axons form recurrent branches that ascend diagonally back into the cortex to superficial layers (Lorente de Nó, 1922). Layer III pyramidal cells, therefore, have the opportunity to connect with cells in all layers of the cortex (Figure 2.11). A major difference compared with the layer IV projections is that they are not confined to the barrel-column and send projections several barrels away within the cortex (Gottlieb and Keller, 1997). There is evidence that the connections tend to be oriented more strongly along the rows of barrels than across the arcs (Bernardo *et al.*, 1990b). When individual connections are traced along the barrel row, layer III to layer III connections can span three to seven barrels.

### 2.4.2.3    *Layer V connections*

Layer V is particularly highly developed in the somatosensory cortex. Two sublaminae, Va and Vb, can easily be distinguished on the basis of cell density, cell type, connectivity and receptor expression (Mercier *et al.*, 1990; Bodor *et al.*, 2005; Schubert *et al.*, 2006a). In addition, the intrinsic membrane properties of cells in the same layer (and sublaminae) can also differ. Some cells fire spikes regularly in response to a somatic current injection (regular spiking [RS]) while others respond with a burst of spikes (intrinsic bursting [IB]) (Section 3.1.3).

The main differences between the sublaminae are in their inputs and outputs. Cells in layer Vb receive a connection from the thalamic afferents from VPm, which send a collateral to them on passing up to the layer IV barrel. Layer Va cells receive a far smaller input from this source but do receive a connection from layer IV, which is not shared by the layer Vb cells. The main differences between the RS and IB cells, apart from their intrinsic membrane properties, are again that the IB cells do not receive direct VPm input and receive their connections from intracortical sources, while RS cells do receive thalamic input. This is not to say that IB cells are exclusively in layer Va and RS cells exclusively in Vb, as there is a clear mixture in the sublaminae. Finally, one more generalization that can be made is that RS cells receive stronger inhibitory inputs than IB cells (Schubert *et al.*, 2001). Having made these general points, it is useful to consider the detailed evidence more closely.

Layer V pyramidal cell connections are even more widespread laterally within the cortex than those of layer II and III (Figure 2.12). Layer V cells interconnect extensively within the layer as well as projecting back to layers II/III and down to layer VI cells. The lateral connections to other barrel-columns tend to be to adjacent rows rather than along the rows, in contrast to supragranular cells (Bernardo *et al.*, 1990b). The IB cells tend to receive a higher percentage of connections from other barrel-columns than RS cells, but both receive an input from other columns. Perhaps surprisingly, the major source of intracortical transcolumnar input to IB cells is from layer VI (Schubert *et al.*, 2001), closely followed by layers IV and V. Layer VI provides the main source of intracolumnar input to IB cells, whereas layers IV and V are the main source for RS cells. Most canonical circuits for the cortex have tended to emphasize the connection from layers II and III to layer V as a major step in cortical processing. However, layer VI is a major source of input, and layers II/III connections, while

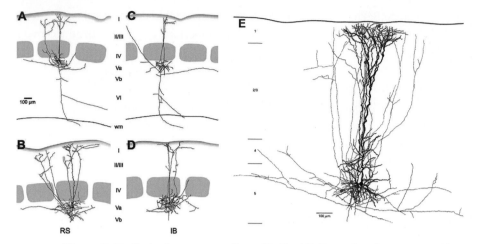

**Figure 2.12.** Projection patterns of layer V cells. A,B. Examples of reconstructed layer Va regular spiking (RS) cells that have horizonatal axons within layer V and vertical and diagonal connections to supragranular layers. C,D. Examples of layer Va intrinsic burster (IB) cell axon trajectories. (Reproduced from Schubert *et al.* [2006b], with kind permission of the authors and Oxford University Press.) E. Example of the axonal arbors of two synaptically coupled layer V cells. In both cases, axons course horizontally within layer V and send vertical projections toward and including layer I. Circles denote the location of unidirectional connections. NB: more connections are made between the adjacent cells on the apical than on the basal dendrite. (Reproduced from Markram *et al.* [1997], with kind permission of the authors and Cambridge University Press.)

present, only form approximately 30% of the input to layer V neurons (Schubert *et al.*, 2001).

### 2.4.2.4    *Layer VI connections*

Layer VI provides the back projection to VPm in the barrel cortex. Approximately 50% of layer VI cells project to the thalamus (Gilbert and Kelly, 1975; Zhang and Deschenes, 1997). In addition, layer VI contains a number of stellate cells and modified pyramidal cells, including inverted pyramids with their apical dendrites oriented away from the pial surface (Figure 2.13D). Most conventionally oriented pyramidal cells do not send their apical dendrites closer to the surface than layer IV (Figure 2.13 A–C). Layer VI cells provide extensive intracortical connections within layer VI and throughout the other cortical layers (Figure 2.13D,E).

Layer VI is conventionally recognized to be composed of two sublaminae, designated VIa and VIb. Together with the Cajal–Retzius neurons of layer I, layer VIb forms the primordial plexiform layer (Marin-Padilla, 1978), which represents the earliest cells in the developing cortex. Layer VIa cells migrate into this area

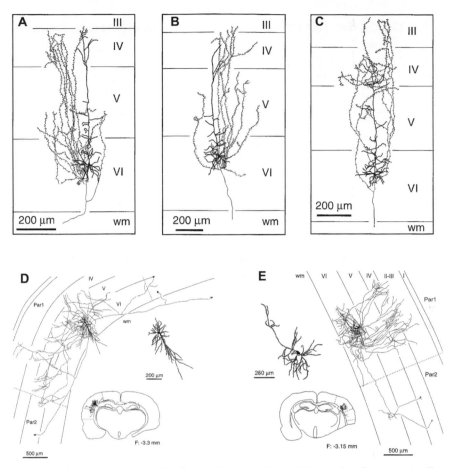

**Figure 2.13.** Layer VI cell axonal trajectories. A–C. Examples of recurrent collaterals formed by layer VI corticothalamic neurons. Note that the axons and apical dendrites only reach as far as layer IV and only in C do the axons reach into layer III. D. Inverted pyramidal cell in layer VIa sends widespread connections to primary and secondary parietal cortex (Par1 and Par2, respectively) mainly within infragranular layers. E. Horizontal pyramidal cells send strong parallel streams of axons vertically to layer IV and III (wm, white matter). (Adapted from Zhang and Deschenes [1997], with kind permission of the authors and the Society for Neuroscience.)

later. In general, the VIa neurons form connections with the thalamus, and in barrel cortex layer VIa has a higher density of cells solely projecting to VPm, while layer VIb cells can connect with both VPm and POm (Zhang and Deschenes, 1997).

Corticothalamic cells have extensive recurrent axonal arbors that project within the confines of a column back into layer V, IV and occasionally III (Figure 2.13A–C). Some cells have been observed to make particularly dense

Table 2.1. *Classification of inhibitory interneurons; neurogliaform and Cajal–Retzius interneurons are not included*

| Cell type | Target structure[a] | Calcium-binding proteins | | |
|---|---|---|---|---|
| | | Calbindin | Parvalbumin | Calretinin |
| Bipolar | Dendrites | | | + |
| Double bouquet | Dendrites | + | | + |
| Bitufted | Dendrites | + | | + |
| Small basket | Soma | + | + | |
| Large basket | Soma | + | + | |
| Nest basket | Soma | + | + | |
| Chandelier | Axons | + | + | |

+, immunoreactivity for calcium-binding proteins.
[a] Main location of the inhibitory cell's synapses.

connections around the IV/V border (Zhang and Deschenes, 1997). A proportion of pyramidal cells can have extensive horizontal connections within layers V and VI and also send connections to SII and the dysgranular zone.

### 2.4.3    *Inhibitory intracortical pathways*

#### 2.4.3.1    *Classification of inhibitory cells*

Inhibitory interneurons form a diverse class of neurons in the cortex, in stark contrast to the relatively few types of excitatory cell. Numerous attempts to classify inhibitory interneurons by morphology, expression of calcium-binding proteins, neuropeptides and spike firing pattern have lead to some useful generalizations, but none can be made entirely without caveats. Table 2.1 describes some of the basic generalizations that can be made for seven of the inhibitory interneuron subtypes. Unfortunately, even with one of the most useful correlations between basket cells and parvalbumin-staining neurons, it needs to be kept in mind that only about half the basket cells produce parvalbumin at all.

A classification based on the axonal projection targets of the interneurons is quite useful because it highlights that different morphologies arise from the need to inhibit different portions of the excitatory cells and hence links form to function (Figure 2.14). Basket cells inhibit the somata of pyramidal neurons while various cell types are directed to different aspects of the dendrites including the bipolar, bitufted and double bouquet cells. The last two cell types are also differentiated by their propensity to contain parvalbumin in the case of the soma-targeting basket cells and calretinin in the case of the dendrite-targeting cells (Section 3.2 has a further description of cell types).

Chandelier                    Bitufted cell                    Bipolar cell

Large basket cell              Martinotti cell                  Double bouquet cell

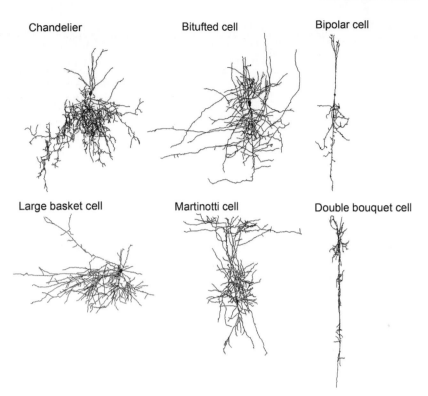

**Figure 2.14.** Examples of the axonal arborizations of six types of cortical inhibitory neuron. Chandelier cells make synaptic contact with axon initial segments and, therefore, often have vertical axon terminations. Bitufted cells make connection with dendrites and the bitufted nature refers to the dendrites rather than the axon pattern. Bipolar and double bouquet cells are both dendrite-targeting cells, and their thin vertical arborization suggests a role in columnar inhibition. Large basket cells make terminations on cells bodies. Martinotti cells send strong vertical projections to layer I of the cortex. (Reproduced from http://microcircuit.epfl.ch/ with kind permission of Henry Markram.)

### 2.4.3.2    *Layer IV inhibitory cells*

Approximately 50% of the neurons in layer IV of the barrel contain parvalbumin, which would suggest that at least half are basket cells of some sort or chandelier cells, a figure that fits with independent estimates (Markram *et al.*, 2004). Like most cells in layer IV, inhibitory cells receive thalamic input from VPm and tend to be more sensitive to it than the excitatory cells in layer IV (Porter *et al.*, 2001). Layer IV inhibitory interneurons tend either to have axons ramifying within the confines of the barrel or to send axons vertically to supragranular layers. The vertical projections can either be confined to the barrel-column or project outside it diagonally, over a radial distance of some

200 μm in the mouse (Porter *et al.*, 2001). The pattern of projections suggests that inhibition is directed to limit excitation within the barrel and to provide a brake on excitation transmitted out of layer IV to layers II/III. In this sense, inhibitory pathways follow the same route as excitatory pathways at this early stage of intracortical processing. The synchrony of inhibition is enhanced by the presence of gap junctions that connect inhibitory interneurons (Beierlein *et al.*, 2003). The layer IV inhibitory neurons also inhibit one another, so that thalamic stimulation leads to an excitatory–inhibitory sequence in postsynaptic potentials in the GABAergic cell. One of the consequences is that inhibitory cells often fire a single spike in response to thalamic stimulation, even though their spike adaptation properties would theoretically allow them to fire many more (Porter *et al.*, 2001).

It has been found that in the rat barrel cortex, layer IV cells have two distinct inhibitory circuits. The circuits are formed by fast spiking cells (FS), which show little adaptation, and the low threshold spiking cells (LTS), which show spike accommodation but have a particularly low threshold response to somatic current injection as a result of the current $I_t$, which is depolarizing and only de-inactivates when hyperpolarized (see Figure 3.8, below). The FS cells are connected together by gap junctions as are the LTS cells, but junctions are not present across cell types (Gibson *et al.*, 1999). While the excitatory interneuron synapses on to FS cells show depressing short-term synaptic dynamics, the LTS cells show facilitation (Beierlein *et al.*, 2003). Consequently, FS cells produce inhibition at a lower frequency of input than LTS cells. Finally, the FS cells are activated by thalamic input whereas LTS cells rarely are (Beierlein *et al.*, 2003).

### 2.4.3.3   Layer II/III inhibitory cells

Layers II and III contain a variety of inhibitory interneurons including basket cells, chandelier cells, double bouquet and bitufted cells (Zhu *et al.*, 2004). The subthreshold receptive fields of these cells show that they receive input from a number of whiskers, although the principal whisker produces the largest EPSP and inhibitory postsynaptic potentials (IPSPs). Chandelier cells tend to have the largest receptive fields but are less excitable than other inhibitory interneurons. This appears to be because the IPSP arrives at the chandelier cell before the EPSPs (Zhu *et al.*, 2004). Since chandelier cells contact the axon initial segments of excitatory cells and have large axonal arbors, they are in a good position to prevent intracortical transmission over a wide area. However, as noted, whisker stimulation is usually not sufficient to activate the chandelier system, at least under conditions of barbiturate anesthesia (Zhu *et al.*, 2004).

### 2.4.3.4    *Layer V/VI inhibitory cells*

Layer V contains two major types of pyramidal cell: the IB cells, which have branched apical dendrites, and the RS cells, with thinner apical dendrites that ascend to the surface before producing an apical tuft that enters layer I. The IB pyramidal cells tend to have less inhibitory control than the RS cells, although some inhibition does originate from other cells in layer V itself. In contrast, the RS pyramidal cells tend to receive inhibition from all layers within the column and some transcolumnar input from layer V (Schubert *et al.*, 2001).

The circuitry for layer Va and layer Vb inhibitory systems differ somewhat. Layer Va cells tend to receive projections from a subset of inhibitory cell that contain cholocystekinin and have presynaptic cannabinoid (CB1) receptors (Bodor *et al.*, 2005). Layer V cells tend to be richer in a different type of inhibitory interneuron that contains parvalbumin but not CB1 receptors. Cannabinoid receptors are thought to be important for invoking a form of presynaptic inhibition known as depolarization-induced suppression of inhibition (Wilson and Nicoll, 2002) whereby cortical pyramidal neurons can disinhibit themselves by releasing endocannabinoids on to presynaptic CB1 receptors on the GABAergic interneuron somatic terminals (Bodor *et al.*, 2005; see also Section 3.3.2).

Layer VI contains the largest proportion of Martinotti cells in the somatosensory cortex (see Markram *et al.*, 2004), and these cells are characterized by their vertically directed axons, which often reach layer I (Lorente de Nó, 1922). A second source of inhibitory input from layer VI comes from the corticothalamic neurons that have ascending axons terminating in layer IV, largely on inhibitory interneurons (White and Keller, 1987; Beierlein *et al.*, 2003). Within layer IV, the corticothalamic neurons can engage either the FS or LTS subcircuits.

### 2.4.4    *Non-specific innervation*

The barrel cortex receives a number of diffuse projections from midbrain and thalamic structures, in common with other cortical areas. The main projections from the midbrain are the noradrenergic pathway from the locus coeruleus (Ungerstedt, 1971), the serotonergic pathway from the dorsal raphe nucleus (Lidov *et al.*, 1980), the dopaminergic projection from the ventral midbrain tegmentum (Lindvall *et al.*, 1974) and the cholinergic projection from the basal forebrain (Mesulam *et al.*, 1983). These projections are denoted as diffuse because they are not topographically organized and the axons project widely over more than one cortical area. However, a degree of specificity is conferred by the specificity of the receptor subtypes involved.

The β-adrenoceptors show a laminated pattern in cortex, having a higher density in layers I–IV than in infragranular locations (Schliebs *et al.*, 1989). In contrast, $\alpha_2$-adrenoceptors are more uniform in distribution (Dunn-Meynell and

Levin, 1993). The adrenergic fibers themselves tend to run parallel to the pial surface in layer I and VI but elsewhere show no particular orientation and cross septal and barrel boundaries at all angles (Simpson *et al.*, 2006). It was originally thought that noradrenaline provided the only catecholaminergic innervation of the cortex; however some dopaminergic innervation is also present. The dopaminergic innervation is largely focused on the frontal cortex, but a small projection does occur to layer VI of parietal cortex (Descarries *et al.*, 1987).

The serotonin innervation of the cortex is not topographically organized, but because $5HT_{1B}$ receptors are located on the presynaptic terminals of thalamo-cortical afferents in layer IV, staining for $5HT_{1B}$ does show a strong barrel pattern (Bennett-Clarke *et al.*, 1994). It is beyond the scope of this chapter to discuss the many 5HT receptor subtypes present in cortex, but suffice to say that both subtypes 1 and 2 effects have been observed in rat sensorimotor cortex (Foehring *et al.*, 2002). Interestingly, inhibitory interneurons appear to be a target for serotonergic innervation, with hyperpolarizing mediated by $5HT_{1A}$ receptors and depolarizing effects by $5HT_2$ receptors (Foehring *et al.*, 2002).

Cholinergic receptors are restricted to muscarinic types in the adult brain, though presynaptic nicotinic receptors and acetylcholinesterase do appear on thalamocortical afferents during the first two weeks of postnatal life (Chapter 4). Both $M_1$ and $M_2$ muscarinic receptor are present in somatosensory cortex (Skangiel-Kramska *et al.*, 1992) with $M_1$ being highest in density in layers II/III, lowest in VI and moderate elsewhere (Schliebs *et al.*, 1989). In general, receptor subtype actions in barrel cortex have not been investigated extensively but acetylcholine clearly plays an important role in sensory processing and plasticity (Maalouf *et al.*, 1998).

In addition, a further diffuse projection arises from the intralaminar nuclei (Herkenham, 1980). Electrophysiological studies show that widespread evoked responses can be elicited in cortex by stimulating the intralaminar nuclei (Dempsey and Morison, 1943; Olausson *et al.*, 1989). In agreement with this, Golgi-stained material shows widespread bilateral projections from the intralaminar nuclei to cortex (Scheibel and Scheibel, 1967) and autoradiographic tracer injections show widespread layers V and VI innervation (Herkenham, 1980). However, the intralaminar nuclei appear to be a heterogeneous group and projections may be more specific than once believed (Berendse and Groenewegen, 1991). The centrolateral nucleus of the intralaminar group does appear to project to layers I and V/VI of parietal cortex while the centromedial and paracentral nuclei do not. The parafascicular nucleus only projects weakly to somatosensory areas, including layer I (Berendse and Groenewegen, 1991) and in general the posterior intralaminar nuclei are mainly directed at striatum and layer VI of the motor cortex (Deschenes *et al.*, 1995).

## 2.5    Cortical outputs

### 2.5.1    *Corticocortical connections*

Different cortical areas can be arranged in a hierarchy according to which areas project information forward and which areas project information back. Forward projections usually originate in extragranular layers and terminate in layer IV of the higher-order area (Maunsell and Van Essen, 1983). Back projections usually terminate in extragranular layers of the lower-order cortical area. Barrel cortex (SI) is most closely related to two other cortical areas, namely MI and SII. Barrel cortex projects strongly to SII (Fabri and Burton, 1991; Hoffer *et al.*, 2003). Retrograde transport of tracer from SII labels projection neurons in SI that are located in layers III and V but not IV (Chakrabarti and Alloway, 2006). Anterograde transport from single barrel injections produce termination patterns in SII that cover layers III, VI and V (Wright *et al.*, 2000). This partly conforms to the hierarchy seen in visual cortex and would define SII as a higher-order area, but not quite, because extragranular layers also receive the "forward" projection from SI, which is a trait of a back projection. In projections between MI and SI, cells projecting in both directions arise from extragranular layers (Chakrabarti and Alloway, 2006). In addition, there are reciprocal connections between SII and MI, all of which suggests that the three areas are best thought of as equivalent in hierarchy.

The barrel cortex projection to SII is topographic and a mirror image about a line running approximately parallel to the A-row of whiskers. A single barrel projects to a strip of SII, and neighbouring barrels in a row project to the same strip, which is largely overlapped. Barrels in different rows project to different strips in SII. Therefore, within-row information is integrated to a greater extent than between-row information in SII. A similar pattern is seen in MI, and indeed a few cells in barrel cortex project to both SII and MI.

The projections from barrel cortex to MI arise from extragranular layer cells above and below the septal areas (Hoffer *et al.*, 2003). The projection to MI is predominantly from the septal areas (Figure 2.15) rather than the barrel areas (Alloway *et al.*, 2004). No such segregation is found in the barrel cortex projection to SII however, which arises relatively uniformly from cells above and below septae and barrels alike (Chakrabarti and Alloway, 2006). Callosal connections also preferentially project into septal areas rather than barrels (Olavarria *et al.*, 1984).

Given that POm also projects to septal areas, the barrel cortex appears to have two separate circuits to communicate with other cortical areas: the septal circuit, which is bilaterally connected, receives input from POm and connects with MI and SII; and the barrel circuit, which is unilateral, receives input from VPm and connects with SII (Figure 2.16).

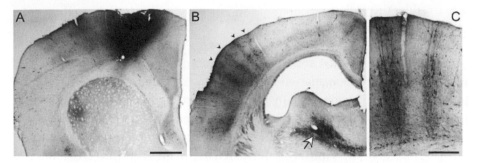

**Figure 2.15.** Anterograde labeling of neurons in septal areas projecting to area I of the motor cortex (MI). A. Location of injection site in MI. B. Coronal section through barrel cortex shows septal columns of the retrograde tracer cholera toxin b and also labels the posterior medial thalamic nucleus (white arrow). Scale bar = 1 mm (A, B). C. Closer view of the cells labeled in septal columns. Scale bar = 250 μm. (Reproduced from Alloway *et al.* [2004], with kind permission of the authors and Wiley.)

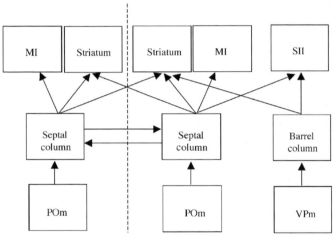

Midline

**Figure 2.16.** Diagram to illustrate the bilateral nature of the connections of the septal columns in the barrel cortex. Note that septal columns connect via the callosum and also send a diffuse bilateral projection to the striatum in addition to the more topographic ipsilateral connection. The barrel-columns also project to striatum, but only ipsilaterally. MI, motor cortex area I; POm, posterior medial thalamic nucleus; SII, second somatosensory area; VPm, ventral posterior medial thalamic nucleus.

*2.5.2    Subcortical somatomotor projections*

The output projections from the cortex are principally either to motor structures such as the striatum, superior colliculus and pons or feedback to sensory structures such as VPm, POm and the trigeminal nuclei. This section will consider the projections to motor structures and Section 2.5.3 will describe the sensory feedback.

A major projection to the pons is derived from layer Vb, where the vast majority of cells can be labeled by a retrograde injection into the pontine nucleus. The pontine nuclei project to the cerebellum, which contains two maps of the body, one in the anterior and one in the posterior lobe. Because most of the layer Vb cells project to the pons, and yet layer Vb also projects to other subcortical targets, it is logical that many of the corticopontine projections must branch to project elsewhere. It has been estimated that approximately 25% of the cells that project to the pons also send a collateral to the superior colliculus in the rat (Mercier *et al.*, 1990).

The corticopontine projection is organized in a topographic manner, but as with the corticocortical projections to MI and SII there is greater convergence along rows than between rows (Leergaard *et al.*, 2000). Projections from the same row form overlapping concentric ovoid loops of terminations in the pons when viewed from the ventral surface. Projections from barrels in the same arc in adjacent rows project to the same concentric loop but are displaced somewhat along the length of the loop (Leergaard *et al.*, 2000). There is also a small satellite projection more medial in the pons, which is also topographically organized and may be related to the dual somatosensory representation in the cerebellum.

The projection to the striatum is largely derived from cells located in layer Va (Mercier *et al.*, 1990; Wright *et al.*, 1999). However, a narrow tier of cells in Vb also project to the striatum, though nowhere near the number that project to the pons (Mercier *et al.*, 1990). The projection to the striatum is topographically organized with individual barrel-column outputs corresponding to arcs of terminal arbors in the striatum that, in coronal section, follow the same line as the lateral contour of the nucleus. The topography is organized so that barrels located in the same row project to the same arc in the striatum with anterior barrels displaced ventrally, while different rows of barrels project to different arcs in the striatum arranged parallel to one another such that the A-row lies laterally and the E-row medially (Wright *et al.*, 1999, 2000; Leergaard *et al.*, 2000). As with the pontine projection, a dual map is formed in the striatum, one lying medial to the other and both topographically organized. There is greater overlap of the barrel representation within rows than between rows, as previously noted for motor cortex, SII and pontine projection from barrel cortex.

Finally, a third corticostriatal projection also exists specifically from the septally located layer V cells, which project more diffusely than the projections described above and furthermore project bilaterally (Wright *et al.*, 1999, 2000). Since the septal locations in the cortex receive contralateral input from the barrel cortex, this pathway appears to be part of a bilateral coordination system

(Figure 2.16). It is worth noting that the motor cortex also receives input from the septally located layer V cells.

### 2.5.3    *Subcortical somatosensory projections*

The cortex projects back to the somatosensory thalamic nuclei (VPm and POm) via layer V and VI cells, which have largely been treated in Section 2.4.2. The back projection to VPm is topographically organized (Bourassa *et al.*, 1995; Land *et al.*, 1995; Wright *et al.*, 2000) with little overlap from adjacent barrels (Wright *et al.*, 2000). Because retrograde transport is confined to the anterograde transport pattern, it seems likely that the cortico-cortical projection is back to the appropriate thalamic barreloid (Land, 1995; Wright *et al.*, 2000).

The projection to POm originates from layer V and, where small injections have been used, appears to come from the septal areas rather than the barrel areas (Wright *et al.*, 2000). The cortical influence on this nucleus is considerable, as discussed in Section 2.3.4. The cortico–POm projection is not as highly topographic as the projection to VPm, but nevertheless does show topographic order, with the terminations forming rods running rostrocaudally in POm (Hoogland *et al.*, 1987; Wright *et al.*, 2000).

The cortex also projects back from layer V cells to the trigeminal nuclei (White and DeAmicis, 1977; Welker *et al.*, 1988) where the terminations are largely made in the septal areas between the barrelettes in principalis and interpolaris and in laminae III–V in caudalis (Jacquin *et al.*, 1990). The projection is almost entirely contralateral, although a small ipsilateral component has been observed (Jacquin *et al.*, 1990). The termination pattern of cortical inputs has been termed "honeycomb" by Jacquin and colleagues and is most pronounced in contralateral caudalis and interpolaris and ipsilateral principalis. The back projection from cortex to brainstem is reciprocally topographically organized in the mouse (Welker *et al.*, 1988) and rat (Jacquin *et al.*, 1990) as it is for the back projection to thalamus.

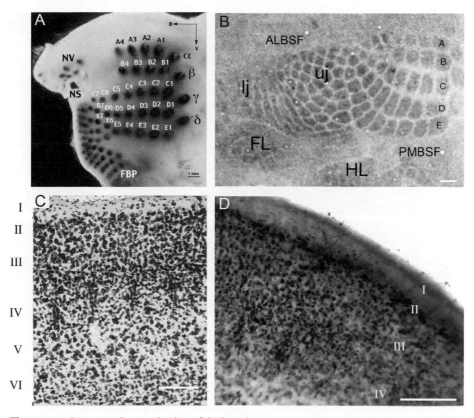

**Figure 1.1.** Somatotopic organization of the barrel cortex. A. A section through the muzzle of the rat reveals the pattern of vibrissae follicles arranged in five rows labeled A to E. The vibrissae are conventionally numbered from 1 at the back and increasingly higher numbers toward the nose (left). (Reproduced with kind permission of S. Hairdarlui and E. Ahissar.) B. The same pattern is replicated in barrel cortex. This cytochrome oxidase-labeled section through layer IV of the somatosensory cortex reveals barrels organized in five rows. The posterior medial barrel subfield (PMBSF) is on the right and corresponds to the large vibrissae that are actively whisked. The anterior lateral barrel subfield (ALBSF) is to the left and represents the smaller vibrissae around the upper jaw (uj) and nose region and lower jaw (lj). Other components of the body can also be seen such as the forelimb (FL) and hindlimb (HL). (A, B reproduced from http://www.neurobio.pitt.edu/barrels/ pics.htm.) C. A cross-section through the cortex reveals the six-layer structure and the barrels in layer IV, which appear like staves of a barrel. (Nissl stain adapted from Woolsey and Van der Loos [1970] with kind permission of Elsevier and the authors.) D. Nissl stain through barrel cortex showing the barrels and a pyramidal neuron labeled with biocytin located at the top of layer III.

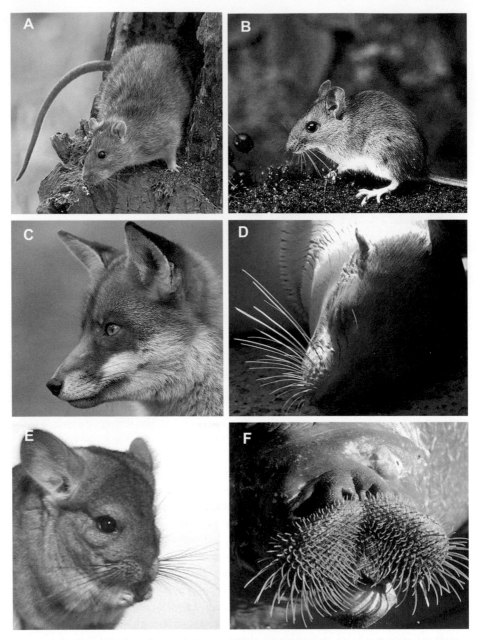

**Figure 1.3.** Many species of animals have whiskers. A. The rat is a common laboratory species for studying barrel cortex (*Rattus norvegicus*). (Courtesy of Stephen Round, reproduced with kind permission.) B. The mouse is a valuable laboratory species that can be genetically manipulated and is frequently used to study barrel cortex (pictured is the common wood or field mouse *Apodemus sylvaticus*, a cousin of the laboratory mouse, which is derived from the house mouse *Mus musculus*). C, D. Foxes (C) along with other carnivores such as sea lions (D) have whiskers but are unlikely to have barrels because other carnivores such as cats do not. E. The chinchilla has whiskers and barrels. F. The walrus has an impressive set of whiskers but it is not known whether this species has barrels.

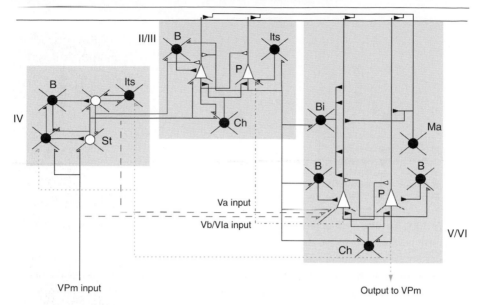

**Figure 3.11.** Multilayer cortex based on connected single layer cortex (see Figure 3.10). Each grey box contains cell types connected in a fashion that conforms to the single layer stereotype. B, basket cell; lts, low threshold spiking cell; St, stellate cell; Ch, chandelier cell; P, pyramidal cell; Bi, bipolar or bitufted (dendrite-targeting) cell; Ma, Martinotti cell. Inhibitory interneurons are black ended and excitatory neurons are white ended.

Leftmost panel. Layer IV contains reciprocally connected spiny stellate cells and basket cells. Basket cells provide feedforward perisomatic inhibition from the thalamic input (VPm) and feedback inhibition to the excitatory stellate cells. Low threshold spiking cells do not receive thalamic input but reciprocally connect with stellate cells. The excitatory output of this layer projects to layers II/III.

Middle panel. Layers II/III contain reciprocally connected pyramidal cells. Basket cells provide feedforward perisomatic inhibition from the layer IV input (spiny stellate projections) and feedback inhibition to the excitatory pyramidal cells. Low threshold spiking cells do not receive layer IV input but reciprocally connect with pyramidal cells. Chandelier cells receive layer IV excitatory input and project to the axon initial segment of the pyramidal cells. The excitatory output of this layer from the pyramidal cells projects to layers V/VI.

Rightmost panel. Layers V/VI are illustrated as one for simplicity even though layer Va and Vb and layer VI in general are diverse in pyramidal cell subtypes. Again basket cells provide feedforward perisomatic inhibition from the layers II/III input (spiny stellate projections) and feedback inhibition to the excitatory pyramidal cells. Chandelier cells receive layers II/III excitatory input and project to the axon initial segment of the pyramidal cells. Note that bipolar/bitufted cells are dendrite-targeting cells with axons traversing the layers. Note also that Martinotti cells project to layer I.

Intracortical connections are superimposed on the three layers. The lines below the three panels represent the more complex superimposed intracortical excitatory connections and do not have obvious correlates in the single layer model. Red, thalamic input connects directly with layer Vb and layer VIa cells, and layer IV cells connect with layer Va cells. Blue, feedback connections from layer V project to layers II/III. Green, corticothalamic neurons back project to inhibitory cells in layer IV.

Note that an absence of connections in this diagram should not be taken as a known lack of connection. The main pathways are illustrated in a simplified form to combine information from the single layer model with known cortical pathways to cellular subtypes (Sections 3.4.4–3.4.6 and 3.6.1).

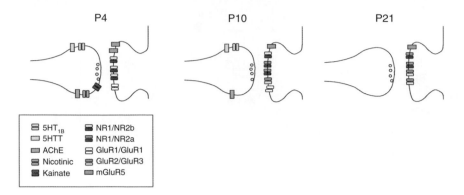

**Figure 4.11.** Development of pre- and postsynaptic receptors at thalamocortical synapses. On the fourth postnatal day (P4) in the rat, the presynaptic terminal has a variety of receptors and transporters present including serotonin receptors ($5HT_{1B}$), serotonin transporter (5HTT), nicotinic cholinergic receptors (NR) and acetylcholinesterase (AChE) in addition to kainiate receptors. These are progressively lost over the next few weeks of postnatal life (compare with P21). The postsynaptic side develops from mainly NR2B-containing NMDA receptors (P4) to mainly NR2A-containing (P10+), while AMPA receptors increase in number including the calcium-impermeable GluR2-containing types (P21). Note that postsynaptic kainate receptors are not included on this type of synapse because evidence points to their location on separate thalamocortical connections (Bannister *et al.*, 2005).

# 3

# Cellular and synaptic organization of the barrel cortex

The cerebral cortex is well known for its complexity. At least 20 different cortical cell types can be classified with ease, and by many accounts this would represent a conservative estimate. Recent studies have used gene expression to identify cell types within the cortex and revealed a high degree of cell diversity (Sugino *et al.*, 2006). It is not the purpose of this chapter to describe every nuance of cell type exhaustively, and indeed there are many excellent accounts elsewhere (Peters and Jones, 1984; Markram *et al.*, 2004; Sugino *et al.*, 2006). Instead, a brief summary of the salient features is given in the following sections as a prelude to describing their synaptic properties and some of the general features of cortical circuitry to emerge from studies in recent years. Neurons in the cortex are almost entirely glutamatergic and thus excitatory, or GABAergic and thus inhibitory (Section 3.3). The following two sections look at the excitatory and inhibitory cell types.

## 3.1    Excitatory cells

There are three main types of excitatory cell in the cortex: the spiny stellate, the star pyramid and the pyramidal cell. The star pyramid is intermediate in form between the stellate and pyramidal cell. The main features of the three cell types are described below, beginning with the spiny stellate and star pyramidal cells and ending with the diversity of pyramidal cell types in individual cortical layers.

### 3.1.1    *Spiny stellate cells*

Spiny stellate cells are characterized by, and indeed named after, their star-shaped dendritic pattern. They occur in layer IV of primary sensory cortex

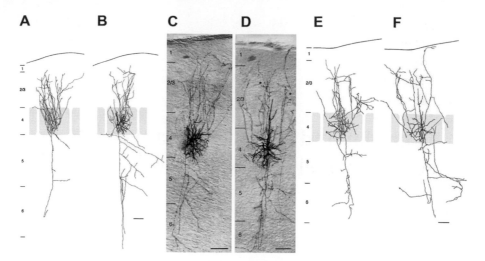

**Figure 3.1.** Stellate cells and star pyramidal cells in layer IV of barrel cortex. A,B. Camera lucida drawings of two spiny stellate cells (relative to the location of the barrels shown in light grey). C. Micrograph of the synaptically coupled pair of spiny stellate cells shown in A and B labeled with biocytin. Note the asymmetric bias of the dendrites. D. A synaptically coupled pair of star pyramidal cells. E,F. Camera lucida drawings of the two star pyramidal cells shown in D. Note the symmetric basal dendrite orientation and the vertical apical dendrite that does not reach as far as layer I. Scale bars = 100 µm. (Adapted from Lubke *et al.* [2000], with kind permission of the authors and the Society for Neuroscience.)

including somatosensory cortex. In the barrel cortex, most spiny stellate cells are located on the edge of the barrels and are modified in form such that their dendrites are preferentially oriented toward the center of the barrel rather than the septum (Figure 3.1), so they are asymmetric stellate cells. However, other stellate cells toward the center of the barrel and in the septal areas are more symmetrical in their dendritic spread (Harris and Woolsey, 1979; see Figure 2.11D).

The axons of spiny stellate cells mainly run in a columnar orientation (Figure 3.1). The main projection ascends toward layer I with arborization in layers II, III and IV (Lubke *et al.*, 2000). However, spiny stellates also project down toward layer VI, with a small number of axon branches that bifurcate sparingly to innervate layers V and VI. For a consideration of the intrinsic circuitry of stellate cells see Section 2.4.2.

### 3.1.2   Star pyramids

Approximately 20–25% of the cells in layer IV of rat barrel cortex are star pyramids (Lubke *et al.*, 2000; Staiger *et al.*, 2004). They differ from spiny stellates in that they have an ascending main apical dendrite that is longer than the rest of the radially arranged dendrites, and they differ from pyramidal cells in that their cell bodies are not overtly pyramidal and their apical dendrite is relatively short, does not reach layer I and is branched sparingly (Figure 3.1). The basal dendrites of star pyramids are symmetrical, in contrast to the anisotropy of the spiny stellate cells (Lubke *et al.*, 2000).

The axons of star pyramids project vertically to layers II/III and IV and a few branches project down to layers V/VI. Star pyramidal cells connect with cells in neighboring barrels, though most of their axonal projection lies within the column (Staiger *et al.*, 2004). Comparison of the axonal pattern of spiny stellates and star pyramids shows that the star pyramidal axons are oriented more diagonally and ramble more than those of the stellate cells (compare Figure 3.1A,B with 3.1E,F). For a description of the intrinsic circuitry of the star pyramid cells see Section 2.4.2.

### 3.1.3    *Pyramidal cells*

The pyramidal cell name refers to the triangular shape of the soma, which is apparent in Nissl-stained material, with the point of the pyramid usually oriented toward the pial surface. Studies of pyramidal cells using Golgi-staining methods have led to several attempts to define the cell class using soma size, dendritic arborization pattern and spine density (Feldman, 1984). However, the pyramids are so diverse in these details within the cortex that a better method of defining them is simply to say that they have a main apical dendrite. The apical dendrite is usually thicker than the others and stays untapered or unbranched far enough along its course that it can easily be distinguished from the other dendrites. The proximal portion of the apical dendrite can be seen in some Nissl-stained material, with Golgi staining and intracellular dyes as well as under infra red differential interference contrast or Dodt optics in living slices. The main apical dendrite is a common feature despite the diversity of size, dendritic arborization pattern and even main axial orientation of the pyramidal cells.

The diversity of the layer II pyramidal cells is a case in point. Because they lie close to the surface of the cortex and their apical dendrite often cannot run vertically, they often give the impression of being squashed beneath the pia by comparison with layer III pyramids (Figure 3.2). Some layer II pyramids have apical dendrites that actually run horizontal to the direction of the vertical column, parallel to the pial surface; others have a short primary apical dendrite that branches almost immediately on leaving the cell body. Most of the dendrites of layer II pyramidal cells occupy a range of angles from horizontal to vertical, with few projecting downward. Many cells have a strong asymmetry, where the dendrites will project in a horizontal or diagonal direction further on one side than the opposite side. This can allow them to be located in one barrel-column but reach across horizontally into the adjacent barrel-column.

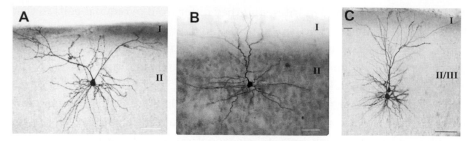

**Figure 3.2.** Supragranular layer pyramidal cells. A. A layer II cell labeled with biocytin and located in mouse barrel cortex. Note that the apical dendrite bends diagonally almost immediately on exiting the soma. B. A layer II cell labeled with biocytin in a Nissl-counterstained section. Note how the apical dendrite branches just above the soma before entering layer I. Scale bar = 50 μm (A,B). C. A synaptically coupled pair of pyramidal cells located in the lower half of layers II/III in rat barrel cortex. Note the clear apical dendrites projecting to layer I. Scale bar = 100 μm. (B is reproduced from Feldmeyer *et al.* [2006], with kind permission of the authors and the Physiological Society.)

The axons of layer II cells project vertically to layer I, where they can run for long distances of several barrels and downward into layer III and V. There is some evidence for the projection to layer V being more prominent in cells of layers II/III lying above the barrel wall (Dodt *et al.*, 2003).

Layer III pyramidal cells have a strong apical dendrite that reaches layer I. The depth of the soma within the cortex, therefore, determines the length of the dendrite. Like layer II cells, the termination of the dendrite in layer I can give rise to several branches, but unlike layer II pyramids there is more opportunity for the dendrite to produce side branches (Figure 3.2). Consequently, the apical dendrite often has many horizontal, or more often diagonal, side branches emanating before it finally bifurcates nearer layer I. The basal dendrites are arranged in a star-like form. The basal dendrites of cells close enough to layer IV reach down into layer IV where the thalamic afferents terminate, and thereby these dendrites can receive direct thalamocortical synaptic input.

The axons of layer III cells project widely within layers II/III and V, both within the column and to neighboring barrels (Bernardo *et al.*, 1990a, b; Feldmeyer *et al.*, 2006). Layer III cells also send axons down to the white matter on course for other cortical areas including SII. Recurrent collaterals can emanate from the descending axon and rise back up to layers II/III along a diagonal trajectory that takes it into a neighboring barrel.

Layer V pyramidal cells are generally far larger than their layer II or III counterparts. There are two main forms of layer V pyramidal cell, defined by a covariation of their morphology and intrinsic membrane properties (see

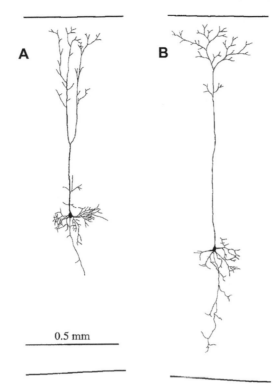

**Figure 3.3.** Morphological subtypes of layer V pyramidal cell. A. An intrinsic burster pyramidal cell with a highly branched apical dendrite. B. A regular spiking pyramidal cell with relatively symmetric basal dendrites and an unbranched apical dendrite ascending to layer I before branching. (Reproduced from Zhu and Connors [1999], with kind permission of the authors and the American Physiological Society.)

Section 3.4.1 for a fuller account of intrinsic membrane properties). Tufted pyramidal cells have a relatively thin apical dendrite that ascends to the surface with little if any branching until it reaches layer I, where it forms an apical tuft (Figure 3.3). These cells are designated RS because when injected with a depolarizing somatic current pulse they fire spikes that are regularly spaced in time. The second type of pyramidal cell has a single thick apical dendrite that branches several time before reaching layer I. These cells are designated as IB because a depolarizing somatic current injection produces a short high-frequency burst of spikes that ends abruptly, presumably through activation of calcium-dependent potassium channels. The RS and IB pyramidal cells are independent in a number of ways including the relative paucity of thalamic and inhibitory synapses on IB cells compared with RS cells and differences in the level of intercolumnar connectivity and plasticity.

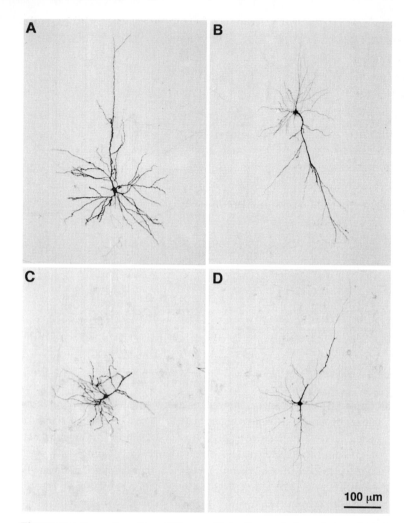

**Figure 3.4** Examples of layer VI pyramidal cell morphology. A. Standard short pyramidal cell labeled with biocytin. The apical dendrite ascends to layer IV. B. Inverted pyramidal cell where the apical dendrite descends within layer VI. C. A horizontal pyramidal cell. D. A bipolar pyramidal cell with an ascending and descending major dendrite. (Reproduced from Zhang and Deschenes [1997], with kind permission of the authors and the Society for Neuroscience.)

In general, layer V pyramidal cells are projection neurons and innervate a variety of subcortical and cortical targets (Section 2.5). They also send recurrent collaterals up into layers II/III of the cortex within the column and diagonally to many neighboring barrels. Layer V cells also send a strong projection to layer VI and interconnect with one another within the layer (Section 2.4.2).

Layer VI has a variety of pyramidal cell morphological subtypes and layer VIb in particular has been termed the polymorph layer for this reason. Most layer VI pyramidal cells have a main ascending dendrite that reaches only as far as layer IV. Some layer VI pyramids are inverted while occasionally cells lie horizontal along the axis of the layer (Figure 3.4). The horizontal pyramidal cells can have basal dendrites that ascend to layer IV. The apical and basal dendrites, therefore, swap roles in horizontally versus vertically oriented layer VI pyramids and this emphasizes the requirement for layer VI and layer IV integration for these cells. Layer VI cell axons project to thalamic and cortical targets (Section 2.5). Intracortically, layer VI axons project in a wide variety of forms. Many send axons vertically to layers V and IV, and many have extensive horizontal arbors within layer VI itself.

## 3.2    Inhibitory cells

There are numerous subtypes of inhibitory cell in the cortex, and full diversity almost defies any summary. In addition to differences in axonal arbors, soma and dendritic morphology, there are differences in the secondary neuro-peptide transmitter they produce, their calcium-binding proteins, intrinsic membrane properties, electrical coupling and glutamate receptor subtypes (Gibson *et al.*, 1999; Markram *et al.*, 2004). Most inhibitory cells inhibit excitatory cells but they also make autapses on themselves and synapse on to other inhibitory cells (Section 3.6). However, inhibitory cells all have GABA as a primary neurotransmitter and they all have a far lower spine density than excitatory cells, hence the designation aspinous or perhaps more accurately sparsely spinous. It is useful to classify the cells according to where they form synapses on their target cells as this is likely to relate to their function. Basket cells make synapses on the somata of pyramidal cells; chandelier cells form synapses on the initial segment of the axon, and a third class that includes bitufted cells have synapses on dendrites. A brief description of each type is given in the following sections.

### 3.2.1    *Soma-targeting inhibitory cells (basket cells)*

Basket cells have a characteristic axonal termination pattern that tar-gets the soma and proximal dendrites of pyramidal cells and interneurons. Their axons are sparsely branched giving off small pericellular basket-shaped elaborations at several intervals along their length. There are three main types of basket cell, known as small, large and nest types.

Small basket cells are distinguished from large basket cells by a local arbor-ization pattern in the vicinity of its own dendritic range and by their curved axons. Consequently, they tend to arborize within a column rather than across cortical columns. Inhibitory interneurons often express a secondary transmitter in addition to GABA, which is always a neuropeptide. In the case of small basket cells this neuropeptide is vasoactive intestinal peptide.

Large basket cells differ from small basket cells in sending axons to innervate somata in different columns of the cortex. They can be present in layers III to V of the cortex and project to different layers of the cortex. Figure 2.14 shows the characteristic termination pattern of a layer III basket cell, which, as described by Cajal (Ramon y Cajal, 1911), outlines the pyramidal cells they innervate. The dendrites of large basket cells are usually multipolar but can often contain a descending dendrite as if it was an inverted pyramid (though one with few spines).

Nest basket cells are intermediate in form between large and small basket cells. They have longer axons than small basket cells but not the reach of large basket cells. Despite this, they have less dendritic length per dendrite than either small or large basket cells (Wang *et al.*, 2002). Most but not all of the axonal contacts made by nest basket cells lie within the same column or layer. In part contradiction of the classification method adopted here, nest basket cells do have some terminals connecting to the apical dendrites as well as the proximal basal and somata of pyramidal cells (Wang *et al.*, 2002). Finally, nest basket cells do not normally contain the calcium-binding protein calretinin (Chapter 2), in common with the small and large types of basket cell.

### 3.2.2    *Axon-targeting inhibitory cells*

Chandelier cells are clearly a separate interneuron class because they alone project to axons within the cortex. The branches of the cell are covered in vertically oriented short termination branches that form the candles of the chandelier (Figure 2.14). These terminations contact the initial segment of pyramidal cell axons as they exit the soma. By hyperpolarizing the axon at this point, the chandelier cell can "veto" the output of the cell, while leaving the cellular processing intact. In so far as back-propagating action potentials are required for synaptic plasticity, chandelier cells can prevent them occurring.

Because the cortex is extensively interconnected with reciprocal excitatory connections, targeting the output of the excitatory cells is a particularly effective way of reducing intracortical positive feedback. Chandelier cells contact numerous targets (60–80) and can be found in all layers. They do not respond as strongly to whisker input in cortex as other interneurons but do respond strongly once the overall cortical excitation increases (Zhu *et al.*, 2004), suggesting that they may function to keep overall cortical positive feedback within limits.

### 3.2.3    Dendrite-targeting inhibitory cells

Double bouquet and bitufted cells have vertically oriented axons that run from layer II to V and tend to be confined to narrow bundles, often referred to as a horsetail (Figure 2.14). The double bouquet is formed by the dendrites that project in two sets, one dorsal and one ventral to the soma. The lateral spread of dendrites are generally no wider than the spread of the axons. Double bouquet cells, therefore, appear to be involved in columnar processing. They innervate spines and the smooth surface of the dendrites of pyramidal cells. Double bouquet cells occur in layers II/III. They do not produce the calcium-binding protein parvalbumin, nor neuropeptide Y and somatostatin.

Bitufted cells are similar to double bouquet and bipolar cells in that they have primary dendrites emerging from opposite ends of the soma and are oriented vertically. However, unlike the narrow vertical dendrites of bouquet and bipolar cells, bitufted cells have a wider distribution of dendrites to neighboring columns and preferentially to other layers. Bitufted cell dendrites also mainly project vertically toward the pial surface rather than projecting up and down the column. Bitufted cells project to dendrites of their target cells (Figure 2.14). They are located in layers II/III and IV in barrel cortex and probably correspond to the LTS cells that form gap junctions with other LTS but not other inhibitory cell types. Bitufted cells do not stain for parvalbumin.

Bipolar cells can be found in layers II to V of the cortex. They tend to have rather simple dendrites, with one ascending and one descending primary dendrite emerging from the soma to branch rather sparsely. The axons are vertically oriented and, enigmatically, a subset of bipolar cells form asymmetrical synapses on dendrites and spines of pyramidal cells (Peters and Kimerer, 1981). A second group of bipolar cells usually express both GABA and vasoactive intestinal peptide and form symmetric synapses on dendritic shafts (Peters and Harriman, 1988).

### 3.2.4    Other categories of inhibitory interneuron

Martinotti cells are inhibitory cells that typically project vertically to form terminal arbors in layer I (Fairen et al., 1984; Wang et al., 2004). Initially, Martinotti referred to a cell with an ascending non-bifurcating axon that only branched once it reached layer I (Martinotti, 1889, 1890) and while such cells clearly exist and have been consistently described (Marin-Padilla and Marin-Padilla, 1982), other variations exist based on the theme (Wang et al., 2004). The dendrites of Martinotti cells can be bipolar in nature, and in deeper layers the descending dendrite can be more elaborate to give the impression of an inverted pyramidal cell (Figure 2.14). The ascending axon sends collaterals to several layers while projecting to layer I and so can contact cell bodies and dendrites of cells in those layers. However, because layer I mainly contains the distal arborization of apical dendrites, the layer I projections of the Martinotti cells mostly contact dendrites. The rare axosomatic connections in layer I are with the few surviving Cajal–Retzius cells in that layer. Axons can project over a far wider area than a single barrel-column (up to several millimeters) and so Martinotti cells, together with the large basket cells, provide a substrate for cross-columnar inhibition. Given that they project to distal apical dendrites, their influence includes inhibiting excitatory inputs on pyramidal cells in that layer, for example projections from the ventromedial nucleus of the thalamus and back projections from other cortical areas.

Cells in all layers from II to VI have Martinotti cells. Layer VI Martinotti cells send a strong projection to layer IV as well as layer I, to complement the excitatory projection from layer VI to layer IV (Wang *et al.*, 2004). Presumably, this is important for controlling the thalamic input to cortex. Martinotti cells contain the neuropeptide somatostatin. There is some evidence that there are subtypes of Martinotti cells with a subset that fires LTS and another that shows stuttering firing patterns of spikes (Oliva *et al.*, 2000; Ma *et al.*, 2006).

Cajal–Retzius cells are important during development and are among the first cortical cells in place. They are not present by virtue of migration but as a constituent of the preplate (Chapter 2). Initially they form connections within layer I and what becomes the subplate during migration (Marin-Padilla, 1978). They have extensive horizontal axons within layer I, often along one major axis, but can also look bipolar in form. The main dendrite does not taper but has a lumpy appearance, making it look like a rudimentary club. Much thinner branches can protrude from the main dendrite, often vertically. The axons project mainly within layer I, and like the Martinotti cells axons can travel millimeters (Radnikow *et al.*, 2002). The Cajal–Retzius neurons are thought to target the apical dendritic tufts of pyramidal cells.

The final form of inhibitory interneuron to describe is the neurogliaform cell. These cells are smaller and far more symmetrical than most neurons and have short beaded dendrites that branch close to their point of emergence from the cell body. The axon of the cell is highly branched and gives the impression of a tight tangle of fibres or, as Cajal described it, a spider's web (Ramon y Cajal, 1922). This cell type has been described in the barrel cortex based on the dendritic rather than the axonal pattern (Zhu *et al.*, 2004). The axonal pattern is difficult to view, presumably because the very thin axons are difficult to fill with tracers. Neurogliaform cells make contact with the dendrites of target cells.

## 3.3    Synaptic transmission

A considerable body of work on cortical synaptic transmission has accumulated from studies on barrel cortex and somatosensory cortex in general, and while there is little reason to believe that synaptic transmission works any differently in somatosensory cortex compared with any other cortical area, the converse argument is that what is learned here may serve as a good model system for understanding cortical synapses in general. Before dealing with the dynamic nature of synaptic transmission in Section 3.4, first we review some of the basic features of excitatory and inhibitory transmission. Other cortical transmitter systems are dealt with elsewhere (Section 2.4.4).

A relatively pure EPSP can be produced in barrel cortex by stimulating the thalamic input to a layer V pyramidal cell. The EPSP rise time is on average approximately 1 ms and the fall time approximately 37 ms (Gil and Amitai, 1996). Similarly, the layer IV to II/III pyramidal cell connection can produce an EPSP with a rise time of 0.8 ms and decay time constant of 12.7 ms (Feldmeyer *et al.*, 2006).

The duration of the EPSP can be curtailed dramatically by the presence of a disynaptic IPSP, such that the EPSP lasts less than 5 ms (Figure 3.5). The example shown demonstrates that IPSPs can even precede the EPSPs, though it should be noted that in general the EPSPs occur first by 1–2 ms. The IPSCs triggered in layer IV RS cells shortly after the onset of the excitatory postsynaptic current have a strong effect on the amplitude and duration of the excitatory component (Gabernet *et al.*, 2005). The time course of the IPSP is relatively slow and can last for 50–100 ms (Zhu and Connors, 1999), typically peaking about 20 ms after stimulus (Gil and Amitai, 1996), which means that temporal summation of late arriving EPSPs are also strongly regulated by inhibition. Figure 3.5 shows the effect of a higher frequency input to a cell that evokes inhibition for the first response but that fatigues for subsequent responses. It has been estimated that the integration window of cortical RS cells (Section 3.4.1), which is the time during which a second synaptic input can increase the total EPSP amplitude, is as little as 1 ms when inhibition fully operates but increases to closer to 20 ms after repetitive 10 Hz stimulation (Figure 3.5).

The input from the ventrobasal nucleus of the thalamus to layer IV excitatory and inhibitory cells has been studied in some detail. The thalamic input on to excitatory cells is far weaker than the input on to inhibitory cells (Bruno and Sakmann, 2006; Cruikshank *et al.*, 2007), which means that excitatory input to layer IV needs to be highly synchronous among thalamocortical inputs to overcome the feedforward inhibition. The consequences and functional relevance of the relative phase and strength of excitation and inhibition are explored in Section 5.2.1.

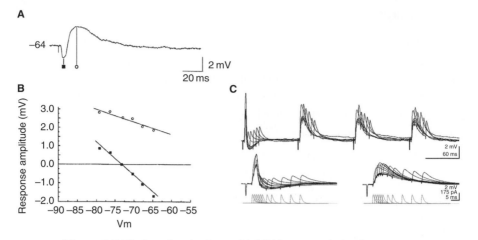

**Figure 3.5** Timing of excitation and inhibition at cortical cells. A. Intracellular post synaptic potentials recorded from a cortical neuron showing a biphasic response. B. The amplitude of the positive (circle) and negative (square) peaks shown in A are plotted for different membrane holding potentials. The negative peak reverses at approximately −75 mV (and is, therefore, probably an inhibitory postsynaptic potential [IPSP]) and the positive peak at approximately 0 mV (if extrapolated). Note that the IPSP can occur before the excitatory postsynaptic potential [EPSP]. (Reproduced from Gil and Amitai [1996], with kind permission of the authors and the Society for Neuroscience.) C. The top trace shows an intracellular recording of four synaptic responses to stimuli delivered at 10 Hz. Several repetitions are superimposed. During the synaptic stimulation, current is injected to produce artificial EPSPs. The two middle traces show the first and last synaptic responses from the top trace on an expanded timescale. The bottom trace shows the current amplitude and timecourse of the artificial EPSPs relative to the timescale of the middle traces. Note that the IPSP after the first stimulus strongly decreases the effectiveness of the artificial EPSPs. (Reproduced from Gabernet *et al.* [2005], with kind permission of the authors and Elsevier.)

The following sections (3.3.1 and 3.3.2) describe the receptors involved in excitatory and inhibitory events before looking in more detail at the short-term dynamics of cortical synapses between different pairs of cell types (Section 3.4).

### 3.3.1   *Excitatory synaptic transmission*

It is widely accepted that glutamate is the major excitatory transmitter in the cerebral cortex, which is not to say that aspartate cannot be involved but rather that glutamate certainly is. Early evidence for the role of glutamate as a transmitter came from electron microscopy studies using antibodies raised against glutamate to allow it to be visualized. Glutamate proved to be enriched in terminals at asymmetric synapses (Storm-Mathisen *et al.*, 1983). The amount of glutamate present was shown to be proportional to the number of vesicles present (Kharazia and Weinberg, 1994). Later evidence showed that the specific glutamate transporter BNPI later renamed VGLUT1 was localized at vesicles (Bellocchio *et al.*, 1998) including those in cerebral cortex (Fremeau *et al.*, 2001), confirming glutamate as the major excitatory transmitter. This conclusion is entirely commensurate with the fact that all the fast excitatory synapses studied so far in cortex activate glutamate receptors. Glutamate receptors fall into two main classes, the ionotropic and the metabotropic receptors. The main ionotropic receptors are the α-amino-3-hydroxy-5-methyl-4-isoxazoleproprionate (AMPA), NMDA and kainate receptor-controlled channels (for a review see Hollmann and Heinemann [1994]) and the main metabotropic glutamate receptor (mGluR) subtypes are 1, 2, 3 and 5 (for a review see Conn and Pin [1997]).

In the adult, low-frequency synaptic transmission at thalamocortical synapses is largely mediated by AMPA receptors. This is partly because the NMDA and kainate receptor components of transmission are downregulated during development (Chapter 4) and partly because the strong inhibitory component activated by thalamocortical input to layer IV creates an IPSP that largely negates the NMDA receptor component. The IPSPs have similar kinetics to the NMDA component of the EPSP; both tend to reach their peak amplitude at approximately 20–30 ms after the initial stimulus. Therefore, the IPSPs in layer IV are timed to coincide with the NMDA EPSP. The NMDA receptor is particularly sensitive to hyperpolarization produced by IPSPs because it is voltage sensitive and conducts far less at hyperpolarized potentials (Mayer *et al.*, 1984). Consequently, sensory stimulation of the whiskers leads to short-latency responses in layer IV cells that are unaffected by iontophoresis of NMDA receptor antagonists (Armstrong-James *et al.*, 1993).

Layer IV spiny stellate cells are interconnected by excitatory synapses within layer IV. Evoked EPSPs between spiny stellates activate AMPA and NMDA receptor components. The NMDA component accounts for approximately 40% of the overall charge transfer, although the peak amplitude of the depolarization is, of course, much less than for the earlier AMPA component (Feldmeyer *et al.*, 1999). The NMDA receptors located on spiny stellate cells in layer IV of the mouse barrel cortex tend to contain a high level of the NR2C subunit (Binshtok *et al.*, 2006). The lower voltage sensitivity of NR2C-containing NMDA receptors may help to explain the presence of longer-latency sensory responses to whisker stimulation in layer IV (Armstrong-James *et al.*, 1993).

Layer IV to layers II/III synapses also show a mixture of AMPA and NMDA components (20%), only slightly less than that of the spiny stellate cells (Feldmeyer *et al.*, 2002). When sensory responses are elicited in cells of layers II/III, they can often be entirely blocked by iontophoresis of NMDA receptor antagonists (Armstrong-James *et al.*, 1993), in common with visual cortex (Fox *et al.*, 1989). This is probably to be expected as the highest density of NMDA receptors are found in layers II/III of barrel cortex (Monaghan and Cotman, 1985; Jaarsma *et al.*, 1991). The other main density for NMDA receptors occurs in layer Va and this may be related to non-specific thalamic projections to this layer (Herkenham, 1980; Fox and Armstrong-James, 1986).

Pre- and postsynaptic mGluRs are present in the cortex. In monkey prefrontal cortex, mGluR1α and mGluR5 are mainly postsynaptic with some presynaptic expression and they occur in pyramidal cells as well as in parvalbumin-positive interneurons (Muly *et al.*, 2003). However, mGluR1α has very low levels of expression in rat cortex and, where present, appears located in inhibitory interneurons rather than pyramidal cells (Petralia *et al.*, 1997). Stimulating mGluR1α with exogenous agonists can cause rhythmic synchronous inhibition through the LTS inhibitory cells (Beierlein *et al.*, 2000). The receptor subtypes mGluR2, mGluR3 and mGluR5 are expressed in all layers in the adult, but differentially in layer IV during development. A barrel pattern can be discerned with mGluR5 staining in neonatal animals, though this becomes less distinct from postnatal day 14 (P14) onward (Blue *et al.*, 1997; Munoz *et al.*, 1999).

The metabotropic receptors play a role in plasticity (Chapter 6) but also in excitatory transmission. Decreases in extracellular calcium concentrations produced by rapid synaptic transmission can reduce EPSP amplitude by decreasing quantal amplitude size. The group I mGluRs are responsible for sensing this as they respond to both extracellular calcium concentration and, of course, glutamate (Hardingham *et al.*, 2006). The action of group I mGluRs is presumably by phosphorylation of AMPA receptors. There is also some evidence that mGluR2/3 subtypes affect synaptic transmission by enhancing NMDA receptor function (Tyszkiewicz *et al.*, 2004). These effects have not so far been specifically tested in barrel cortex.

### 3.3.2    *Inhibitory synapses*

The inhibitory transmitter in the barrel cortex is GABA. In addition, a number of neuropeptides may be coreleased by particular subtypes of inhibitory cell. GABAergic transmission is mediated by ionotropic GABA$_A$ and metabotropic GABA$_B$ receptors. The GABA$_A$ receptor is a chloride-conducting channel that mediates the majority of fast GABAergic transmission in the cortex. The metabotropic GABA$_B$ receptors act to open potassium channels and inhibit dendritic calcium channels. They are further divided into GABA$_{B1a}$ and GABA$_{B1b}$, which lie pre- and postsynaptic to GABAergic synapses, respectively (Perez-Garci *et al.*, 2006). The GABA$_A$ receptor subtype appears to play a greater role in controlling the dynamic responses of neurons than the GABA$_B$, perhaps because of its faster kinetic responses, but both receptor subtypes are involved in controlling receptive field size in the barrel cortex (Kyriazi et al., 1996a, b). $GABA_C$ receptors do not appear to be present in barrel cortex (Salin and Prince, 1996). For reviews on GABA receptor subtypes see Rabow et al. (1995), Couve et al. (2000) and Sieghart (2000).

The GABA receptors play a major role in shaping the spatial and temporal responses of the excitatory cells in the cortex as well as simply controlling the excitability of what might otherwise be a catastrophic level of excitatory positive feedback within the cortex. Tonic inhibition is evident in the barrel cortex from the responses of neurons in vivo to iontophoresis of GABA antagonists in the absence of any intentional stimulation; application of $GABA_A$ antagonists led to an increase in spontaneous activity, which after a short time led to epileptiform burst discharges (Fox et al., 1996a; Kyriazi et al., 1996b). Tonic inhibition appears greater in layer V than in other layers of the somatosensory cortex, which may be because the $GABA_A$ receptor heteromer of layer V pyramidal cells contains the $\alpha_5$-subunit (Yamada et al., 2006).

Tonic and evoked inhibition can be modulated in layer V cells by a mechanism known as depolarization-induced suppression of inhibition (DSI). Excitation of layer V cells leads to release of endocannabinoids, which decrease spontaneous IPSPs and evoked IPSPs (Bodor et al., 2005). Cannabinoid receptors are present on inhibitory presynaptic terminals (Marsicano and Lutz, 1999) and cannabinoid antagonists enhance IPSP in layers II/III and V of the cortex (Trettel and Levine, 2002; Dale et al., 2007). There is evidence that DSI is mediated by suppressing somatic rather than dendritic inhibition (Trettel et al., 2004), which could implicate basket cells in the process.

Inhibition mechanisms differ between subtypes of layer V cell. A subset of large pyramidal cells in layer Vb receive little inhibition from cannabinoid-producing inhibitory cells and, therefore, do not exhibit DSI. In contrast, layer Va appears, in general, to express the highest density of cannabinoids receptors (Bodor et al., 2005) and does exhibit DSI (Figure. 3.6). One further distinction can be made between IB cells, which receive little inhibition either from within their own column or from surrounding cortical columns, and RS cells, which do (Chagnac-Amitai and Connors, 1989; Chagnac-Amitai et al., 1990; Schubert et al., 2001).

Inhibitory cells express a variety of neuropeptides that otherwise find employment in the enteric nervous system, including somatostatin, vasoactive intestinal peptide, cholocystekinin and neuropeptide Y. In addition, some GABAergic cells express nitric oxide synthase, which is the synthesizing enzyme nitric oxide. Although these cotransmitters are useful for identifying interneuronal subtypes, relatively little is known of their function in the cortex at the time of writing (Toledo-Rodriguez et al., 2005).

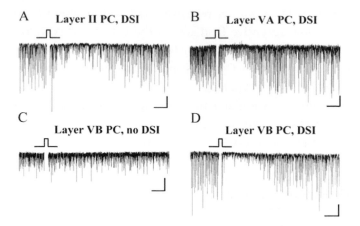

**Figure 3.6** Examples of depolarization-induced suppression of inhibition (DSI). A. Layer II neurons exhibit DSI. The current is injected into the soma for 1–2 s at the time indicated by the pulse. The spontaneous inhibitory postsynaptic currents are inhibited for 15–20 s after current injection (time scale bar = 5 s; amplitude scale bar = 50 pA). B. Layer Va cells also exhibit DSI. C,D. While most layer Vb cells do not exhibit DSI (C), some do (D). (Reproduced from Bodor *et al.* [2005], with kind permission of the authors and the Society for Neuroscience.)

## 3.4    Short-term dynamics

Some aspects of synaptic function can be studied by looking at the response of a neuron to low-frequency stimulation, which is similar to looking at the impulse function of an otherwise quiet system. However, synapses are seldom at rest and in a system like the barrel cortex where the rodent purposely sets its whiskers into rhythmic motion in order to investigate objects in the environment, it is particularly pertinent to study the response of synapses to repetitive stimulation. It was originally noted in the motor cortex (Thomson *et al.*, 1993), and soon after in the somatosensory cortex (Markram and Tsodyks, 1996), that repeated stimuli at an excitatory connection on to a pyramidal cell produces a larger response for the first stimulus followed by diminished peak amplitude EPSP for subsequent stimuli. This form of synapse is common between excitatory cells in the cortex and is known as a depressing synapse (Figure 3.7). The converse is also found, where the response to a rapid train of pulses is to increase the EPSP amplitude gradually to successive stimuli; this is known as a facilitating synapse (Figure 3.7). Both short-term depression and facilitation can be observed in sensory responses evoked during artificial whisking (Derdikman *et al.*, 2006).

In general, the short-term dynamics of the synapse depend on three main factors: the age of the animal, the identity of the pre- and postsynaptic cells and the recent plasticity at the synapses. Synapses between excitatory cells are

**A**    **B**

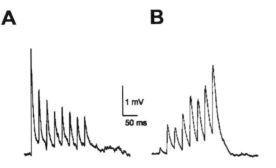

**Figure 3.7** Examples of short-term dynamics at different corticocortical synapses. A. Example of a depressing synapse made between a regular spiking and a fast spiking inhibitory cell in layer IV. Note how the first excitatory postsynaptic potential (EPSP) is the largest in amplitude and subsequent EPSPs are smaller when stimulated at 40 Hz. B. Example of a facilitating synapse made between a regular spiking cell and a low threshold spiking layer IV cell. Stimulation at 40 Hz evokes a small EPSP at first but subsequent EPSPs increase in amplitude. (Reproduced from Beierlein *et al.* [2003], with kind permission of the authors and the American Physiological Society.)

generally depressing in young animals and can become facilitating with development (P14–P28), as with the development of layers II/III to layer V connections and the interconnections between pyramidal cells in layer V (Reyes and Sakmann, 1999). The identity of the pre- and postsynaptic cells involved is also a factor. While thalamocortical connections on to LTS inhibitory interneurons in layer IV are facilitating, the same synaptic input on to RS cells in the same layer is depressing (Beierlein *et al.*, 2003). Presumably, particular circuits in the cortex operate within specific frequency ranges in order to perform their function. Last, regarding plasticity, it is possible to convert facilitating synapses into depressing synapses by inducing long-term potentiation (LTP) at the synapses with a spike-pairing protocol (Markram and Tsodyks, 1996). This process also occurs in vivo in response to alterations in sensory experience (Finnerty *et al.*, 1999) and would, therefore, be expected to produce a variety of short-term dynamics in different cells.

The main synaptic pairs in which short-term dynamics have been studied to date are described in the following sections, together with the possible functional significance of their dynamic properties. However, first it is necessary to describe briefly three electrophysiologically characterized cell types.

### 3.4.1    *Regular spiking, fast spiking and low threshold spiking cells*

Cortical neurons can be classified by their pattern of action potential generation in response to somatic current injection and the duration of their action potentials (Figure 3.8). There are three main types: RS cells show spike

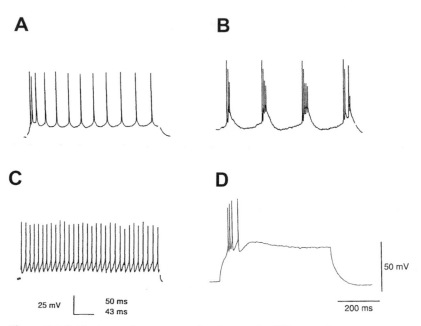

**Figure 3.8** Intrinsic membrane properties characterize different cell types in the cortex. A. Response of a regular spiking cell to a step current injection. The action potential rate shows rapid accommodation followed by sustained regular frequency firing. B. Current injection into an intrinsic burster cell causes oscillatory behavior in the membrane where the depolarizations result in bursts of action potentials that decrease in amplitude during the burst. C. The fast spiking cell shown here is typical of inhibitory interneurons. Time scale bar = 50 ms (A, B), 43 ms (C). (Adapted from Agmon and Connors [1992], with kind permission of the authors and the Society for Neuroscience.) D. A low-threshold spiking cell shows a burst of spikes in response to sustained depolarization initiated from a low-voltage threshold (holding potential –81 mV). Note that unlike the intrinsic burster cell, the spikes increase in amplitude during the burst rather than decrease. This cell had a bitufted cell morphology. (Reproduced from Kawaguchi [1995], with kind permission of the author and the Society for Neuroscience.)

accommodation and include most excitatory cells and some inhibitory cells; FS cells have action potentials of short duration and fire a rapid non-adapting stream of action potentials when a current pulse is injected; and LTS cells have a particularly low threshold for evoking action potentials because they can produce a low threshold calcium current and correspond to a subset of bitufted inhibitory interneurons (see Figure 2.14). The short-term dynamics of the interconnections between these cell types are different, as described below.

### 3.4.2    Short-term dynamics of excitatory connections on to excitatory cells

Where it has been studied, almost all connections from excitatory cells on to layer IV and VI RS cells are depressing (see Table 3.1) both in young rats

Table 3.1. *Short-term dynamics of excitatory to excitatory connections with respect to age in the rat*

| Presynaptic neuron | Postsynaptic neuron | Postnatal age (days)[a] | | Reference[b] |
|---|---|---|---|---|
| | | P13–P21 | P28+ | |
| Thalamocortical | IV (RS) | Depressing | Depressing | Beierlein *et al.*, 2003; Gil *et al.*, 1997; |
| IV (RS) | IV (RS) | Depressing | – | Petersen, 2002 |
| IV | II/III | Depressing | Mixed | Feldmeyer *et al.*, 1999; Hardingham and Fox, 2006 |
| II/III | II/III | Mixed | Mixed | Reyes and Sakmann, 1999; Feldmeyer *et al.*, 2006 |
| II/III | V | Mixed | Facilitating | Reyes and Sakmann, 1999 |
| V | V | Depressing | Facilitating | Reyes and Sakmann, 1999 |
| VI (RS) | VI (RS) | Depressing | – | Beierlein and Connors, 2002 |

RS, regular spiking cell; II–VI, layers.
[a] Short-term dynamics in young and older rats.
[b] Original evidence.

(P13–P21) and older adolescent animals (P28+). As noted above, excitatory connections between layer V cells change from depressing to facilitating over this young to older period of development (Reyes and Sakmann, 1999). However, while there is a trend for layer II/III cells to make a transition from depressing to facilitating with development, their synapses end up as a mixture of facilitating and depressing connections (Reyes and Sakmann, 1999). Layer IV connections on to layer II/III pyramidal cells are also mixed in the adult while they are more uniformly depressing in the younger animal (Feldmeyer *et al.*, 1999; Hardingham and Fox, 2006). In fact, LTP in the IV to II/III pathway can convert facilitating synapses to depressing synapses (Hardingham and Fox, 2006), which suggests that the lifelong plasticity present in this layer ensures a variety of short-term dynamics based on the recent plasticity of the input pathways. Therefore, excitatory to excitatory pathways comprise a mixture of facilitating and depressing responses in adults.

### 3.4.3    *Factors controlling short-term dynamics*

Synapses tend to be depressing if the release probability of the presynaptic terminals are high and the number of release sites per synaptic bouton is low (typically unity at small synapses). This is because the initial transmitter release probability following a long pause (10 s or so) is close to unity and, therefore, requires replacement of vesicles at the limited number of docking sites of most of the synapses before a similar response amplitude can be generated again. If a second presynaptic depolarization arrives during this recovery period, the probability of release is far lower than before and the peak EPSP produced is smaller. Even if the terminal does not release transmitter on depolarization, some depression to subsequent stimuli can occur through inactivation of calcium channels (Thomson and Bannister, 1999). Theoretically, postsynaptic factors can also come into play, such as desensitization of AMPA channels and circuit effects such as shunting inhibition. While these do occur in the cortex, they cannot explain the classic depressing effect at 20 Hz at this depressing synapse, while presynaptic fatigue can (Thomson et al., 1993). The desensitization of AMPA channels typically occurs too rapidly to account for changes in peak EPSP beyond the difference between the first and second pulse in a train.

Conversely, if release probability is low, then most synapses will not release their vesicles to the first action potential and, provided the second pulse arrives within about 50 ms, there will be an opportunity for paired-pulse facilitation through accumulation of calcium in the presynaptic terminal with subsequent action potentials. Low release probability, therefore, favors facilitating short-term dynamics.

### 3.4.4    *Thalamocortical and layer IV inputs on to inhibitory cells*

Thalamic inputs on to the RS spiny stellates (Table 3.1) and FS inhibitory interneurons (Table 3.2) of layer IV are strongly depressing even in older animals. However, a subtype of cortical interneurons present in layers IV and II/III known as the LTS cell is facilitating to the RS excitatory input (Beierlein and Connors, 2002). The FS and LTS inhibitory interneurons seem to form two separate circuits within the cortex because they are also connected together via gap junctions that are specific to their own subtype (Section 3.5). Hence LTS cells are joined to LTS cells by gap junctions but LTS and RS cells are not (Gibson et al., 1999; Beierlein et al., 2003).

This is an example where the particular cell types involved dictate the nature of the short-term dynamics rather than developmental stage or the recent plasticity of the synapse. In other words, the LTS cell circuits are inherently facilitating (Figure 3.9). The LTS cells also have facilitating synapses on to the RS cells. Consequently, thalamic input will serve to activate the RS/FS system at low frequency, but if the RS cells fire at a higher frequency, perhaps owing to fatigue of the strongly depressing FS cell input, the LTS cells will produce an increasing level of inhibition. This means that the layer IV RS cells are covered for negative feedback control over two different frequency ranges.

Table 3.2. *Short-term dynamics of connections made by and on to inhibitory interneurons in the rat*

| Presynaptic neuron | Postsynaptic neuron | Excitatory or inhibitory synapse | Short-term dynamics | Reference[a] |
|---|---|---|---|---|
| Thalamocortical | IV (FS) | Excitatory | Depressing | Beierlein and Connors, 2002 |
| IV (FS) | IV (FS) | Inhibitory | Depressing | Beierlein *et al.*, 2003 |
| IV (FS) | IV (LTS) | Inhibitory | Depressing | Beierlein *et al.*, 2003 |
| IV (RS) | IV (LTS) | Excitatory | Facilitating | Beierlein *et al.*, 2003 |
| IV (RS) | IV (FS) | Excitatory | Depressing | Beierlein and Connors, 2002 |
| IV (LTS) | IV (RS) | Inhibitory | Facilitating | Beierlein *et al.*, 2003 |
| IV (LTS) | IV (FS) | Inhibitory | Facilitating | Beierlein *et al.*, 2003 |
| II/III (pyramidal) | II/III (BTC) | Excitatory | Facilitating | Reyes *et al.*, 1998 |
| II/III (pyramidal) | II/III (MPC) | Excitatory | Depressing | Reyes *et al.*, 1998 |
| Corticothalamic | IV (FS) | Excitatory | Facilitating | Beierlein *et al.*, 2003 |
| Corticothalamic | IV (LTS) | Excitatory | Facilitating | Beierlein *et al.*, 2003 |

BTC, bitufted cell; FS, fast spiking; LTS, low threshold spiking; MPC, multipolar cell; II–IV, layers.
[a] Original evidence.

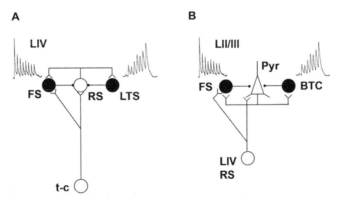

**Figure 3.9** Repeated cortical circuits in layers IV and II/III of the barrel cortex. A. The connections of the ventral posterior medial thalamic nucleus thalamocortical afferent (t-c) fibers with layer IV of the cortex. A regular spiking (RS) cell and two types of inhibitory cell (fast spiking [FS] and low threshold spiking [LTS]) are shown. The thalamic to FS and the RS to FS synapses are depressing. However the RS to LTS synapse is facilitating as is it is an inhibitory feedback connection. (Data from Beierlein *et al.* [2003].) B. A similar circuit to that shown in A is present in layers II/III. The layer IV to FS and pyramidal (Pyr) to FS synapses are depressing while the pyramidal to bitufted cell (BTC) and its inhibitory back connection are facilitating. (Data from Reyes *et al.* [1998].)

### 3.4.5    *Layer IV and layers II/III input to layer II/III inhibitory cells*

A similar circuit exists within layers II/III to that described above for layer IV (Figure 3.9). The layer IV input to pyramidal cells is depressing, in common with the main excitatory input to layer IV RS cells from the thalamus. However, the layer II/III cells then provide facilitating input to bitufted cells and depressing input to multipolar cells (Reyes *et al.*, 1998). Therefore, in the same way that low-frequency input activates the pyramidal cell to multipolar (FS) cell circuit, the bitufted cell takes over inhibition at the higher frequencies and thereby ensures the pyramidal cells are covered at both parts of the frequency range.

### 3.4.6    *Corticothalamic recurrent collateral to layer IV inhibitory cells*

Corticothalamic neurons project from layer VI back to the VPm in the thalamus and hence influence the ascending sensory information from VPm to layer IV; however, they also send projections directly to layer IV via the recurrent collaterals of the corticothalamic axons. Anatomical and physiological evidence suggest that the recurrent collaterals preferentially terminate on inhibitory cells within layer IV rather than on excitatory cells (White and Keller, 1987; Beierlein *et al.*, 2003). Both LTS and RS inhibitory cells are contacted, and each shows distinctly different short-term dynamics: the layer VI to layer IV RS synapse is depressing whereas the layer VI to LTS synapse is facilitating (Beierlein *et al.*, 2003). In the same way that a dichotomy of inhibitory circuit exists within layer IV for feedforward connections, so too are the feedback projections from layer VI separated into two circuits with differing short-term dynamics.

The layer VI to layer IV FS pathway differs from the VPm to layer IV FS pathway in two respects: first, the latency of response is less for thalamocortical inputs than for corticothalamic recurrent collaterals; second, the response latency increases with increasing stimulation frequency for thalamocortical inputs while it decreases for corticothalamic recurrent collaterals (Beierlein *et al.*, 2003). The latency shift is a property of axonal conduction rather than synaptic transmission. This feature complements the different frequency responses of the synapses involved. The thalamocortical input to layer IV is more effective and has shorter latency at lower frequencies while the corticothalamic recurrent collaterals are more effective and have shorter latency at higher frequencies.

There is a bias in the way the thalamic input connects to FS rather than LTS cells in layer IV, which means that the LTS cells receive their input from intracortical excitatory pathways within layer IV and layer VI; both of which

are facilitating. The general picture to emerge from this organization is, therefore, one of feedforward excitation operating at lower frequencies and relying
on RS inhibitory feedback, while feedback excitation from layer VI operates at
higher frequencies. It is not known at present what functions the two circuits
might subserve, except to note again that they cover different frequency ranges
and the balance between the two is, therefore, dependent on overall levels of
cortical excitatory activity. It has also been found that cholinergic input differentially activates LTS cells while inhibiting FS cells (Xiang *et al.*, 1998), which
again suggests that the facilitating synapses are important during behavioral
states associated with cortical activation, or what used to be known as high
cortical tonus. It is also the case that the LTS cells tend to target dendrites while
FS cells target perisomatic regions (Kawaguchi and Kubota, 1997; Xiang *et al.*,
1998), giving the LTS cells a role in modulating integration of excitatory synaptic
input rather than vetoing the output spike generation at the soma.

## 3.5    Electrical synapses

Electrical synapses are formed by gap junctions between cells and are
known to exist between several similar cell types during early postnatal development. For example, 70% of cells are dye-coupled at P1–P4 in the rat cortex
(Connors *et al.*, 1983). However, extensive gap junction connections have only
recently been found to exist in adult cortex, where they occur between similar
subtypes of inhibitory cells. While evidence in favor of cells being electrically
coupled via gap junctions comes from dye injections and electron microscopy
studies of dendritic and axonal appositions between cells, confirmation can
only really be achieved by observing electrical coupling in dual intracellular
recordings. Therefore, although gap junctions had been posited to exist in
neocortex as long ago as 1972, the techniques have only recently been developed that could verify their existence (Sloper, 1972; Galarreta and Hestrin,
2001).

In layer V, FS basket cells have been shown to be electrically coupled by dual
intracellular recording. In layer IV of barrel cortex, FS and LTS subtypes of
inhibitory cells have been found to be electrically coupled within their own
subtype but very rarely with other subtypes (Gibson *et al.*, 1999). While good
evidence exists for basket cells to be coupled and LTS cells to be coupled, it is not
known whether chandelier cells are coupled. In layers II/III of rat barrel cortex,
basket cells have been shown to be coupled by gap junctions and GABAergic
synapses or both (Tamas *et al.*, 2000). The gap junction coupling appears to be
weaker in layers II/III compared with layer IV or V (Tamas *et al.*, 2000).
Theoretically, gap junctions could form a large syncytium of inhibitory neurons

over wide areas of cortex. Inhibitory interneurons only connect with one another via gap junctions within 200 μm of one another, but because each cell is electrically coupled to 20–50 others, the network formed can be quite large (Amitai *et al.*, 2002). It is not known whether the gap junction networks extend beyond barrel-column boundaries.

Gap junctions are formed by various connexins including connexin (Cx) 26, 32, 33, 34 and 36. In visual cortex, mRNA for connexins has been detected in electrically coupled bipolar (Cx32, Cx36), fusiform (Cx36), stellate (Cx 26, Cx36) and basket cells (Cx26, Cx36) (Venance *et al.*, 2000). In the mouse barrel cortex, connexins have been observed in parvalbumin-containing inhibitory cells, which are most likely to be basket cells. Approximately half the parvalbumin-containing cells are double labeled with Cx36 and almost all the other with either Cx32 or Cx34 (Priest *et al.*, 2001). Electron microscopy of Cx36 localization in mouse barrel cortex has shown that the membrane appositions containing the connexin are mainly localized on dendrites (Liu and Jones, 2003). It is likely that Cx36 is the main cortical connexin.

The function of gap junctions appears to be to help to synchronize the activity of inhibitory neurons in the cortex. In layers II/III of rat barrel cortex, gap junctions can act in concert with GABAergic synapses to produce rapid synchronization of action potentials between basket cells (Tamas *et al.*, 2000). The synchrony can follow quite high frequencies in the gamma oscillation band (30–70 Hz). Basket cells contain Cx36, and indeed synchronous activity of inhibitory networks is weaker in animals lacking Cx36 (Deans *et al.*, 2001).

Gamma oscillations occur in human electroencephalograph recordings (Gross *et al.*, 2007) and can self-organize in the presence of carbochol and kainate in superficial layers of auditory cortex (Buhl *et al.*, 1998). They also occur in rat barrel cortex, where they precede periods of exploratory whisking (Hamada *et al.*, 1999). The function of gamma oscillations are not known, but these data suggest that they function to cause widespread inhibition of some cortical circuits immediately before movement, perhaps to prevent inappropriate responses while the animal is preparing patterns of motor activity in readiness for execution.

While the evidence for gap junctions between inhibitory interneurons is well established, it is currently less clear whether they exist in substantial numbers between excitatory cortical neurons. Attempts at modeling epileptic activity in cortex have predicted the existence of electrical connections between pyramidal cells (Traub *et al.*, 2005). In rat auditory cortex, RS pyramidal cells in layers II/III can exhibit spikelets, which are the attenuated image of an action potential produced in a different cell and produced in the RS cell via a gap junction connection between RS cells (Cunningham *et al.*, 2004). It is not known at present whether such connections exist in adult barrel cortex, but the lack of evidence over several decades of cortical recording suggests not.

## 3.6    Organization of synaptic circuits

Barrel cortex is a complex structure composed of several layers, each receiving a diverse set of subcortical and intracortical connections. As described above, there are over 20 different cell types present in the cortex and interconnected in various ways. Are there any simplifying principles that allow a pattern of synaptic organization to emerge from this complexity? One guide to the synaptic organization of the neocortex comes from a consideration of the basic connectivity of the hippocampus (Somogyi et al., 1998). The hippocampus is composed of a single layer of pyramidal neurons rather than the multiple layers of pyramidal cells found in neocortex. Hippocampus is similar to the primitive forms of neocortex present, for example, in reptiles. Reptilian cortex contains a single layer of pyramidal cells, albeit not as uniformly aligned as in hippocampus, bounded on either side by fiber layers (Luis de la Iglesia and Lopez-Garcia, 1997). Reptilian cortex is strongly connected to the striatum and it can be argued that it is analogous to layer V in the mammalian cortex (Lanuza et al., 2002). The thalamic input to reptilian cortex terminates in layer I, which contains the apical dendrites of the pyramidal cells (Hall and Ebner, 1970). This is similar to neocortex in so far as several thalamic nuclei do project to layer I there too, although of course the main termination is in layer IV in mammals, a layer that is absent in reptilian cortex. In the barrel cortex, layer I projections arise from VPm, POm and the ventromedial thalamic nucleus, the last of which has an exclusively layer I termination site (Sections 2.3.2 and 2.3.4). The intrinsic and synaptic physiology of the reptilian cortex is also similar to that of neocortex (Connors and Kriegstein, 1986; Kriegstein and Connors, 1986). Therefore, given that some similarities exist between neocortex and single layer cortex, the following section considers its organization before returning to the subject of multilayer cortex.

### 3.6.1    Single layer cortex

One way to think of neocortex is as multiple versions of a single layer archetype superimposed on one another. The single layer cortex is shown in Figure 3.10 (Somogyi et al., 1998). Here we describe the single layer version before exploring how this maps on to the neocortical circuit elements, which not only contain variations within layers but also have connections between layers and between columns as described in previous sections (2.4.2, 2.4.3 and 3.4).

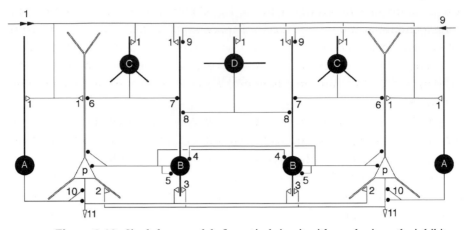

**Figure 3.10.** Single layer model of a cortical circuit with emphasis on the inhibitory cell connections on to pyramidal cells. 1. Extrinsic excitatory input, originating, for example, from the ventral posterior medial thalamic nucleus for layer IV. 2. Interconnections between pyramidal cells. 3. Pyramidal cell connections on to inhibitory cells. 4. Basket cell (B) connections on to basket cells. 5. Basket cell autapses. 6, 7. Dendrite-targeting inhibitory cell (C) connections on to pyramidal cells (6) and (7). basket cells. 8. Specialized GABAergic cells (D) make contact mainly on to other inhibitory cells. 9. Extrinsic GABAergic input to the layer (e.g. layer IV inhibitory input to layers II/III). 10. Axoaxonic connections are made by chandelier cells (A) on to pyramidal cells. (Reproduced from Somogyi *et al.* [1998], with kind permission of the authors and Elsevier.)

The main features of the circuit described in Figure 3.10 are as follows.

- thalamic and intracortical connections (1) connect to the pyramidal cells (p) via apical dendrites (1)
- the pyramidal cells interconnect with one another via recurrent collaterals that terminate on the basal dendrites (2)
  soma targeting inhibitory cells (basket cells [B]) terminate on the pyramidal cells, but also on other basket cells (4)
- basket cells receive thalamic and cortical input (1)
  axon-targeting cells (chandelier cells [A]) terminate on pyramidal cell axon initial segments (10)
- axon-targeting cells receive thalamic and intracortical input (1)
  dendrite-targeting inhibitory cells (bitufted cells [C]) terminate on pyramidal (6) and basket cell dendrites (7)
- dendrite-targeting cells receive thalamic and intracortical excitatory input (1)
- A class of inhibitory cells (D) receiving thalamic and cortical input (1) terminate mainly on other soma-targeting inhibitory cells (8).

The most obvious difference with the barrel cortex is the lack of a cell type corresponding to spiny stellate cells. However, pyramidal cells occur in layers I–VI of the cortex and do interconnect with other pyramidal cells in the same layer and with soma-targeting inhibitory cells. As noted above, all of the connections within this subcomponent of the circuit show depressing short-term dynamics.

The circuit as illustrated does not distinguish between thalamic and cortical inputs. In keeping with the simplified scheme, both cortical and thalamic inputs terminate on apical dendrites of pyramidal cells in layer IV; however, in barrel cortex, they also terminate on basal dendrites and, in fact, a significant thalamic input arrives in layer V on the basal dendrites of layer Vb cells.

The axon-targeting cells in the single layer cortical circuit correspond to the chandelier cells in the neocortex. Chandelier cells exist in all layers of the cortex and, therefore, this is a general feature that is preserved between hippocampus and neocortex. Chandelier cells are likely to receive input from other cortical neurons, and indeed their large receptive fields suggest that this is the case. Therefore, the general scheme is correct provided their input (synapse labeled 1 on A) is considered intracortical.

There are several types of dendrite-targeting inhibitory interneuron, including double bouquet, bipolar and bitufted cells. In the simplified model, they are considered to be organized within the single layer of the cortex; however in neocortex, including barrel cortex, they tend to project vertically up and down the cortical column and, therefore, need to be taken into account within a more complex picture of cortical processing.

One further cell type could be included in the basic circuit without loss of generalization; the Martinotti cell of the cortex is similar to the OL-M cell of the hippocampus (Sik *et al.*, 1995), which projects vertically and is another dendrite-targeting inhibitory cell. In the barrel cortex, Martinotti cells contact apical dendrites in layer I (Section 3.2.4). It is not known whether the Martinotti cells with their somata located in layer V only contact layer V apical dendrites, and Martinotti cells with their somata in layer III only contact layer III cell apical dendrites, which might be in keeping with a duplicated single layer model. However, it seems unlikely given the extensive axonal arbors of the Martinotti cells.

### 3.6.2    Multilayer cortex

How does the single layer model relate to the multilayered nature of the neocortex. Perhaps the most straightforward comparison is with layers II/III of the cortex (Figure 3.11; color version as Plate 3). All the circuit elements present in the basic circuit exist in layers II/III. The main input to layer II/III cells is from

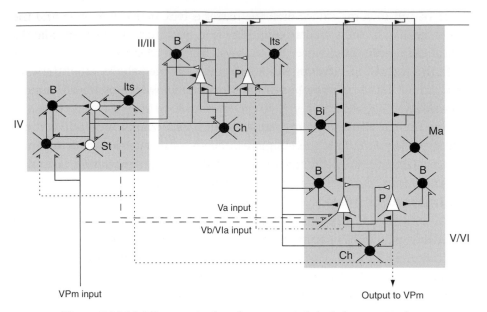

**Figure 3.11** Multilayer cortex based on connected single layer cortex (see Figure 3.10). Each grey box contains cell types connected in a fashion that conforms to the single layer stereotype. B, basket cell; Its, low threshold spiking cell; St, stellate cell; Ch, chandelier cell; P, pyramidal cell; Bi, bipolar or bitufted (dendrite-targeting) cell; Ma, Martinotti cell. Inhibitory interneurons are black ended and excitatory neurons are white ended.

Leftmost panel. Layer IV contains reciprocally connected spiny stellate cells and basket cells. Basket cells provide feedforward perisomatic inhibition from the thalamic input (VPm) and feedback inhibition to the excitatory stellate cells. Low threshold spiking cells do not receive thalamic input but reciprocally connect with stellate cells. The excitatory output of this layer projects to layers II/III.

Middle panel. Layers II/III contain reciprocally connected pyramidal cells. Basket cells provide feedforward perisomatic inhibition from the layer IV input (spiny stellate projections) and feedback inhibition to the excitatory pyramidal cells. Low threshold spiking cells do not receive layer IV input but reciprocally connect with pyramidal cells. Chandelier cells receive layer IV excitatory input and project to the axon initial segment of the pyramidal cells. The excitatory output of this layer from the pyramidal cells projects to layers V/VI.

Rightmost panel. Layers V/VI are illustrated as one for simplicity even though layer Va and Vb and layer VI in general are diverse in pyramidal cell subtypes. Again basket cells provide feedforward perisomatic inhibition from the layer II/III input (spiny stellate projections) and feedback inhibition to the excitatory pyramidal cells. Chandelier cells receive layer II/III excitatory input and project to the axon initial segment of the pyramidal cells. Note that bipolar/bitufted cells are dendrite-targeting cells with axons traversing the layers. Note also that Martinotti cells project to layer I. (See color plate section.)

layer IV and to some extent directly from the thalamus (VPm, POm and the ventromedial thalamic nucleus). However, in cortex, both the thalamic and the cortical inputs do terminate on basal as well as apical dendrites.

Mapping the single layer model on to layer V is also relatively straightforward in so far as all the cellular elements and contacts are again present. However, obviously the apical dendrites of the cortical cells span across layers II, III and IV and so the circuit elements providing inhibition to the layer V cells are not necessarily organized with their somata in layer V. Basket cells do tend to connect within their own layer and receive much of their excitatory input from within the layer, but, as noted above, bitufted and bistratified cell types do not confine either their axonal or their dendritic ramifications within the layer.

Layer IV has no analogue in the hippocampus nor in the reptilian cortex and might be considered a mammalian invention. However, there are still some similarities in some of the basic circuit elements involved that should be mentioned. For example, the spiny stellate cells are not unlike the pyramidal cells in their position within the cortex. Spiny stellates interconnect with other spiny stellates in the same way as pyramidal cells interconnect. Spiny stellates also have reciprocal connections with FS inhibitory cells that provide them with perisomatic inhibitory projections. This is the circuit that exhibits depressing short-term dynamics and is similar to the depressing inhibitory circuit with pyramidal cells in layers II/III.

If the barrel cortex is considered as multiple superimpositions of the single layer cortex plus the addition of layer IV, one further level of complexity that needs to be added is the interconnections between the layers. We have largely dealt with this in Section 2.4.2; however, it may be worthwhile relating it here to the single cortical layer model. The connections from layer IV can be considered as an intracortical input to the pyramidal cells and terminate not only on apical dendrites but also on basal dendrites of layer III cells. Layer Va receives input from layer IV while layer Vb appears not to, emphasizing that the two

---

**Caption for Figure 3.11 (cont.)**

Intracortical connections are superimposed on the three layers. The lines below the three panels represent the more complex superimposed intracortical excitatory connections and do not have obvious correlates in the single layer model. Thalamic input connects directly with layer Vb and layer VIa cells, and layer IV cells connect with layer Va cells (— · — ·). Feedback connections from layer V projects to layers II/III (– · · – · ·). Corticothalamic neurons back project to inhibitory cells in layer IV (. . . .). Note that an absence of connections in this diagram should not be taken as a known lack of connection. The main pathways are illustrated in a simplified form to combine information from the single layer model with known cortical pathways to cellular subtypes (Sections 3.4.4–3.4.6 and 3.6.1). (See color plate section.)

subdivisions should be considered as two individual "single layers" in the basic circuit. The connection from layer III to layer V preferentially terminates on basal dendrites and, therefore, conforms to the basic single layer model if the connection is considered as synapse (labeled 2 in Figure 3.10) on to a pyramidal cell. In fact, it is noteworthy that the layer III cells do this despite the fact that the apical dendrites of the layer V cells are far closer than the basal dendrites for efficiency of coupling. Similarly, the excitatory connections between layer V and VI and vice versa are in keeping with the single layer cortex, it is just that the layers are on top of one another rather than aligned in a row as they are in the hippocampus. The layer VI projection back to layer IV again has no analogue within the single layer cortex because there is no analogue of layer IV at all. Therefore, the preferential terminations of layer VI corticothalamic projection neurons on inhibitory cells within layer IV is another neocortical specialization.

Finally, the extrinsic input from the thalamus terminates in layer I of the single layer model, while in cortex it terminates mainly in layer IV. However, if layer IV is removed from the cortex along with the thalamic projection to that layer, the thalamic innervation of layer I is left, which is similar to the thalamic innervation of the molecular layer of the single layer hippocampus. As noted before, the exception to this simplification is that thalamus also projects to the border of layer V/VI.

In conclusion, many salient features of the barrel cortex circuit are captured within the single layer model, particularly where the inhibitory connections are concerned. A simplification is achieved by considering a single type of extrinsic excitatory input to the pyramidal and inhibitory cells (labeled 1 in Figure 3.10). In understanding many of the important features of cortical processing, this simplification needs to be expanded to describe the organization involved in connections between cortical layers, between cortical columns, between cortical areas and, in the case of barrel cortex, within septal and barrel streams emanating from layer IV.

# Development of barrel cortex

This chapter describes the formation of the barrel cortex from the birth of the cells through to maturation of synaptic circuits. Special consideration is given to formation of the distinctive somatotopic pattern in the barrel field that has captured the imagination of so many scientists over the years. Pattern formation is, of course, a field within developmental science in its own right, of which formation of the somatotopic pattern in the barrel field is an interesting example. Somatotopic pattern formation per se is, therefore, treated in a section on its own. Barrel formation, however, does not raise the same issues and could just as easily be concerned with the formation of a single barrel as with a pattern of barrels. For these reasons, pattern formation and barrel formation are treated in separate sections. Of course the cellular aggregates composing the barrels themselves also make a pattern (Chapter 1), but as we shall see the pattern is present in the thalamocortical afferents before they reach layer IV where the barrels form, and in some circumstances the pattern itself can form in the thalamocortical afferents without the barrels forming. Therefore, the sections on pattern formation concentrate on the origin of the pattern itself, including the role of the peripheral innervation (Section 4.2), while the sections on barrel formation concentrate on the behavior of the cellular aggregates that compose the walls of the barrels (Section 4.3).

Section 4.4 on synapse formation charts the enormous progress in this field in recent years, particularly in the understanding of thalamocortical synapse development. Although the functional significance of several aspects of thalamo-cortical development seems clear (for example AMPA channel insertion into synapses or "AMPA-fication" of synapses), others still remain a mystery (e.g. the transient expression of acetylcholinesterase on the presynaptic thalamocortical terminals). In the latter cases, the chronology of events is described in an attempt to give some insight into their possible role in development of this system.

One other consideration needs mentioning before embarking on a tour of barrel cortex development, and that is the slight difference between the developmental ages of rats and mice. Rats and mice have been the subject of most of the developmental studies on barrel cortex. However, the mouse is born shortly after embryonic day 19 (E19) while the rat is born shortly after E21. This means that P0 (the first postnatal day) comes two days earlier in the mouse than the rat, a period of little consequence were it not for the fact that the barrel cortex develops very rapidly over a period of days. It would appear that development occurs at approximately the same rate in the two species because the cellular aggregates that form the barrels appear on P5 in the mouse and P3 in the rat (i.e. 24 days from conception in both). Therefore, in order to keep results in the two species in register, the species is mentioned when an age is mentioned in each case. Here, we start at the beginning with a general description of corticogenesis.

## 4.1    Premaps and clones

### 4.1.1    *Progenitor cells*

Cortical neurons and glial cells are derived from progenitor cells. The defining characteristic of a progenitor cell is that one of the two progeny after a mitotic division remains a progenitor cell while the other differentiates further to become a particular type of neuron or glial cell. Thus, the population of progenitor cells remains constant while the cortical cells are generated.

In the cortex, the progenitor cells are radial glial cells, which have a process at the surface of the marginal zone (Figure 4.1C) and their cell body in the ventricular zone, which lines the lateral ventricles (Figure 4.1A). The radial glial cells generate neurons by asymmetric division in the ventricular zone (Noctor *et al.*, 2004). This process yields a neuron and the original progenitor radial glial cell. A second variant on this process can also occur. In some cases the progenitor cell produces a cell that is itself a progenitor, which migrates vertically up the radial glia to the subventricular zone lying between the ventricular zone and the intermediate zone (Figure 4.1C). In the subventricular zone, the intermediate progenitor makes one final symmetric division to create two postmitotic neurons (Noctor *et al.*, 2004).

An individual progenitor cell can give rise to many cortical cells. Early studies showed how cells produced from the same progenitor tended to form columns of cells within the cortex. For example, one could imagine many cells within a barrel-column being derived from the same progenitor. The observation was

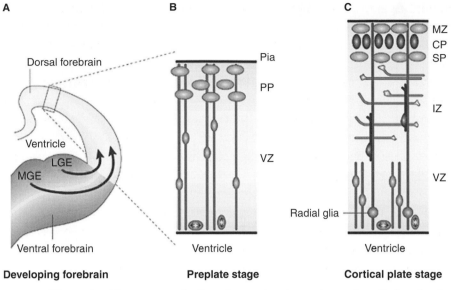

**Figure 4.1.** Two sources of cells and two migration pathways for cells forming the neocortex. A. In the developing forebrain, neurons are born in the medial and lateral ganglionic eminences (MGE and LGE, respectively) and migrate toward the cortex, arriving orthogonally to the radially oriented ventricular migration route (B); the MGE cells provide the interneurons of the cortex. B. At preplate stage, neurons are born in the ventricular zone (VZ) and migrate dorsally to form the preplate (PP) cells of the cortex, which subsequently differentiate into the marginal zone (MZ) and the subplate (SP). C. In the cortical plate stage, neurons continue to be born in the VZ and migrate up radial glia via the intermediate zone (IZ) to form the cortical plate (CP), from which they differentiate out and form the layers in reverse from VI to II. (Reprinted from Nadarajah and Parnavelas [2002], with kind permission of the authors and Macmillan Publishers Ltd.)

made by infecting progenitor cells with a virus carrying a marker gene (Luskin *et al.*, 1988). When the cell divided the virus was partitioned between the two cells and the marker gene could be seen in all the progeny of that cell. Figure 4.2 shows a column of cells within the cortex of a neonatal mouse. The idea that clonally related cells could form a column provided evidence for the concept that the identity of cortical areas and indeed even individual columns might be prespecified in the sheet of progenitor cells. One puzzling observation at the time that argued against this theory was that while many clonally related cells were located close to one another in columns others were found a relatively long way apart in different cortical areas (Walsh and Cepko, 1988).

The resolution of this issue came when it was realized that there were two sources for the generation of cortical cells, one source in the ventricular zone

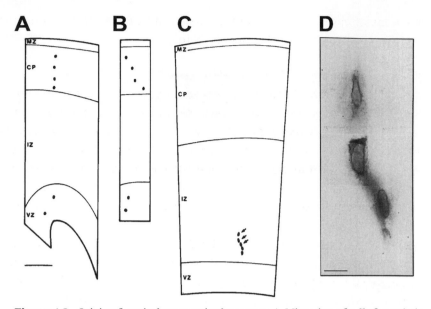

**Figure 4.2.** Origin of cortical neurons in the mouse. A. Migration of cells from their birth place in the ventricular zone (VZ), through the intermediate zone (IZ) to the cortical plate (CP) just below the marginal zone (MZ). B. An example of clonally related cells located in a single cortical column. C,D. Clonally related cells migrating through the IZ (C); the three cells arrowed are shown and at higher magnification in (D). Scale bar = 100 μm (A–C), 10 μm (D). (Reprinted from Luskin *et al.* [1988], with kind permission of the authors and Elsevier).

(Figure 4.1) and another in the lateral and medial ganglionic eminence (Lavdas *et al.*, 1999). The radially arranged cells migrate from the ventricular zone to the cortical plate (Figure 4.1) along radial glia (Rakic, 1971). The widely dispersed cells migrate along a less direct path from the medial eminence through the subventricular zone that traverses the radial glia (Lavdas *et al.*, 1999). The developmental issue raised by this finding is that the medial ganglionic eminence can produce cells for many different cortical areas and it becomes important to know how this is controlled and to understand the implications for area specification (Valcanis and Tan, 2003). The functional issue raised by this finding comes from the observation that the laterally displaced cells generated by the lateral and medial ganglionic eminence are inhibitory (Lavdas *et al.*, 1999) while the radially displaced cells from the ventricular zone are excitatory. The tangentially migrating inhibitory cells perform one further function, which is to create a permissive environment for the thalamocortical axons to grow through the developing striatum and pallidum to reach the cortex (Lopez-Bendito *et al.*, 2006). The following sections explore the degree to which the layers and columns of cortex are determined by such intrinsic factors and describe the degree to which extrinsic factors play a role.

### 4.1.2    Columnar and layer development

Much of the development of the barrel cortex takes place before birth. The neurons are generated between approximately E15 and E17 in the mouse and the last cells are in place by P7. Between these two times, cells are generated in the ventricular and subventricular zone and migrate along radial glia into the area that will become the cortex (Figure 4.1). Eventually, the archetypical plan of the barrel cortex is formed with six layers, but before that occurs, a number of intermediate layers can be distinguished, each with its own nomenclature. The arrival area for migrating cells is known as the cortical plate. Initially, before any migration has occurred the same area is known as the preplate, which gives rise to two developmentally important layers of cells, the marginal zone and the subplate. The marginal zone contains the Cajal–Retzius cells, which produce reelin, a protein important for radial migration (Rice and Curran, 2001). In reelin knockouts, the cortex develops upside down. The subplate contains the earliest migrating cells and lies below the marginal zone, where it plays a role in organizing afferent pathways projecting to the cortex (Ghosh and Shatz, 1992).

Cells migrating from the proliferative zones arrive in the cortical plate, lying between the subplate and the marginal zone. The adult layers of the cortex form out of the cortical plate as the newly arrived neurons differentiate into particular cell types. The layers tend to form in an inside-out fashion, so that layer VI cells arrive in the cortex first and layer II cells arrive last. Layer I forms out of the marginal zone, which is already in place before migration into the cortical plate and has few cells. In the rat barrel cortex, layers V and VI have differentiated at birth, while layer IV contains cells not yet differentiated from the cortical plate cells. Layer IV is apparent during P2, while layers II and III are clearly present at P4. Migration of cells is complete by about the end of the first postnatal week in the rat and mouse (Figure 4.3).

The timing of layer development was discovered for a variety of cortical areas by [³H]-thymidine labeling (Luskin and Shatz, 1985). This method relies on incorporation of radiolabeled thymidine into cells during replication of DNA, a process that only occurs to any extent during mitotic division. It was found that giving the [³H]-thymidine on a specific day led to labeling of cells in a particular layer when the fully formed cortex was studied postnatally. In this way the "birthday" could be determined for cells in particular cortical layers. In the rat, neurons destined for layer VIb were, on average, born on E14, VIa on E15, V on E17, III on E19 and II just before birth on E20 (Miller, 1985).

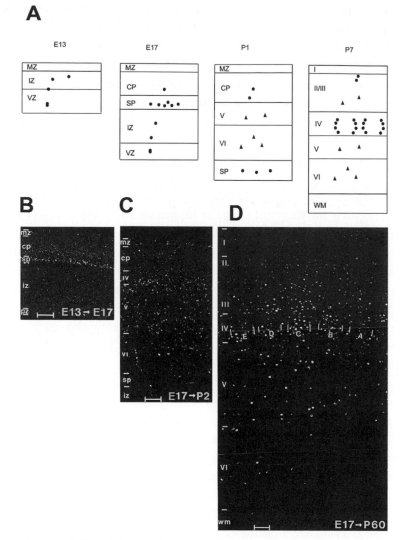

**Figure 4.3.** The timing of migration and layer formation in the rat barrel cortex.
A. Diagrammatic representation of the main events and approximate timings of
cortical neurogenesis and migration. On the 13th day of gestation (E13), cells begin to
migrate from the ventricular zone (VZ) through the intermediate zone (IZ) and offload
below the marginal zone (MZ), which itself already contains a sparse contingent of
cells (Cajal–Retzius cells). On E17, cells destined to become the middle layers
(mainly layer IV) begin to migrate. Subplate cells are in place on E17. On the first
postnatal day (P1), just 24 hours after birth, layer V and VI have condensed out of the
cortical plate and layer IV is still undifferentiated. By P7, the layers have essentially
formed with the last few layer II cells finally reaching their destination. Almost all
the subplate cells have perished at this point. B–D. Autoradiographs of cortical

One of the developmental questions raised by the observation that birth date is correlated with layer location is whether the identity of each layer is determined by the progenitor cell counting the number of divisions it makes; in other words, does it divide three times to make layer VI cells and then the next four divisions produce layer V cells and so on, eventually making the final divisions to form layer II cells? Alternatively, do the migrating neurons differentiate into particular subtypes as a result of local cues within the emerging cortex?

### 4.1.3    Tabla rasa *concept*

The issue of cell fate determination is central to many questions in development. Is a cell destined to differentiate into a specific cell type because of an internal genetic clock or is it pushed toward one fate or another by extrinsic cues? In general, we know that particular cell types produce factors that diffuse locally to cause differentiation of their neighbors along particular paths. For example in the spinal cord, the diffusible factor shh, produced by the gene *sonic hedgehog*, from the notochord and floor plate causes differentiation of cells in the ventral spinal cord into motor neurons (Ericson *et al.*, 1995, 1996). But the question then becomes one of what determines the fate of the controlling cells and so the question is pushed back in time into a series of classic "chicken and egg" questions until one arrives at the first cell.

The issue in cortical development arises from the fact that the ventricular zone is arranged broadly as a premap of the cortex, with each cortical area arising from a different area of the ventricular zone. Therefore, the fate of individual cortical areas could theoretically already be determined by the time the ventricular zone has formed. Alternatively, it is possible that the ventricular zone gives rise to an isomorphic cortical sheet of cells that only differentiates after migration has occurred. Differentiation could be controlled by a number of

---

**Caption for Figure 4.3 (cont.)**

sections where the cells have been labeled with [$^3$H]-thymidine. B. Cells labeled at E13 and the sections prepared at E17. At this stage, the postmigratory cells are located in the cortical plate and subplate. Labeled cells continue to migrate through the IZ. C. Cells labeled four days later at E17 and visualized at postnatal day 2 (P2) reveal labeling in the emerging layers IV and V. Few cells are labeled in the subplate. This implies that the layer IV and V cells are born later than the subplate cells. D. Visualizing the cells labeled at E17 later in a P60 animal when the supragranular cells are formed shows that many are born at E17. (Adapted from Miller [1995], with kind permission of the author and Wiley).

organizing cells secreting factors that diffuse and act at varying concentrations to produce different cortical areas. Similarly, sets of projections to the cortex might arrive and produce differentiation along a particular path depending on the nucleus from which they originated. On the one hand we have a vision of the early cortex as a *tabla rasa* waiting to be written upon by extrinsic factors and on the other as the product of a premap originally contained in the progenitor cells. These ideas have been tested in the barrel cortex by transplantation studies.

### 4.1.4    Transplant studies

Two transplantation experiments have been performed to date to answer the question of whether or not the cortical area is predetermined by the end of migration. In one case, the presumptive barrel cortex was transplanted to the area normally occupied by the visual cortex to see whether it still formed barrels. Such a result would favor the premap hypothesis. In the other case, visual cortex was transplanted to the area normally occupied by the barrel cortex to see whether it was capable of forming barrels. Such a result would favor the *tabla rasa* hypothesis.

It was found that visual cortex can form barrels if it is transplanted into the region that normally develops barrels (Schlaggar and O'Leary, 1991). Visual cortex taken from late embryonic animals can be transplanted into the neonate barrel cortex region before the barrels form. It is possible to see the barrels form in the transplanted area alongside barrels forming in the area previously destined to be visual cortex (Figure 4.4). This observation implies that the cortex is a *tabla rasa*, at least until some postnatal timepoint. The converse experiment where protobarrel cortex is transplanted into visual cortex does not yield barrels. As will become clear in Section 4.3, the thalamic afferents play an important role in barrel formation and so this is not entirely surprising in retrospect.

The conclusions drawn from the barrel transplant studies are in accord with earlier experiments showing how somatosensory cortex could develop vision-processing properties. By routing the output from the retina into the somatosensory thalamus, the somatosensory cortex was made to receive visual information during development (Metin and Frost, 1989). The surgery involved in this study was more complicated than that required for the cortical transplant studies. First, the natural input from the spinal cord and dorsal column nuclei pathways were cut to prevent the ventrobasal complex from receiving its normal somatosensory connections. Second, one of the normal targets of the retina (the superior colliculus) was ablated to allow visual input to project to the ventrobasal complex. The result was that the somatosensory cortex developed as if it were the visual cortex to some extent (i.e. the neurons responded to visual stimuli).

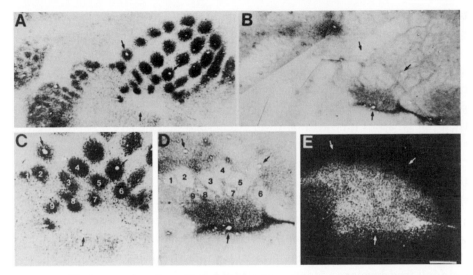

**Figure 4.4.** Formation of barrels in visual cortex transplants. A. Acetylcholinesterase is used to mark the location of thalamic axons that form the somatotopic pattern in a transplant of occipital (visual) cortex into the parietal area. B. Peanut agglutinin (PNA) labels the boundaries of the barrels in an adjacent serial section to (A). C. The section in (A) at higher magnification. D. Barrels numbered in (C) stained with PNA. E. The transplanted area identified with fluorescent marker. Arrows in (C–E) correspond and identify the same area. (Reprinted from Schlaggar and O'Leary [1991], with kind permission of the American Association for the Advancement of Science and the authors; copyright 1991, American Association for the Advancement of Science.)

The cortex appears to be extremely versatile during development, supporting the *tabla rasa* hypothesis. In the case of sensory cortical areas like the barrel cortex, the thalamic input clearly plays a major role in shaping the cortical area into its final form. The question arises of whether the thalamus exerts its influence by the behavior and organization of the ingrowing thalamic axons or by the sensory information they carry. The following two sections explore the details and limitations of these interactions more closely.

## 4.2    Pattern formation

### 4.2.1    Theories of pattern formation

Correlated neuronal activity is capable of influencing the development of sensory maps to some extent. The time correlation of neuronal activity is highest for neighboring areas of the peripheral receptor sheet and lower for distant areas. Areas that are some distance apart on the peripheral surface have a higher chance of being activated independently of one another. Therefore, time correlation among a set of afferents can provide a signal that determines which inputs should be wired as close neighbors and which inputs should be wired as distant neighbors. A mechanism for interpreting these signals is known to exist. The NMDA receptor, and voltage-gated channels in general, are able to detect correlated activity provided that it takes several inputs acting together (i.e. in correlation) to depolarize the neuron sufficiently to allow the NMDA channel to conduct. If a particular set of afferents is successful repeatedly in depolarizing the neuron, then the synapses they act upon will strengthen and survive (Chapter 6 gives specific details of this "Hebbian" synaptic mechanism). This has lead to the rubric "neurons that fire together wire together." Conversely, axons that do not activate the cell at the same time will tend not to strengthen their synapses and, perhaps through a time limit, eventually disappear.

One of the most striking examples of how correlated activity can organize a pattern comes from studies on three-eyed frogs. Of course normal frogs have two eyes, but if an extra eye is transplanted into the developing tadpole, then the adult frog develops a functional third eye, which innervates the brain along with the normal two. Normally, each eye projects in an entirely crossed pathway to the contralateral optic tectum in the frog. If the native eye is forced to innervate the optic tectum on one side along with the extra eye, then the two sets of afferents effectively compete with one another for space in the tectum. Activity tends to be correlated for afferents from the same eye but uncorrelated for afferents from different eyes. Correlated activity tends to aggregate the afferents and keep them separate from the uncorrelated afferents. Therefore, the afferents from the two eyes form two separate sets of stripes in the tectum (Constantine-Paton and Law, 1978). If the mechanism that detects the correlated activity is blocked in the developing tectum (i.e. the NMDA receptors are blocked with 2-amino-5-phosphovalerate), then the stripes desegregate into an even distribution of normal and extra eye afferents (Cline et al., 1987).

Correlation-based models of map development are able to explain some aspects of map development and not others. For example, it is not possible to explain the orientation of the barrel map in this way. Identical sets of correlation patterns would lead to the same near-neighbor relationships in a barrel map that was rotated by any angle around an axis located anywhere in the barrel field or outside it. Similarly, the somatotopic pattern would maintain the same neighbor relations if it were a mirror image reflected in any line passing through any part of it. From a theoretical point of view, it is necessary to have positional and orientation cues at least in addition to correlation-based cues to form the somatotopic pattern in its stereotypical form. One way in which this might be done is by having chemical gradients within the cortex to specify front and back, medial and lateral. For a two-dimensional map, two sources in two different locations would provide sufficient orientation.

If it is possible to have positional cues within the cortex, the question arises of whether the somatotopic pattern might be formed entirely from a complex of such cues. Perhaps there could also be a signal for forming the rows of barrels. There are many examples in development of repeated units being formed by a mutually induced pattern of gene expression, such as that forming segments in segmented animals, for example, via homeobox genes (Gehring, 1987, 1993). The bare necessities for such a system are that a diffusible factor initially creates a chemical gradient across the tissue that induces production of a critical factor in a set of cells at a particular concentration. If the critical factor produces differentiation in the cells, the local area becomes defined (Figure 4.5).

In practice, there is likely to be more than one type of control signal, and the behavior of receptor induction for the diffusible factor can add further complexity to the process. For example, if a second factor is also produced by the cells that is inhibitory to production of the first factor but that diffuses more easily, then lateral inhibition will sharpen the concentration peaks of first factor (Figure 4.5; Turing, 1990). There are certainly many examples of concentration gradients producing patterns in developing organisms, such as the patterns on butterfly wings or the digits on the forelimb bud (Carroll *et al.*, 1994; Monteiro *et al.*, 2001), in addition to self-organizing domains within chemical reactions (Tabony, 1994; Glade *et al.*, 2002).

Positional cues are generated by a variety of factors such as fibroblast growth factor 8 (FGF8), Emx2 and Pax6 in the developing cortex. Normally, FGF8 is produced at the anterior pole of the developing cortex. An experiment where an ectopic source of FGF8 was produced at the posterior pole caused a partial duplication of barrels behind the normal barrel field (Fukuchi-Shimogori and Grove, 2001). The orientation of the extra-barrel map was opposite to that of the endogenous map, suggesting that the gross orientation of the barrels is indeed specified by a positional cue. Formation of a partial set of barrels may have been a consequence of the occurrence of two unequal sources of FGF8 in the brain.

One further aspect of somatotopic pattern formation needs to be considered, and that is the extent to which the signal for pattern formation is intrinsic to the cortex and the degree to which it arises in the thalamic afferents growing into the cortex. It is feasible that the somatotopic pattern in the thalamus, which develops earlier in the thalamus than cortex, is simply stamped on the cortex. For this to occur, the thalamic afferents would need to maintain their neighbor relationships as they grow from thalamus to cortex. Alternatively, the somatotopic pattern might be set up in the cortex by a system of chemical diffusion gradients and the thalamic afferents corralled into the appropriate locations by a system of cell adhesion molecules that are inhibitory to axon ingrowth in septal locations and facilitatory in protobarrel locations. To answer the

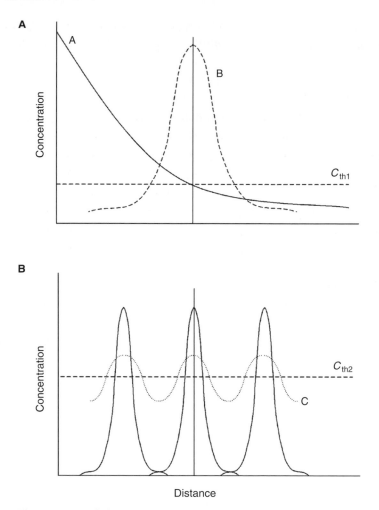

**Figure 4.5.** Defining location with concentration gradients. A. In a theoretical case, the concentration of a factor generated at the origin diffuses through the tissue and the concentration falls to a critical value at concentration threshold 1 ($C_{th1}$). This induces production of a second factor B and hence determines the site of factor B in one dimension. B. If factor B also induces cells to produce more factor B at locations, again defined by its concentration falling to a critical threshold at some distance from the source, several side bands will occur at regular distances from the central source. If an inhibitory factor C is also produced by the same cells, with the property that it diffuses more widely than factor B and, crucially, inhibits factor B production below a critical threshold (indicated by the dotted line $C_{th2}$), then the location of each peak of substance B will become sharper. This is essentially the reaction–diffusion model of Turing (1990; see text) applied to a developmental problem.

questions raised in this section, it is necessary to consider the timing and
interdependence of peripheral and central pattern formation in the barrel
system.

### 4.2.2    Thalamic afferents

Axons grow from the thalamus to the cortex at the same time as the
cortical neurons migrate from the ventricular and subventricular zone to
the cortical plate though the intermediate zone (Figure 4.2). At E16 in the rat,
the thalamic axons can be seen leaving the thalamus. By E17, thalamic axons
run orthogonal to the radial glia in the intermediate zone until they reach a
location beneath the prospective barrel cortex. By E18, the axons can clearly be
seen to turn and enter the lower layers of the cortex (Catalano *et al.*, 1996). At
birth (P0), the cortical plate has differentiated to a certain extent and layers V
and VI can be distinguished from the cortical plate. At this point, the thalamic
afferents have grown into the lower cortical layers and some have reached the
point of the cortical plate where layer IV will be the next layer to differentiate.

A question arises of how the thalamic axons find their way to the cortex. One
mechanism appears to depend on the early corticofugal projections of the
subplate cells, which send fibers into the internal capsule as early as E14 in
the rat (Molnar *et al.*, 1998). These fibers make contact with the thalamocortical
afferents as they grow toward the cortex and could help to guide them to the
correct area. This is known as the handshake hypothesis because the fibers
traveling in both directions appear to shake hands as they make contact before
growing past one another. The thalamocortical axons do not seem to maintain
any obvious nearest neighbor relationships within the tract (Bernardo and
Woolsey, 1987). It is, therefore, conceivable that the subplate projections are
important for maintaining topographic order within the thalamocortical afferents as they make an 180 degree twist in the internal capsule in order to
translate the anterior–posterior organization of thalamic rows into a lateral to
medial organization of cortical rows (Bernardo and Woolsey, 1987).

A rough patterning can be discerned in the thalamic afferents as they grow
into the cortex during P0 (Erzurumlu and Jhaveri, 1990). It had originally been
thought that the cortex was already prepared into a somatotopic pattern before
the thalamic afferents arrive because the somatotopic pattern could be seen
using lectin markers before the barrels had formed (Cooper and Steindler, 1986).
Lectins bind to extracellular component of glial cells located in the septum as
early as P3 and so could provide a signal to guide the thalamic afferents into
barrels. However, increasingly more sensitive anatomical methods using DiI
labeling (Erzurumlu and Jhaveri, 1990; Catalano *et al.*, 1996) and acetylcholinesterase staining (Schlaggar and O'Leary, 1994) demonstrated that the thalamic

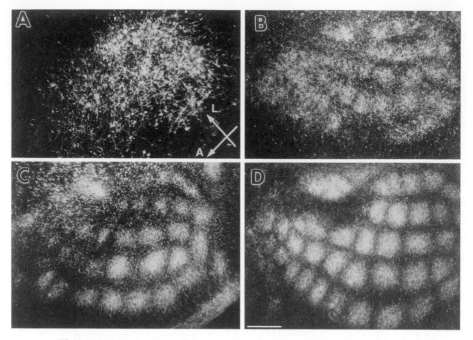

**Figure 4.6.** Formation of the somatotopic pattern within thalamocortical afferents in the rat. A. At one day after birth, it is difficult to discern a pattern in the thalamo-cortical afferents, labeled here with DiI (1,1′-dioctadecyl-3,3,3′,3′-tetramethylindo-carbocyanine perchlorate). B. At two days, a pattern has emerged but is indistinct. C, D. At three days (C) the barrels are more distinct and by four days the adult pattern and form is clear (D). Scale bar = 275 μm (A–C), 300 μm (D). (Reprinted from Erzurumlu and Jhavari [1990], with kind permission of the authors and Elsevier.)

afferents show a somatotopic pattern by the end of the first 24 hours after birth (P0/P1), fully two days before the lectin pattern evolves. These studies suggest that the thalamic afferents already carry the pattern information as they arrive in cortex rather than cortex containing the pattern beforehand, a finding which is in agreement with the barrel transplantation studies cited above (Figure 4.4).

The full somatotopic pattern forms properly during the first postnatal week. If the infraorbital nerve carrying afferents from the whisker follicles into the brainstem is cut during development of the barrels, the development of the system appears to be frozen in time and can, therefore, be studied later in the mature animal. When the nerve is cut on P2, the pattern of thalamic afferents forms a system of five major rows rather than barrels in the posterior part of the barrel field. This observation implies that there are two stages to development, the first of which is segregation into rows and the second for rows to separate out into barrels. This sequence can be seen in the thalamic afferents during development (Figure 4.6) and it raises the question of whether some refinement of the somatotopic pattern occurs in cortex during development despite the origin of the pattern appearing to be carried by the afferents. Before addressing this question again (Section 4.2.4), it will be useful to discuss where and how the somatotopic pattern originates.

### 4.2.3    Influence of the periphery

The prodigious rate of development in the rodent means that it only takes days for the whole barrel pathway to develop. Despite this limitation, it has been possible to observe a sequence of pattern formation beginning with the periphery and working inward to the cortex. The bipolar neurons in the trigeminal ganglion send one axon toward the brainstem and one toward the periphery. The central projection arrives relatively early in development in the rat, at E12, but shows no patterning at this stage. The peripheral projection reaches and innervates the developing mystacial pad in the rat at E14 (Erzurumlu and Killackey, 1983) at about the same time as the follicle pattern is emerging in the epithelium. The somatotopic pattern itself only emerges in the brainstem a week or so later at E21 (Erzurumlu and Killackey, 1983). Therefore, the primary afferents are exposed to the peripheral pattern in the follicle well before the axons form a pattern in the brainstem. As discussed above, the pattern forms in the thalamocortical afferents in the cortex at P0/P1 in the rat (Schlaggar and O'Leary, 1994). This means that the information for forming the pattern at each stage could be derived from the periphery and could cause the central pattern provided the periphery is capable of influencing the central pattern.

Evidence that the peripheral pattern influences the central pattern comes from several sources. First, mutants with extra whiskers form extra barrels (Welker and Van der Loos, 1986). Second, infraorbital nerve section before the central pattern is formed prevents formation of barrelettes in the brainstem and hence elsewhere in the neuraxis (Killackey and Belford, 1980; Henderson et al., 1993). One mechanism by which the signal could be transmitted from the periphery to influence central pattern formation is if the primary afferents depended upon a trophic factor. If the central and peripheral innervation is initially somatotopically organized by a vital trophin that is produced by the afferents innervating the follicles, then the axons innervating the area between the follicles would atrophy, causing a loss of innervation to the central projection of the same neurons. The loss of innervation to a set of neurons in the brainstem in such a fenestrated pattern would then give rise to an uneven distribution of cells in the brainstem corresponding to the somatotopic pattern.

There is some evidence in favor of this theory because the primary afferents are critically dependent on neurotrophins during development. Sectioning the infraorbital nerve or selected follicle nerves causes nerve degeneration in neonates. However, lesion-induced degeneration can be reversed in a sectioned nerve by application of brain-derived neurotrophic factor (BDNF) or neurotrophin-3 (Calia *et al.*, 1998). Conversely, overexpression of nerve growth factor in the mouse mystacial pad leads to increased survival of neurons in the trigeminal ganglion (Davis *et al.*, 1997). The trophic dependence of the primary afferents affects neuronal survival in the trigeminal nuclei and the thalamus. Peripherally applied neurotrophins reduce cell death in nucleus principalis, abolishing the formation of a somatotopic pattern there (Henderson *et al.*, 1994) and further upstream in the thalamus (Baldi *et al.*, 2000).

### 4.2.4   *Activity dependence*

There are clearly theoretical limits to what features of a somatotopic map can be organized by neuronal activity. Activity cannot organize orientation or location of the barrel cortex because these factors are independent of the time correlation of near-neighboring neurons (Section 4.2.1). But could there be any aspect of pattern development that is organized by neuronal activity? Two approaches have been used to address this question. In one type of study, cortical activity was blocked during development by use of tetrodotoxin or 2-amino-5-phosphonopentanoic acid (AP5) (Figure 4.7) or by creating NMDA receptor (NR1) knockout mutants (Chiaia *et al.*, 1992; Schlaggar *et al.*, 1993; Iwasato *et al.*, 2000); this addresses the question of whether any cortical activity is required for pattern formation. In the other type of study, activity in the infraorbital nerve was blocked by tetrodotoxin during development of the barrel cortex (Henderson *et al.*, 1992); this addresses the more specific question of whether activity from the periphery is required for pattern formation. The unanimous verdict from both types of experiment is that the pattern develops normally as judged by staining with CO (a pre- and postsynaptic marker) or acetylcholinesterase (a presynaptic marker). This implies that the gross morphology of the pattern is not dependent on neuronal activity in the neocortex.

Earlier studies on the role of activity in the visual system had shown the importance of neuronal activity for forming normal receptive fields in sensory cortex (Stryker and Harris, 1986). The possibility remains, therefore, that while the formation of a somatotopic pattern itself is not activity dependent other features of development in the cortex are activity dependent. There is some evidence for this in the barrel cortex. If transmission mediated by excitatory amino acids is blocked from P0 in the cortex and the receptive fields studied when the animal is mature, short-latency responses to single whisker stimulation are widespread over many inappropriate barrels instead of being confined to the principal barrel for the stimulated whisker (Fox *et al.*, 1996a). As described in Chapter 5, short-latency responses are thought to be indicative of direct

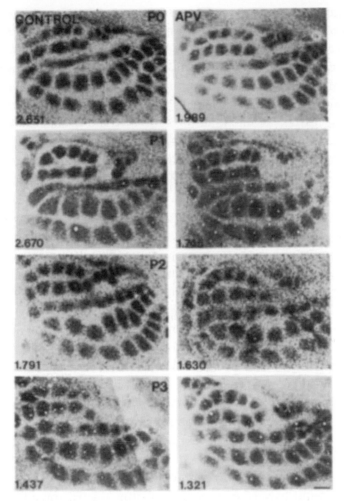

**Figure 4.7.** Effect of follicle ablation during development (postnatal days 0–3 [P0–P3]) on barrel formation in the rat barrel cortex. Left column. Ablating the C-row of follicles on P0 leads to a small fused C-row of barrels forming in the mature animal. A similar effect occurs with ablation at P1, but by P2 it is too late to have prevented some differentiation of barrels within the row. By P3 there is little effect. The inset numbers show the area of the D-row barrels relative to the C-row (in a normal animal D/C is approximately 1.3). Right column. The C-row follicle lesions are repeated on the same days but the developing cortex is treated with APV (2-amino-5-phosphovalerate), which partly prevents the loss of cortical territory by the C-row barrels (see text). Scale bar = 400 μm. (Reproduced from Schlaggar *et al.* [1993], with kind permission of the authors and Macmillan Publishers Ltd.).

thalamocortical activation of layer IV cells (Armstrong-James and Fox, 1987). The thalamocortical arbors tend to overlap several barrels at P0 to P2 before being reduced to one barrel during the first postnatal week (Rebsam *et al.*, 2002). Therefore, an activity-dependent mechanism may normally be responsible for eliminating errors in thalamocortical projections during development. The erroneous connections may be collaterals of correctly formed projections to the appropriate barrel, which would explain why the overall pattern still appears normal in these animals. Consistent with this interpretation, studies in NR1 knockout mice, which have no NMDA receptor function in the cortex, exhibit a somatotopic pattern and thalamocortical axon collaterals that reach beyond the borders of the barrels and have wider termination patterns than those of control animals (Lee *et al.*, 2005). Other anomalies in projections also arise in APV-treated cortex such as a failure for horizontal connections projecting within extragranular layers to orient preferentially along rows of barrels (Dagnew *et al.*, 2003). The picture that emerges is of a two-stage developmental process where an activity-independent pattern formation mechanism is fine-tuned by an activity-dependent mechanism during the first postnatal week.

Interestingly, activity-dependent mechanisms continue to play a role in fine-tuning the cortical map several days after the somatotopic pattern has emerged in brainstem and thalamus. For example, if the infraorbital nerve is sectioned on P2, it affects the somatotopic pattern in the cortex without affecting the pattern in the brainstem (Woolsey, 1990). This implies that a signal is transmitted from the periphery to the cortex, through an already formed somatotopic pattern, to influence pattern formation in the cortex. Evidence that neuronal activity forms part of the transmitted signal comes from studies where a row of follicles are ablated and the cortex treated with APV. Normally, this procedure leads to a narrow fused row of barrels corresponding to the ablated row of whiskers (Figure 4.7). However, in APV-treated cortex, the barrels form relatively normally and the corresponding row is not narrow (Schlaggar *et al.*, 1993). This finding implies that the activity-independent system will normally form barrels unless prevented from doing so by the over-riding influence of an activity-based mechanism. The exact receptor system remains to be discovered for this process as a cortical NMDA receptor knockout does not prevent the activity-based mechanism from allowing the formation of a narrow fused row of barrels in the cortex when a single row of follicles are ablated (Datwani *et al.*, 2002). One possibility is that AMPA receptors or metabotropic glutamate receptors could be involved (Section 4.3) but these issues remain to be resolved. Even though pattern formation is activity independent and can even be hampered by activity-based mechanisms, barrel formation does show activity dependence, as discussed in the following sections.

## 4.3    Barrel formation

### 4.3.1    *Organization of cellular domains*

The thalamic afferents are organized in a rudimentary somatotopic pattern as early as the end of P0 in the rat, but the cells of layer IV do not form into barrels until P3 in the rat (P5 in the mouse). The mature barrel consists of a relatively cell-sparse core region surrounded by a wall of two or three neurons thickness around the outside where the cell density is far higher (Chapter 1). This mature state develops from an initially homogenous and undifferentiated cortical plate at the time the thalamic axons have first arrived to grow in to the future layer IV. Between P0 and P3 in the mouse, the cells change their distribution and organize their dendrites so as to orient them toward the center of the barrels where the thalamic afferents are clustered.

In the mouse, Nissl-stained sections show that the barrels first become evident through a decrease in cell density in the barrel hollow. At this stage, the barrels are much smaller than in the adult (Rice and Van der Loos, 1977). During maturation, the barrel field increases as a proportion of the total cortical surface. So although a pattern is present before barrel formation, a great deal of growth and tangential expansion must occur before the adult form of the barrel cortex is reached. At the time of writing, it is not known what causes the walls and hollows to form, but the process may result from the proliferation of axonal arbors within the barrel hollow, which by occupying more space themselves deny space to the cortical cells. A second factor may be that dendrites form on the hollow side of the barrel wall neurons and not on the other side. This asymmetry could push the cell bodies into the wall as the dendrites grow. Other factors involved in hollow formation may include selective cell death within the barrel hollow and/or active migration of the cells toward the barrel walls. The roles of these potential mechanisms in barrel formation remain to be determined.

Lesions to the periphery have a smaller effect on the emergence of normal barrel morphology after inception of the cytoarchitectonic pattern. However, even though barrels may form if a single row of whiskers is damaged on P3, the row of barrels corresponding to the damaged row will take up less space than the neighboring rows. This competitive battle for space is partly activity dependent as the loss of space by the barrels corresponding to the ablated follicles is reduced when glutamatergic transmission is blocked during barrel formation (Schlaggar *et al.*, 1993). The behavior of the dendrites is also dependent on normal peripheral activity, because if the C-row of whiskers is damaged at around P3 in the mouse, the dendrites do not orient themselves toward the center of the barrel but stretch out more uniformly to

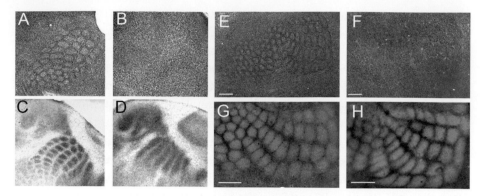

**Figure 4.8.** Cellular barrel pattern formation and thalamocortical afferent pattern formation are dissociated in metabotropic glutamate receptor 5 (mGluR5 [A–D]) and protein kinase A regulatory subunit RIIβ [E–H] knockouts. A. The cellular pattern is present at postnatal day 6 (P6) in the wild-type, B but not the mGluR5 knockouts (A, B Nissl stain). C. The thalamocortical afferent pattern is present in the wild-type mouse and D. normal rows can be seen for the axons of mGluR null mutants, though the rows do not differentiate into a barrel pattern (C, D axons stained by 5HT immunohisto-chemistry) (Reprinted from Hannan *et al.* [2001], with kind permission of the authors and Macmillan Publishers Ltd). E. The cellular pattern in wild-types (P16) F. is absent in RIIβ knockouts; the barrels are poorly formed and indistinct (E, F Nissl stain). G. The thalamocortical afferent pattern is normal in wild-types (P7). H. and RIIβ knockouts. (G, H, 5HT transporter staining) (Reproduced from Inan *et al.* [2006], with kind permission of the authors and the Society for Neuroscience.)

reach the neighboring rows of barrels (Harris and Woolsey, 1981). The question arises of how the thalamic afferents influence the development of the cortical neurons during this period, and this question is addressed in the next section.

### 4.3.2    *Interaction of thalamic afferents with neurons*

Perhaps the starkest evidence that the cortical cells need to be instructed to form barrels comes from studies where particular mutations have led to the abolition of a neuronal pattern despite the presence of a somato-topic pattern in the thalamic afferents (Figure 4.8). The first indication of this came from studies of the barrelless mouse (Welker *et al.*, 1996), which it tran-spires is a natural adenylyl cyclase type I (ACI) null mutant (Abdel-Majid *et al.*, 1998). The barrelless mouse has no barrels in the cortex although the somato-topy of the whisker representation is preserved. Similarly, later studies showed that a knockout of phospholipase C (PLC) $\beta_1$-subunit also prevents the cytoarch-itectonic differentiation of layer IV into barrels despite the thalamic afferents forming a normal somatotopic pattern (Hannan *et al.*, 2001). A number of mutants have subsequently been documented to lack cytoarchitectonic barrels, including knockouts of mGluR, PLCβ$_1$, the Ras GTPase-activating protein SynGAP and the protein kinase A (PKA) regulatory subunit RIIβ (Figure 4.8). It is likely that the effect of these knockouts are all connected because they disrupt a common set of signaling pathways. By some means, the signaling pathway must allow the thalamic afferents to shape the morphological development of the layer IV cells via receptor-linked biochemical mechanisms (Section 4.3.3).

Although thalamocortical afferents can exhibit a somatotopic pattern while the cells do not, the converse is not true. Mutations that cause the thalamic afferents to lose their clustered and segregated barrel form have no somatotopic pattern in the afferents or in the cells of layer IV. For example, the monoamine oxidase knockout mouse lacks both thalamocortical and cytoarchitectonic barrels (Cases *et al.*, 1996). In this case, an antagonist to serotonergic receptors can rescue the barrels. This finding implies that an excess of serotonin disrupts the thalamic afferents from forming barrels. Given that a somatotopic pattern is necessary but not sufficient for forming the cellular pattern of barrels, the question becomes one of how do the thalamic afferents signal to the cells to form the barrels? While this question is not answered as yet, there are a number of clues emerging from recent work on signaling pathways, as described in the following section.

### 4.3.3    *Signaling pathways*

Although neuronal activity per se appears not to play a role in pattern formation, the fact that mutation in receptor-signaling pathways can affect barrels from forming does suggest a role for activity in this process. Thalamocortical axons use glutamate as a transmitter, which make it a likely candidate for signaling pattern information between pre- and postsynaptic cells.

Two glutamate receptors have been implicated in barrel formation so far, the NMDA receptor and the metabotropic receptors. If the NMDA receptor is knocked out in just the cortex, the CO-staining pattern of barrels can still be seen. However, if a Nissl stain is used to examine the formation of the cytoarchitectonic barrels, the somatosensory cortex appears uniform (Iwasato *et al.*, 2000). This implies that NMDA receptor activation is necessary for translation of the thalamocortical afferent pattern into the cytoarchitectonic pattern. Mice lacking mGluR5 show row formation but not barrel formation in the thalamo-cortical axons (Figure 4.8) and lack cytoarchitectonic barrels (Hannan *et al.*, 2001). There are several intracellular signaling pathways by which both NMDA and mGluR5 could be involved in barrel formation.

Both NMDA receptors and mGluR5 can control calcium signaling in the postsynaptic spine, which theoretically gives access to a very large number of intracellular signaling pathways. Fortunately, the possible signaling pathways involved can be restricted by observations made on a number of other mutants without barrels. The original barrelless mouse is a naturally occurring ACI null mutant, and so lacks this calcium-dependent enzyme. Further evidence that ACI is involved comes from studies of knockouts for the catalytic and regulatory subunits of PKA. Barrels do not form if the RIIβ subunit of PKA is knocked out, although the somatotopic pattern is present (Inan *et al.*, 2006) (Figure 4.8). Therefore both NMDA receptors and mGluR5 could affect barrel formation by ACI effects on PKA. To test this further, it would be important to study a cortex-specific ACI knockout to see whether ACI is required in cortex or brainstem to allow the development of the somatotopic pattern. The role of PKA in early development of thalamocortical synapses is discussed in Section 4.4.1

There is evidence that the PLC $\beta_1$-subunit is critically involved, most probably downstream of mGluR5, in differentiation of the barrels. This enzyme is located within the barrels but not the barrel walls of developing mouse barrel cortex in a clear somatotopic pattern (Hannan *et al.*, 2001). In PLC $\beta_1$-subunit knockout mice, the axonal pattern forms normally but the cytoarchitecture of the barrels does not form at all. Since phosphoinositol hydrolysis activated via mGluR5 is dependent on PLC $\beta_1$-subunit in the barrel cortex, it is possible that these two molecules are sequentially linked in a signaling pathway that controls barrel differentiation (Hannan *et al.*, 2001) although the downstream effector molecules are not yet known.

The other transmitter that might be involved in translating the thalamic pattern to the cortical barrels is serotonin. Intriguingly, thalamocortical axons transiently express a serotonin-uptake transporter and label for serotonin during early development (Lebrand *et al.*, 1998). This raises the possibility that, in addition to glutamate, thalamocortical afferents could release serotonin during barrel development. Mutations affecting serotonin levels such as monoamine oxidase knockouts certainly disrupt barrel formation by affecting the branching of the thalamocortical afferents (Cases *et al.*, 1996). However, it appears that activity-dependent vesicular release of serotonin is not required for barrel formation because knocking out the vesicular monoamine transporter VMAT2, which is expressed by thalamocortical neurons, does not affect barrel development. Knocking out the serotonin transporter does prevent barrel formation by depleting the cortex of serotonin (Persico *et al.*, 2001). These findings suggest that thalamocortical afferents require but do not release serotonin for normal barrel formation. Consequently, the mechanism for relaying the somatotopic pattern from thalamocortical afferent to postsynaptic layer IV cells seems to be

activated via glutamate receptors. The precise mechanism remains to be determined, but it is a fair assumption that it will involve processes important for
development of glutamatergic synapses, and that topic is treated in the next
section.

## 4.4    Synaptic development

### 4.4.1    Thalamocortical synapses

If synaptic activity is important for barrel formation in the cortex and
the barrels form early in the first postnatal week, then synaptic transmission
should be functional during the first postnatal week. In studies where synaptic
transmission has been studied in slices of barrel cortex, it is certainly possible to
detect synaptic responses in the cortical plate neurons as early as P0 (Kim *et al.*,
1995), but the responses are easily fatigued. Despite this, synaptic transmission
is possible owing to a number of specializations that exist at this age. First, most
of the synaptic current is carried by NMDA receptors in the first few postnatal
days. Currents in these NMDA receptors can last for 300 ms or more, which
produces a far more sustained depolarization of the neuron than could be
achieved by AMPA currents. Second, there are few functional inhibitory
synapses at this age to attenuate the response (Section 4.4.3). Third, neurons
have very high input impedance compared with adult neurons (several giga-
ohms), which means that very small currents are able to cause considerable
depolarization. Fourth, many excitatory cells have gap junctions at this age,
which may spread excitation between cells receiving few chemical synaptic
input (LoTurco *et al.*, 1991; Yuste *et al.*, 1992; Kim *et al.*, 1995).

The number of these weak but specialized immature synapses is relatively
low during the period of barrel formation (Figure 4.9). The number of synaptic
spines, the number of multiple synapses at varicosities and synapse density all
increase rapidly after barrel formation between P6 and P20 (Micheva and
Beaulieu, 1996; White *et al.*, 1997). Similarly, many of the physiological changes
in thalamocortical synapses occur following barrel formation; for example, silent
synapses disappear between P5 and P8 (Isaac *et al.*, 1997). Therefore, a case can be
made that some of the early synapses pioneer for those that come later.

How do thalamocortical synapses mature during barrel formation? It is
known that in the rat the proportion of current carried by AMPA channels
increases between P0 and P5. The mechanism for this is likely to be the conversion of silent synapses to active synapses (Figure 4.10). Between P2 and P5, a
significant proportion of synapses are silent, that is they show postsynaptic
responses to stimulation of the thalamocortical afferents only if the cell is

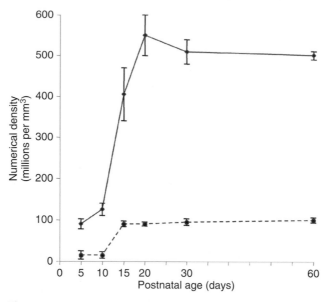

**Figure 4.9.** Development of inhibitory and excitatory synapses in rat barrel cortex. The density of synapses is estimated from electron microscopy of sections and plotted for symmetrical synapses (solid line) and asymmetric synapses (dashed line). (Adapted from Micheva and Beaulieu [1996] and printed with kind permission of the authors and Wiley.)

depolarized because the synapse only contains NMDA channels and not AMPA channels. If the cell is depolarized during presynaptic stimulation, AMPA-mediated postsynaptic currents appear after a short delay of a few minutes (Isaac *et al.*, 1997). The mechanisms is thought to be NMDA-dependent inser-tion of AMPA channels into the postsynaptic membrane (Hayashi *et al.*, 2000; Malinow and Malenka, 2002). By P8 or P9, the ability of thalamocortical synapses to show LTP is practically absent and coincides with the loss of silent synapses activated by thalamic inputs.

The process of changing from a silent to a functional synapse appears to require ACI. In barreless mice lacking functional ACI, synapse development is arrested in a state where they contain some AMPA receptors but far fewer than in normal animals. The surface expression of GluR1, which is an AMPA receptor subunit with a PKA phosphorylation site, is reduced in barreless animals (Lu *et al.*, 2003). This suggests that the ACI/PKA pathway is simultaneously involved in early synapse maturation and barrel formation (Figure 4.8) either in parallel or in series.

The process of changing from a silent to a functional synapse also appears to require BDNF. In somatosensory cortex of BDNF knockout mice, silent synapses

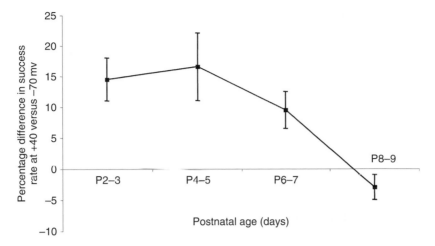

**Figure 4.10.** Developmental decrease in silent synapses at the thalamocortical synapse. The difference in the success rate for evoking an excitatory postsynaptic current in a cortical cell at $+40$ mV (NMDA currents present) versus $-70$ mV (NMDA currents absent) by stimulating thalamocortical afferents is plotted for animals at different ages. The proportion of NMDA-only synapses decrease substantially after the first seven postnatal days. (Adapted from Isaac *et al.* [1997] and printed with kind permission of the authors and Elsevier.).

are more abundant than in wild-type mice (Itami *et al.*, 2003). In the age range P8–P12, failure rates at synapses for AMPA transmission were 0.9 for homozygous null mutants compared with 0.26 for age-matched wild-type animals. Furthermore, it was not possible to convert silent synapses to active synapses in the BDNF knockouts using an LTP protocol without the inclusion of exogenous BDNF at low concentrations (Itami *et al.*, 2003). These results demonstrate a role for BDNF in maturation of the thalamocortial synapse. At present, it is not clear whether BDNF plays a permissive or instructive role in synapse development.

The presynaptic side of the thalamocortical synapse also matures at the same time as AMPA insertion. Thalamocortical arbors form synapses on spines and dendritic shafts (Micheva and Beaulieu, 1996; White *et al.*, 1997) and increase in complexity during the first postnatal week (Senft and Woolsey, 1991). Thalamocortical afferents transiently express a number of presynaptic receptors, transporters and enzymes at this early stage of development for the serotonergic, cholinergic and glutamatergic systems. These are described in Figure 4.11 (color version as Plate 4). The glutamatergic receptors are perhaps understandable as the synapse itself is glutamatergic. However, the developing axons appear to be set up to respond to the non-specific projection systems

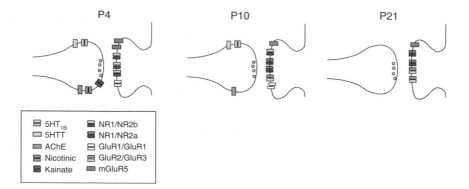

P4                    P10                   P21

| 5HT$_{1B}$ | NR1/NR2b |
| 5HTT | NR1/NR2a |
| AChE | GluR1/GluR1 |
| Nicotinic | GluR2/GluR3 |
| Kainate | mGluR5 |

**Figure 4.11.** Development of pre- and postsynaptic receptors at thalamocortical synapses. On the fourth postnatal day (P4) in the rat, the presynaptic terminal has a variety of receptors and transporters present including serotonin receptors (5HT$_{1B}$), serotonin transporter (5HTT), nicotinic cholinergic receptors (NR) and acetylcholinesterase (AChE) in addition to kainiate receptors. These are progressively lost over the next few weeks of postnatal life (compare with P21). The postsynaptic side develops from mainly NR2B-containing NMDA receptors (P4) to mainly NR2A-containing (P10+), while AMPA receptors increase in number including the calcium-impermeable GluR2-containing types (P21). Note that postsynaptic kainate receptors are not included on this type of synapse because evidence points to their location on separate thalamocortical connections (Bannister *et al.*, 2005). (See color plate section.)

from the basal forebrain cholinergic system and the dorsal raphe serotonergic system. The evidence for their particular involvement in development comes partly from the transient expression of these receptor systems (Figure 4.11). Serotonin is also known to be important for normal barrel field development because high concentrations acting via 5HT$_{1B}$ receptors induce outgrowth in the thalamocortical fibers, which disrupts the somatotopic pattern (Cases *et al.*, 1996; Lotto *et al.*, 1999; Young-Davies *et al.*, 2000). The presynaptic 5HT$_{1B}$ receptors and the 5HT transporter are both expressed transiently during development between P4 and P16 (Mansour-Robaey *et al.*, 1998). The thalamocortical arbors, therefore, remain sensitive to serotonin after the somatotopic pattern has formed but during the period when the branches of the afferents are elaborated.

Acetylcholine is not as clearly implicated in barrel field development as serotonin. Nevertheless, presynaptic acetylcholinesterase shows strong developmental expression. Nicotinic receptors are present as early as P1 and are downregulated between P7 and P10 (Broide *et al.*, 1996). Acetylcholinesterase is present at birth and downregulated between P17 and P21 (Kristt and Waldman, 1982). Because of its presynaptic location, acetylcholinesterase shows a clear somatotopic pattern. It is not clear what the function of the presynaptic receptors might be; however, there is some evidence that glutamate release can be modulated by activation of nicotinic receptors in the prefrontal cortex (Gioanni et al., 1999) as has been demonstrated in the interpedunclear nucleus (Girod et al., 2000). While it is not clear what the function of many of these developmentally regulated modulatory systems is at present, there are clues as to the role of developmentally regulated glutamate receptors.

Kainate receptors show an increase in expression during the first postnatal week (Jablonska et al., 1998). However, the physiological effect of the presynaptic receptor decreases during the same period (Kidd et al., 2002). There are two cases to consider, the presynaptic and the postsynaptic kainate receptors. Presynaptic kainate receptors act to inhibit glutamate release from the thalamocortical terminal, and by so doing limit the amount of excitation produced postsynaptically for repetitive firing patterns. During the early phase of synapse development, synapses are weak and cannot in any case produce a great deal of excitation. However, following the conversion of a significant proportion of silent synapses to their active form, sufficient excitatory drive exists to clearly see the governing effect of the kainate autoreceptor (Kidd et al., 2002). Kainate receptors tend to limit transmission at higher frequencies but to leave transmission at lower frequencies intact. It is feasible that this system limits high-frequency responses toward the end of the first postnatal week until the inhibitory system is better developed. In the second postnatal week, the kainate autoreceptor is downregulated, but inhibition is better developed to control high-frequency responses (Section 4.4.3).

Postsynaptic kainate receptors are also downregulated during the first postnatal week. They exist at separate synapses from those that gain AMPA receptors during unsilencing silent synapse (Bannister et al., 2005) and they generate EPSPs, which have small peak amplitudes but nevertheless transfer a large amount of charge owing to their long duration (Kidd and Isaac, 1999). If LTP is evoked in the thalamocortical pathway during the first postnatal week (Section 6.1.2), it not only unsilences silent synapses but downregulates postsynaptic kainate receptors at their separate synaptic location. Given that kainate receptors are downregulated during development, LTP may activate the same activity-dependent processes that naturally occur during development.

Finally, mGluRs are known to be important for barrel development because the mGluR5 knockout shows thalamic patterning but not barrel formation (Figure 4.8). In particular, the mGluR5 subtype shows a clear somatotopic pattern in normal animals between P5 and P14 (Blue et al., 1997; Munoz et al., 1999). It is clear that many of these receptors are postsynaptic, although presynaptic locus is not ruled out. As described in Section 4.3.3, their mode of action is likely to control activity of the PLC $\beta_1$-subunit and thereby control postsynaptic development of the barrels (Hannan *et al.*, 2001).

### 4.4.2    *Intracortical synapses*

Formation and refinement of thalamocortical synapses are clearly only the first stage in the development of the cortical circuit. After the thalamocortical afferents have imprinted the somatotopic pattern on the cortex, the great complexity of the cortical circuit is generated by a wealth of intracortical connections. The question arises of how intracortical synapses are formed and how their maturation and survival are controlled.

Cells of layers II and III migrate from the ventricular zone to arrive in the cortex later than those forming layer IV. Consequently, layer II/III cells differentiate and form connections slightly later than cells in layer IV. It would seem to make sense that the cortical circuit becomes wired-up in the order in which cells are normally activated by whisker stimulation in the adult animal: that is, layer IV before layer II/III (Chapter 5). In this way, the receptive field processing could be established at one level before it influenced receptive field formation at the next level. Whether by design or chance, this certainly appears to be the case for the layer IV to layers II/III connection, where layer IV synaptic development is advanced by the end of the first postnatal week before the critical period for layer II/III cells begins.

The major excitatory drive from layer IV cells tends to stay within the column and projects to layer II/III cells during the later part of the first postnatal week. Evidence for the timing of synapse formation and receptive field development in these cells comes from studies where putative synapses have been imaged directly (Lendvai *et al.*, 2000). Using two-photon laser microscopy, it is possible to image cells in the living brain if the neurons are made to fluoresce. This is achieved by incorporating green or yellow fluorescent protein into the genome (Trachtenberg *et al.*, 2002) or by introducing the protein with a virus (Chen *et al.*, 2000). This allows the experimenter to see dendrites and processes as small as postsynaptic spines. Between P11 and P15, the spines of layer II/III pyramidal cells extend and retract relatively rapidly compared with the period before or after (Stern *et al.*, 2001). The growth and retraction process is thought to be indicative of synapse formation (Figure 4.12), and, indeed, the recently formed spines can be shown to form synapses (Trachtenberg *et al.*, 2002).

A crucial question is whether the spine dynamics, and, therefore, synapse formation, is activity dependent or simply turned on by a developmental clock at some point. Two observations are germane to this subject; first, if the whiskers are trimmed during the period of increased spine dynamics, then the receptive fields of the layer II/III neurons do not develop normally. Rather

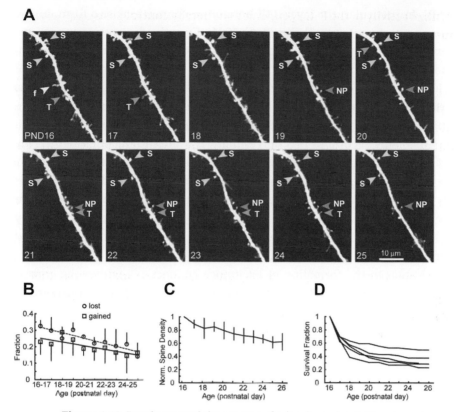

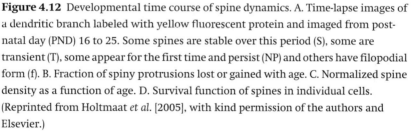

**Figure 4.12** Developmental time course of spine dynamics. A. Time-lapse images of a dendritic branch labeled with yellow fluorescent protein and imaged from post-natal day (PND) 16 to 25. Some spines are stable over this period (S), some are transient (T), some appear for the first time and persist (NP) and others have filopodial form (f). B. Fraction of spiny protrusions lost or gained with age. C. Normalized spine density as a function of age. D. Survival function of spines in individual cells. (Reprinted from Holtmaat *et al.* [2005], with kind permission of the authors and Elsevier.)

than develop with a clear principal whisker and lesser surround receptive field inputs, the cells have undefined connections from many whiskers (Lendvai *et al.*, 2000). This observation suggests that activity is important for guiding synapse formation between P11 and P15 in the barrel cortex. Second, trimming the whiskers can cause spine motility to decrease in areas of the cortex lacking their normal whisker input. This suggests that not only is sensory activity required for guiding selection of the correct connections but it is also required for instigating the process that leads to synapse formation (Lendvai *et al.*, 2000).

Of course the correct alignment of center and surround receptive field components is likely to depend upon more than just the columnar projections from layer IV. In particular, the layer II/III horizontal connections also form during the second postnatal week (Miller *et al.*, 2001). Growth of intrinsic connections depends on an intact periphery. This can be demonstrated by cutting the infra-orbital nerve at P7 in the mouse when the barrels are already formed in layer IV and looking at the development of horizontal fibers in extragranular layers. Under these conditions, horizontal connections do not grow out to link neigh-boring columns within the cortex (McCasland *et al.*, 1992). As usual with experi-ments involving section of this nerve, there is a question about whether the effect is caused by a loss of ascending sensory activity or by some other factor induced by nerve lesion such as neuronal degeneration. From other studies, it is likely that neuronal activity is necessary for the horizontal connections to form properly because either clipping the whiskers or blocking cortical activity with APV prevents the normal pattern of projections from forming (Keller and Carlson, 1999; Dagnew *et al.*, 2003).

In addition to the formation of excitatory connections within the cortex, inhibitory circuits need to develop in order to create a functional cortical system and this is the subject of the next section.

### 4.4.3    *Inhibitory synapses*

As the excitatory connections develop and strengthen in the cortex, it becomes imperative to limit the possibility for positive feedback circuits to form, which could lead to excitotoxic damage. As described above, this problem is helped during the first postnatal week for the thalamocortical synapse by presynaptic kainate receptors. However, for the majority of cortical circuits, excitation is controlled and shaped by inhibition.

Development of inhibition lags behind that of excitation in the cortex during the first postnatal week. If recordings are made from the youngest cells, which lie in the cortical plate, it is possible to record EPSPs but not IPSPs at any age from P0 to P5 (Kim *et al.*, 1995). However, as each layer differentiates out from the cortical plate, inhibition can be detected. For example, IPSPs can be recorded from layer V/VI neurons on P0 in the mouse and from layer IV neurons as it differentiates on P2 (Agmon *et al.*, 1996). Presumably, excitatory connections need to form before inhibitory connections (a) because the inhibitory cells need to be driven by excitatory connections themselves and (b) because excitatory synapses need to strengthen in a manner that depends on depolarization of the cell. In general, inhibition would tend to oppose depolarization and, therefore, make it difficult for excitatory connections to establish a foothold in the cortex. Having low levels of inhibition early on helps this process. However, another specialization exists that also has a beneficial effect for maturing excitatory synapses; IPSPs tend to have a more positive reversal potential in young barrel cortex than they do in adults (Agmon *et al.*, 1996). When $GABA_A$ receptors are activated in young barrel cortex, they tend to move the membrane voltage toward the reversal potential. The reversal potential for $GABA_A$ receptors alters during development from $-26$ mV in mouse cortex at P3–P5 to $-63$ mV in the adult. This means that neonatal cortical neurons would tend to be more depolarized in general and it is conceivable that individual IPSPs may even contribute to depolarizing the cell to some extent (Agmon *et al.*, 1996).

Studies where the number of symmetrical synapses have been counted suggest that from P4 to P32 the number of inhibitory synapses steadily increases (Figure 4.9) to an adult value of approximately 11% of the total number of synapses (De Felipe *et al.*, 1997). The rate of production of inhibitory synapses is initially lower than that of excitatory synapses and may even decrease slightly between P5 and P10 (Micheva and Beaulieu, 1995a). The main production of GABA synapses occurs around P10 to P15 (Micheva and Beaulieu, 1996). Layer IV is the main locus of inhibitory cells in the adult (Chapter 2) and inhibition continues to mature right up to P30 (Micheva and Beaulieu, 1996).

Just as experience has an effect on excitatory connections, so too it affects the development of inhibitory synapses. During early development, a subpopulation of inhibitory synapses on spines can be reduced in number by whisker trimming from birth (Micheva and Beaulieu, 1995b, c). Inhibitory connections on to spines can obviously have a large selective local influence on the excitatory connections on the same spine. Therefore, experience-dependent development of GABAergic connections are likely to have an important functional role in development and plasticity. Interestingly, GABAergic synapses remain plastic into adulthood in mouse barrel cortex (Knott *et al.*, 2002). Overstimulation of a single whisker in an adult mouse leads to an increase in synapses on to spines in general, but the excitatory connections are more transient than the inhibitory ones, which remain up to four days after the initial stimulus regimen (Knott *et al.*, 2002). So far, our understanding of activity-dependent mechanisms controlling excitatory synapse formation and elimination far outweighs our understanding of the analogous processes at inhibitory synapses. One of the questions for the future must be elucidating the mechanism by which the formation and selection of inhibitory connections are controlled.

## 4.5    Conclusions

The barrel cortex develops partly as a product of intrinsic factors inherited from the cortical progenitor cells and partly as a product of the influence of thalamic afferents projecting to it. The thalamic axons impose a topographic pattern on the cortex, which is generated under the control of the peripheral nerves innervating the mystacial pad and guided into position by cortical diffu-sible factors. The primary afferents of the follicles nerves create a pattern because some axons receiving neurotrophic support from the follicles survive while others do not. Neuronal activity is not essential for pattern formation per se although it can play a role in refining the cortical connections, strengthening cortical synapses and guiding cortical receptive field development. Interestingly, the somatotopic pattern that arises in the neurons of layer IV does depends on activity even though the presynaptic pattern does not, and barrel formation, therefore, can be said to be activity dependent.

One of the many challenges for the future is describing the exact signaling pathways involved in forming the barrels. Are dendritic growth and refinement controlled by the synapses and if so what are the signaling pathways? A second major unanswered question is the mechanisms by which inhibitory synapses are controlled and specified. Clearly, inhibitory synapses appear and disappear under the control of sensory activity, but the synaptic mechanisms remain obscure at present. Are inhibitory synapses reacting to what happens to their own excitatory inputs, or is there a synaptic mechanism controlling synaptic strength at the inhibitory synapse as there is at the excitatory synapse? Technical advantages of being able to study the synapses in the thalamocortical slice coupled with the advantage of a clear somatotopic pattern in the barrel cortex make it likely that inroads into developmental questions will continue to be made using this structure.

# 5

# Sensory physiology

This chapter describes how the barrel cortex processes sensory information from a systems viewpoint. Several questions are addressed, such as how information is coded, what processing a cortical column performs and how active touch might work. While considerable progress has been made in recent years in tackling these questions, it is not yet possible to answer them fully. Here we approach sensory processing from the viewpoint that it is possible to shed light on several classic questions in the general field of sensory physiology by studying the barrel system.

One of the classic questions in sensory physiology concerns how information is coded and whether information travels in specialized channels that form labeled lines of information. The issue is particularly pertinent in the barrel system where the very purpose of the anatomical pattern of the whiskers and barrels seems to indicate an affirmative answer. However, while labeled-line processing is a good first-order approximation for the barrel system (Section 5.1), many studies in recent years show how barrel cortex integrates information from different whiskers. The tension between these two ideas has driven many studies in this field and they are treated from two complementary but inverse viewpoints in Section 5.2, which deals with cortical domains driven by single whiskers, and Section 5.3, which deals with receptive fields.

Section 5.4 on dynamic sensory processing looks at the question of how active touch can be understood and the degree to which studies on passive touch (treated in earlier sections of the chapter) can inform this understanding. The idea that the cortical column is a modular unit for processing information is introduced in Section 5.1 and the experimental evidence is addressed in Section 5.2. The complex system of feedback and feedforward systems within the barrel system raises questions about dynamic processing in the cortex, where it forms one part of a number of somatomotor loops; these issues are explored further in Section 5.4. However, we start with a consideration of two of the classic ideas in sensory cortical physiology: cortical columns and labeled-line information processing.

## 5.1    Topography

### 5.1.1    The columnar hypothesis

One of the fundamental tenets of cortical physiology is that the cortex is composed of many repeated elements known as columns. Each column is composed of a vertical array of cells traversing the depth of the cortex from layer I to VI. Within a given cortical area, each column is envisaged as performing a similar transformation function on its thalamic input as every other column. Each column derives its unique identity from operating on a slightly different thalamic input from its neighbor; for example, one column may be responsible for processing information from the index finger while another is responsible for processing information from the thumb. However, the underlying concept is that, whatever the source of information from the periphery, each column essentially performs the same transformation on its input as its neighbor.

When Mountcastle (1957) first introduced the concept of cortical columns, there was little anatomical evidence to support the notion, as it was not yet known that thalamic axons tend to cluster in termination patterns of a few hundred micrometers within cortical layer IV. However, the functional architecture of the cat and monkey somatosensory cortex was apparent enough from electrode recordings for Mountcastle to recognize the columnar architecture anyway (Mountcastle, 1957; Mountcastle et al., 1957; Mountcastle and Powell, 1959). Neurons showed similar receptive field properties in single vertical penetrations within the cortex because vertical penetrations sampled a single column. However, neurons showed different receptive field properties in neighboring penetrations because adjacent vertical penetrations sampled neuronal responses in different columns.

Today, the study of columns has advanced to the point where it can be said that they appear to be composed of 50–80 minicolumns, each with a similar synaptic circuit composed of 80–100 cells. Each cortical column contains approximately 4000–8000 cells and measures approximately 300–500 μm, across (Chapter 1). The size of cortical columns do not vary greatly in brains that vary in size by over three orders of magnitude (Bugbee and Goldman-Rakic, 1983), arguing that larger brains are simply made up of more columns than smaller brains.

At first sight, the barrel cortex appears to be an exemplar of the columnar hypothesis. Not only does barrel cortex have repeating functional units of barrels, each operating on its own thalamic input carrying information from its own principal whisker, but also the anatomical correlate of the column (i.e. the barrel) can be seen in layer IV with simple histochemical stains. In the mouse, barrels are about approximately 100 μm by 200 μm across and contain approximately 2000 cells (Pasternak and Woolsey, 1975). It can be estimated from this that a mouse barrel-column contains approximately 6000 cells. Barrels are larger in the rat, particularly in the posterior medial barrel subfield, and can measure 450–500 μm across including the septal surrounds. It can be estimated using a cell density of 85 000 neurons/mm$^2$ (Ren, 1991) that the larger rat barrel-columns contain 18 000 to 21 000 neurons. Receptive fields in any particular barrel are dominated by responses to one single whisker (Simons, 1985) and a single barrel receives rapid input from just one single whisker (Armstrong-James and Fox, 1987). The evidence has been strong enough to venture the name "barrel-column," meaning the radial column of cells above and below the layer IV barrel.

The columnar hypothesis is a sufficiently good first approximation for how the barrel cortex is organized that we address its function from a columnar viewpoint in this chapter. However, it is worth noting from the outset two clear exceptions that do not fit with the columnar hypothesis. First, the septal areas between the barrels have quite distinct inputs and different intracortical connections from the barrels they surround. The septal areas do not, therefore, conform to the barrel-column model with a different set of inputs and could be considered as a separate cortical area within an area (Kim and Ebner, 1999). Second, it has become increasingly clear that cortical areas operate as one part in a dynamic circuit that includes feedback to subcortical areas (Ahissar and Kleinfeld, 2003), which raises the question of where the unit of function resides, inside or outside the cortex. In other words, is the functional unit a single cortical column or is it the cortical column plus the closed feedback loops it makes with subcortical structures?

### 5.1.2    *Labeled-line processing versus integration*

Cortical columns tend to keep information localized within separate channels. In general, the advantage of parcelating information in this way is that the specificity of receptor activation is preserved from one location to another as it ascends the neuronal pathway. This idea is known as the labeled-line theory of sensory processing (Figure 5.1). The same information is available for integration at every station within the pathway and is not lost en route. In principle, lack of convergence in pathway could allow the individual to become

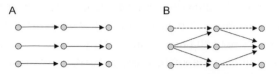

**Figure 5.1.** Labeled-line and distributed processing. A. Labeled-line processing is so called because each receptor signals through a chain of neuronal relays without divergence or convergence. The diagram depicts a receptor layer (left) signaling through one relay to the recipient neuronal layer (right). B. Integrative processing involves mixing information from individual receptors in different channels. The information can be recombined as shown between the middle and recipient neuronal layer (right).

aware of an individual receptor. In practice, the main advantage of a low-convergence pathway is that it results in high spatial acuity. Conversely, a high-convergence pathway results in low spatial acuity for an individual cell. Where convergence occurs early in the somatosensory pathway, it becomes difficult to distinguish between a stimulus at one location and another.

In general, the somatosensory system derives advantages from labeled-line organization because the exact location of a stimulus carries meaningful information. It matters to the organism whether the stimulus is on the left hand or the back of the neck, for example. Similarly, different receptor types code for different types of stimulus such as vibration (Pacinian corpuscles) and pressure (Ruffini nerve endings). In these cases labeled-line organization works well to preserve the identity of the information.

A disadvantage of labeled-line processing is that activation of an individual receptor may not carry any meaning. For example, activation of a single odorant receptor or a single photoreceptor carries very little information without the context supplied by the other receptors within the system. Similarly, in the somatosensory system, interpretation of several types of sensation require considerable convergence of information. For example, to interpret exploratory hand movements, where the receptor surface moves and the object remains stationary, information is integrated from several spatial locations at once.

The whisker system has elements of both labeled-line and integrative organization. Information from a single whisker is preserved from the level of the primary afferents to the barrels within layer IV of the cortex and this forms the labeled-line element. However, as we shall see, there are several places in the subcortical pathways and locations within the cortex where lateral connections between individual whisker representations allow information from neighboring whiskers to be combined, and this forms the integrative element. First, let us consider the anatomical underpinnings of the labeled-line system.

The anatomical organization of the point-to-point projection is described in detail in Chapter 2. The final stage of the pathway into the barrel cortex from the thalamus is highly topographically organized. Practically all the cells in a thalamic barreloid project to the corresponding cortical barrel (Land *et al.*, 1995). The axonal arbors of individual thalamocortical cells project to the center of the barrel. The dendrites of cells sitting in the wall of the barrels are directed inward to make synaptic contact with the thalamocortical arbors (Simons and Woolsey, 1984). The specificity of the topography is partly maintained by the specificity of the axons and partly by the dendrites. The axonal arbors of thalamocortical axons are largely confined within the boundaries of individual barrels (Bernardo and Woolsey, 1987; Jensen and Killackey, 1987). In the rat, a few axonal branches within the barrel "escape" into the septal areas surrounding the barrel wall and some even enter surrounding barrels (Arnold *et al.*, 2001). It has been estimated that approximately 1–2% of the axonal length within layer IV infiltrates neighboring barrels.

A measure of the effectiveness of the thalamic axons can be gauged from physiological measurements. If the shortest latency responses to stimulating individual whiskers are recorded in the cortex and their positions are plotted within the barrel field, short-latency responses are found within the principal barrel for the whisker stimulated and not outside (Armstrong-James and Fox, 1987; Fox, 1992). Since the short-latency responses result from conduction along the fewest number of synapses within the somatosensory pathway, the last section of which is necessarily the thalamocortical axon, this method enables us to see the location of the effective thalamocortical axons. In normal rats and mice, the shortest latency responses of around 5–10 ms are found to be confined to the principal barrel for that whisker (Figure 5.2), implying that the thalamo-cortical axons are functionally confined to their principal barrel.

Studies using a variety of methods have shown that the earliest cortical responses to whisker stimulation are located in the principal barrel. Optical imaging of barrel cortex using voltage-sensitive dyes show principal barrel activation at 10 ms (Petersen *et al.*, 2003). Multielectrode implant recordings in barrel cortex show even shorter latency responses, which are nevertheless confined to the principal barrel (Petersen and Diamond, 2000) (Figure 5.2).

One might easily be led into thinking that the specificity of the thalamocortical topographical projection results in all the cells within a barrel responding to a single whisker. In fact, only about 30% of cortical layer IV barrel cells exhibit a single-whisker receptive field as judged from spike recordings (Ito, 1985; Fox *et al.*, 2003) and almost none do so if subthreshold EPSPs are counted as the receptive field (Zhu and Connors, 1999). The reasons for convergence of whisker information within a single barrel may be attributable to several factors, not

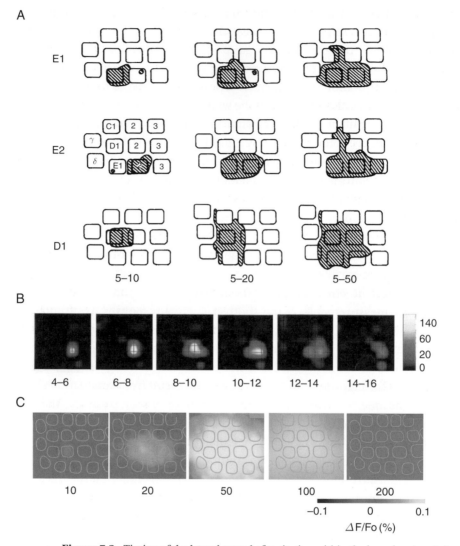

**Figure 5.2.** Timing of the lateral spread of excitation within the barrel cortex. A. In rat barrel cortex, single-unit recording within layer IV shows that responses are initially confined to the principal barrel at 5–10 ms before spreading to near neighbors at times beyond (5–20 ms). Cortical domains are shown for stimulating whiskers E1, E2, or D1 by the shaded areas. (Reprinted from Armstrong-James and Fox [1987], with permission from Wiley.) B. A higher time resolution view of the first 20 ms in this multielectrode recording in rat barrel cortex show the earliest responses at 4–6 and 6–8 ms are confined to the principal barrel. A 400 μm grid is superimposed on the response. (Reprinted from Petersen and Diamond [2000], with kind permission of Society for Neuroscience and the authors.) C. A longer time view in this optical recording shows the full extent of excitatory spread from single-whisker excitation. Excitation spreads to encompass the entire barrel cortex by 100 ms. The field of view is approximately 2 mm. (Reprinted from Petersen *et al.* [2003], with kind permission of Society for Neuroscience and the authors.)

least of which is that many thalamic neurons respond to several whiskers. Neurons in VPm and POm have receptive field sizes estimated to vary between 1 and 20 whiskers (Simons and Carvell, 1989; Diamond *et al.*, 1992a; Nicolelis and Chapin, 1994; Friedberg *et al.*, 1999) and neurons in both nuclei project to the cortex. Clearly this arrangement could result in cortical cells acquiring the surround receptive fields of the thalamic cells.

Furthermore, cells within the cortex in different neighboring barrel-columns project between one another and form another substrate for convergence of whisker information. The septal regions within layer IV also form a network of connections that spread among and surround several barrels (Hoeflinger *et al.*, 1995; Kim and Ebner, 1999) and are, therefore, potentially capable of mixing information from different whiskers.

While labeled-line mechanisms are useful for locating place with minimal processing, this is not necessarily the most salient feature of the information supplied by whiskers. When whiskers are used actively, they move to sample several locations in space multiple times, making location a relative not an absolute measure. Integration of information and relative timing of information from several whiskers are also extremely important in addition to whisker identity. It may well be, therefore, that the value of having an accurate topographic projection from the whiskers through the brainstem and thalamus into the layer IV barrels of the cortex is to preserve the essential elements of whisker timing and place information intact for subsequent intracortical and cortico-subcortical processing.

The mechanisms underlying convergence of information within the barrel cortex are explored in Section 5.3. Suffice to say at this point that there are advantages to both labeled-line and overlapping receptive field methods of representing information and that barrel cortex has elements of both systems. In the following section, we begin to address how the cortex processes information from the thalamus.

## 5.2    Intracortical transmission

Excitatory transmission within the barrel cortex can be studied by applying a brief stimulus to the whisker, which is equivalent to looking at the impulse response of the system to this stimulation. The advantage of this method is that the impulse creates a discrete response in time, which can be followed as a wave of excitation as it travels through the cortex. The methodology has been used classically to assess what is known as the point-spread function of the system, or in other words, to see how stimulation of a single peripheral point spreads out on the surface of the cortex. As we will see, the excitation initially begins in a single barrel-column before spreading out into neighboring barrels. In this sense we can see how the point-spread function evolves in time. In addition, because the neighboring barrels respond to different principal whiskers, we can also see that the information begins as labeled-line processing and progresses to cross-whisker integration. We address the events in the order in which they occur, considering first the thalamocortical response transformation (Section 5.2.1), second the vertical transmission within the column (Section 5.2.2) and, third, the transmission between columns (Section 5.2.3).

### 5.2.1    *The thalamocortical response transformation*

The main termination zone for thalamic axons is in layer IV. The collaterals of thalamocortical axons also form a secondary termination zone at the border of layer Vb and layer VI (Lu and Lin, 1993). This explains why the first cortical neurons to respond to stimulation of the principal whisker are located in layer IV and layer Vb. In layer IV, the average latency for EPSPs following whisker stimulation is 6.9 ms (Wilent and Contreras, 2004) and for action potentials 7.2 ms (Armstrong-James *et al.*, 1992). In layer Vb, the average latency for action potentials is about 8.4 ms (Armstrong-James *et al.*, 1992). A second factor that may affect the short latency of these cells is that layer IV and layer V cells both tend to fire action potentials relatively early on the rising phase of the EPSP, a property not shared by layer II/III cells, for example (Wilent and Contreras, 2004).

Initially it was inferred that thalamic axons require considerable temporal summation to depolarize the excitatory cells in layer IV and only the principal whisker drives thalamic neurons with sufficient temporal synchrony to achieve this (Figure 5.3) (Kyriazi and Simons, 1993; Pinto *et al.*, 1996, 2003). Subsequently it was shown that temporal synchrony is indeed important for driving that thalamic recipient cell because each individual thalamocortical input is relatively weak and only able to depolarize the cells by less than 1 mV on average (Bruno and Sakmann, 2006). Many synchronous thalamic inputs are, therefore, required in order to drive a depolarization sufficient to cause the cell to spike. The thalamic neurons tend to have larger receptive fields than the cortical layer IV excitatory cells. However, principal whisker stimulation produces greater temporal synchrony in thalamic projection cells than that produced by adjacent whisker stimulation. Thalamic neurons respond to their principal whisker with rather similar latencies of between 4 and 6 ms. In contrast, the responses of the same thalamic cells to their surround receptive field components are far more variable at 7–15 ms (Armstrong-James and Callahan, 1991). The result is that the principal whisker produces a more synchronous response in the corresponding thalamic barreloid than the neighboring whiskers do. Because the cortical cells require temporal summation of the input to

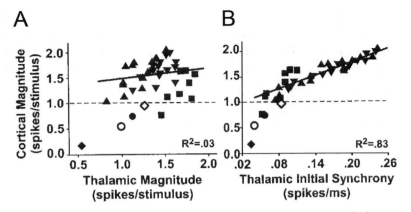

**Figure 5.3.** The relationship between thalamic spike timing and cortical response. A. There is a relatively poor correlation between the magnitude of the cortical and thalamic responses. Above a threshold of approximately 0.8 spikes/stimulus in the thalamus, the relationship is almost flat. B. However, there is a very good correlation between the level of thalamic synchrony and the cortical response above a threshold of approximately 0.06 spikes/ms. (Reprinted from Pinto *et al.* [2003], with kind permission of Oxford University Press and the authors.)

drive them adequately, the principal whisker response tends to be selected from the background of surround whisker responses. This mechanism could be extended to account for other cortical receptive fields properties, for example velocity sensitivity and direction selectivity.

One further mechanism emphasizes the effect of temporal selection. It is known that excitatory cells make connections with one another within the barrel. These excitatory to excitatory cell connections amplify the excitation produced by the thalamocortical afferents (Feldmeyer *et al.*, 1999). Given that synchronous thalamic input is required to depolarize the layer IV cells (Bruno and Sakmann, 2006), excitation is amplified within the barrel if it is triggered by sufficient temporal correlation in the thalamocortical input.

Excitatory positive feedback of this kind would be epileptogenic if uncontrolled, but, as discussed below, inhibitory feedback within the barrel only allows excitation to act for a short time following the initial excitation (Wilent and Contreras, 2004). Figure 5.4 shows a model for how this circuit might work in a layer IV barrel. The inhibitory cells are driven by thalamic axons (Bruno and Simons, 2002; Swadlow, 2003; Gabernet *et al.*, 2005), which means that the thalamic neurons exert inhibition on the excitatory cells via a disynaptic circuit, thereby limiting their positive feedback (Pinto *et al.*, 2003). Owing to the delay imposed by the extra synapse and the inherently slower kinetics of the GABA channels, the excitatory response out-runs the inhibitory response for a short

A                                                    B

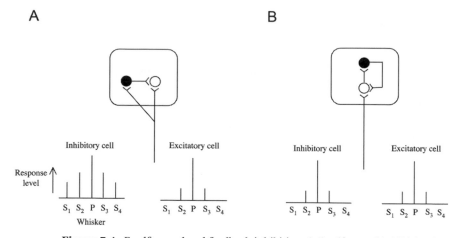

**Figure 5.4.** Feedforward and feedback inhibition. A. Feedforward inhibition is depicted for a layer IV barrel. The thalamocortical input engages both the inhibitory cell (black) and the excitatory cell (white). The inhibitory cell integrates thalamic input in a different way to the excitatory cell and has a larger receptive field (graph lower left) than the excitatory cell. The graphs depict the response magnitude for the cell in response to the principal whisker (central vertical line labeled P) and a number of surround whiskers (labeled $S_1$ to $S_4$). The excitatory cell has a sharper receptive field than the inhibitory cell. B. Feedback inhibition is depicted for an excitatory and inhibitory cell. Because the inhibitory cell receives its receptive field from the excitatory cell, it shares its receptive field properties. This difference in receptive field properties creates a testable theory for receptive field synthesis (Section 5.2.4).

time before disinhibition damps down and abolishes the response. The thalamic input on to the GABAergic cells is more powerful than the input on to the excitatory cells partly because of the fast activation kinetics of their AMPA receptors, which often lack GluR2 subunits, and partly because of the electrotonic location of the synapses near the soma (Cruikshank *et al.*, 2007). This means that the thalamic input requires a higher degree of temporal synchrony to activate the excitatory cells than the inhibitory cells (Bruno and Sakmann, 2006; Cruikshank *et al.*, 2007). If inhibition is decreased by bicuculline, the duration of the excitation is increased (Fox *et al.*, 1996b; Kyriazi *et al.*, 1996b) by widening the time window during which positive feedback can occur.

Following responses in layers IV and Vb, the wave of excitation progresses to layers II/III in the same column, as described in the next section.

### 5.2.2    Vertical transmission within the column

Layer IV cells project profusely to the column directly above the barrel (Feldmeyer *et al.*, 2002). This arrangement tends to ensure that information is initially projected vertically within the column. Extracellular recordings reveal

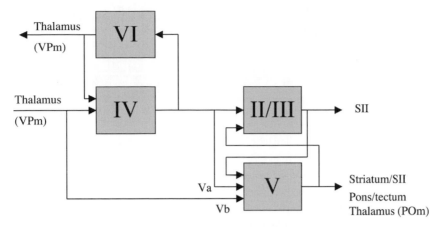

**Figure 5.5.** Simplified cortical microcircuit for a barrel-column illustrating the gateway role of layer IV and the integrative role of layer V. The main input from the ventral posterior medial thalamic nucleus (VPm) is shown as projecting to layer IV and layer Vb. Layer VI creates a short and long feedback loop, the short feedback directly to layer IV and the long loop back to the thalamus. Layer II/III and layer V cells receive input directly from layer IV and create reciprocal feedback loops with one another. Layer V is the main projection layer but layers II/III also projects to other cortical areas.

the sequence of events. Whisker stimulation produces excitation in layer III at an average of 2 ms after excitation in layer IV cells. Excitation in layer II occurs 3.5–4 ms after excitation in layer IV (Armstrong-James *et al.*, 1992). The delay is a combination of the synaptic delay in relay from layer IV to layers II/III and the late production of action potentials on the slowly rising EPSP in layer II/III cells (Wilent and Contreras, 2004). In combination with the layer Vb responses, which occur at almost the same time as those in layer IV, this means that all cells within the column, except those in layers Va and VI, respond to principal whisker stimulation within approximately 4 ms of one another, and before any information is relayed outside the barrel-column. This finding, therefore, supports one of the original tenets of the columnar hypothesis: that information from the sensory periphery is restricted initially within a column (Mountcastle, 1957; Mountcastle *et al.*, 1957).

Layer IV is unique within the cortical layers in sending strong functional excitatory connections to all other layers within the column (Staiger *et al.*, 2000). Layer V is unique within the column in receiving functional excitatory input from all other cortical layers within the column (Staiger *et al.*, 2000). Figure 5.5 shows how the connectivity of layer IV allows this layer to act as the gateway to the whole column and that of layer V places the layer in a position to integrate information from the whole column. However, as described in the next section,

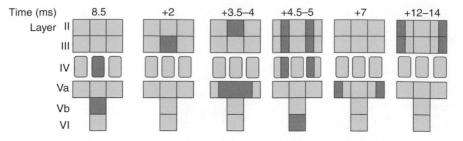

**Figure 5.6.** Flow of excitation within the principal and neighboring barrel-columns. Left to right shows a sequential series of conditions in the principal barrel-column and the immediately surrounding barrels. The dark grey areas define cells that respond at the times shown above each panel. At 8.5 ms after stimulating the principal whisker, cells respond in layers IV and Vb; 2 ms later, cells in layer III respond within the column: 3.5–4 ms later, layer II and layer Va cells respond (the layer Va responses are not confined to the principal barrel); 4.5–5 ms later, cells in layer IV within the column and cells in layers II/III and IV outside the column (near neighbors) respond; finally 12–14 ms later, cells on the far side of the neighboring barrels respond, fully 20 ms after stimulating the principal whisker. (Adapted from Armstrong-James *et al.* [1992].)

there is ample time for information from neighboring barrel-columns to interact between the columnar integration of information and the output of information.

### 5.2.3    *Excitatory transmission between columns*

Beyond the initial wave of vertical transmission, excitation evoked by a brief stimulation of a single whisker is transmitted beyond the boundaries of the barrel (Figure 5.2). The first cells to respond in neighboring barrels are located in layers II/III, IV and V. These cells tend to be closest to the principal barrel and their position is referred to as the nearside of the neighboring barrel (Figure 5.6). The response latency of neurons on the nearside of the barrel occurs approximately 4.5–5 ms after activation of the layer IV principal barrel. In contrast, neurons on the far side of the barrel respond a further 8 ms after that (Figure 5.6). This suggests that there may be direct monosynaptic horizontal projections between the near sides of barrels, but that most projections do not traverse as far as the far side of the immediately neighboring barrel. Although there are some long-range afferents that project further than the near side of the neighboring barrel, their probability of making a connection decreases at greater than the inverse square of distance. Far-side responses, therefore, probably require at least disynaptic connections to transmit excitation beyond the boundaries of the column.

Slice experiments also provide a means of tracing the pathway of intracortical transmission within the cortex. Responses can be seen using voltage-sensitive dyes. Stimulation of the center of a single barrel leads to a similar sequence of activation as seen with whisker stimulation: cells directly superficial to the barrel are first activated within the column, shortly followed by spread into neighboring columns (Laaris and Keller, 2002). The timings of the responses are also similar for lateral spread in a slice, depolarizations tending to occur 3.4 ms after the barrel is directly depolarized, compared with an average action potential latency of 4.5–5 ms after layer IV stimulation for a natural stimulus (Armstrong-James *et al.*, 1992).

A number of anatomical pathways could underlie the horizontal transmission of excitation outside the barrel-column (Chapter 2). Monosynaptic connections are known to exist between layer IV barrel cells and the near side of the neighboring barrel, although they are sparse compared with the same cell's projections within the barrel. Similarly, there are diagonal projections into the neighboring side of the barrel from layer V cells. Potentially diagonal connections could be just as rapid as those from layer IV because layer Vb cells have similar response latencies as layer IV cells (Section 5.2.1). In addition, there are projections from layer II/III cells horizontally into the neighboring barrels. These projections are capable of contacting layer II/III cells and layer IV pyramidal and star pyramidal cells in the neighboring barrel because they project their apical dendrites vertically into layers II/III. Horizontal projections have the greatest reach where they project from layers II/III and V (Bernardo *et al.*, 1990a, b). However some connections are made between layer IV barrel cells across the column. These tend to be connections between pyramidal cells rather than stellate cells (Schubert *et al.*, 2003).

Relay of excitation in the horizontal plane can also be seen using voltage-sensitive dyes in vivo (Petersen *et al.*, 2003). Using this method, it becomes clear that the horizontal spread of excitation travels asymmetrically along the rows and arcs of the barrel field. Approximately 20 ms after stimulation of a single whisker, the area of activated cells extends out to the far side of the barrels in the same row but only to the near side of barrels in different rows (Petersen *et al.*, 2003; Figure 5.2). This effect is presumably a result of asymmetries in the connection densities along rows compared with arcs (Chapter 2).

So far, we have considered the route for intracortical transmission that begins with the column as the source of excitation for cells in surrounding barrels. However, there is at least one further route for transmission, which it is useful to consider as superimposed on the first route. The second major route arises in septal neurons, which we have already noted have extensive horizontal connections around the barrels. Septal cells tend to receive multiwhisker input from the thalamus (Fox *et al.*, 2003). In addition, cells located in layer Va and in layer Vb below the septal regions exhibit multiwhisker responses with latencies that are similar for their principal and surround whiskers (approximately 10–15 ms) and receive a component of their surround receptive field response directly from the thalamus (Section 5.3.1). The septal component of cortical excitation, therefore, arrives marginally after transmission into the near side of the surrounding barrels from the principal barrel but involves a wider area, including the septal areas surrounding the neighboring barrels. It is not known at present how the septal and barrel components of excitation interact. However, given the relatively low connectivity within layer IV between septum and barrel (Bernardo *et al.*, 1990a; Hoeflinger *et al.*, 1995; Feldmeyer *et al.*, 1999), interactions presumably occur via the septal cell connections to extragranular layers.

So far, we have considered the excitatory connections that relay excitation from the principal barrel. At each stage of processing, the excitatory responses are shaped by inhibitory postsynaptic potentials, and this process is described in Sections 5.2.4 and 5.2.5.

### 5.2.4    *Feedforward and feedback inhibition*

Whisker stimulation generates inhibition within the cortex that serves to damp down the excitatory response. Whisker-evoked inhibition is relatively rapid in onset in layer IV cells and, as mentioned above, abolishes the initial EPSP within 5–7 ms of the response onset (Wilent and Contreras, 2004). The observed duration of inhibition varies depending on the method of measurement. Intracellularly, inhibition can be seen as a hyperpolarization occurring immediately following the EPSP and can last for 50–100 ms (Zhu and Connors, 1999; Wilent and Contreras, 2004). The IPSP is often followed by a rebound excitation. Extracellularly, inhibition can be seen if a neuron shows some spontaneous activity (see Figure 5.7) and can last some 20 ms beyond the initial excitation (Simons and Carvell, 1989).

Inhibition is tuned to the same input as the excitatory receptive field, so the principal whisker will always evoke the greatest inhibition and the strongest adjacent whisker the second strongest inhibition and so on (Simons and Carvell, 1989). Barrel cortex shares this property with visual cortex, where IPSPs show the same orientation preferences as the EPSPs (Ferster, 1986). In principle, an identical excitatory and inhibitory receptive field tuning could be achieved by feedback inhibition where the degree of excitatory response determines the degree of feedback inhibition (Figure 5.4). This is the system that operates in the thalamus, where the VPm neurons excite feedback inhibition from reticular neurons; indeed, thalamic reticular nucleus inhibition does curtail thalamic

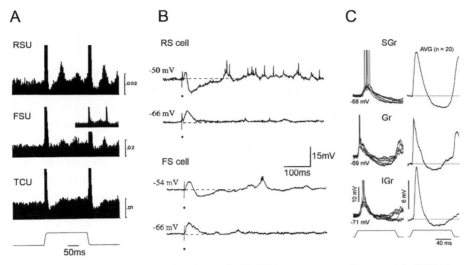

**Figure 5.7.** Whisker stimulus evoked inhibitory postsynaptic potentials (IPSPs) in the barrel cortex. A. Summed poststimulus time histograms for extracellular recordings of spikes from different classes of cell, magnified to show the inhibitory periods as decreases in spontaneous activity. There are two main excitatory responses at the onset and offset of the response. For the regular spike units (RSU) and thalamocortical units (TCU), each is followed by an inhibition. For the fast spiking unit (FSU), the inhibition is less clear. (Reproduced from Simons and Carvell [1989], with kind permission of the American Physiological Society and the authors.) B. Intracellular recordings of RSUs and FSUs at two different potentials reveal the IPSP at –50 mV. (Reproduced from Zhu and Connors [1999], with kind permission of the American Physiological Society and the authors.) C. Excitatory postsynaptic potentials are shown with spikes for supragranular (SGr) granular (Gr, i.e. layer IV) and infragranular (IGr) cells (left); the IPSPs at higher magnification in response to whisker stimulation (right). (Reproduced from Wilent and Contreras [2004], with kind permission of the Society for Neuroscience and the authors.)

excitation to the cortex (Hartings *et al.*, 2000). If a similar system occurs in the cortex, it would suggest that many inhibitory cells would have very similar receptive field properties to the excitatory cells. However, the receptive fields of inhibitory cells have been studied in the barrel cortex in some detail, and their properties differ in a number of important ways from those of the excitatory cells.

Ideally, an inhibitory cell could be distinguished from an excitatory cell by some anatomical method. This is possible when intracellular recordings are made and the cell stained by a marker diffused into the cell from the electrode, such as biocytin. However, it is also possible to distinguish excitatory cells from inhibitory cells extracellularly, on the basis of the duration of their action potentials, which are faster in inhibitory cells than in excitatory cells (Simons, 1978). Using this method of classification, the inhibitory fast-spike units (FSU)

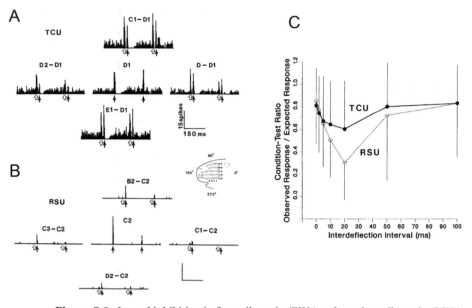

**Figure 5.8.** Lateral inhibition in fast spike units (FSUs) and regular spike units (RSUs). A. Poststimulus time histograms for thalamocortical units (FSUs) are shown for double stimuli involving the principal whisker and a near-neighbor whisker as indicated. The adjacent whisker (in the C, D, or E row) is stimulated first and the principal whisker response can be compared with the single stimulus response to D1 (center). Note that at this interval between stimuli lateral inhibition is not very effective except for D2 stimulation. B. The same type of double stimulation is shown for a RSU and shows much greater lateral inhibition at this interval of the C2 whisker response. C. Timecourse of inhibition in the thalamocortical units (TCU) and RSUs of the cortex. Note that inhibition is stronger in cortex and of similar duration. (Reproduced from Simons and Carvell [1989], with kind permission of the American Physiological Society and the authors.)

have been found to have larger surround receptive fields than the cells with normal spike width (regular spike units [RSU]). Given the difference in receptive field properties of inhibitory and excitatory cells in layer IV, the alternative explanation for the similarity of inhibitory and excitatory tuning is that the excitatory drive for the inhibitory cells comes not from the cortical cells themselves but from the thalamic neurons (Figure 5.4). Therefore, with this theory, the similarity of EPSP and IPSP tuning in an excitatory cell comes from the similarity of tuning of the input to the local excitatory and inhibitory cell population from the thalamus. The receptive fields of the excitatory and inhibitory cells are not identical because the thalamic inputs are summed differently by the RSUs and the FSUs (Figure 5.8).

This model of intracortical inhibition within layer IV is known as feedforward inhibition (Figure 5.4) because the extrinsic thalamic input drives the inhibition rather than the intrinsic cortical cells. There is considerable evidence for the existence of feedforward inhibition. First, inhibitory cells in the cortex receive direct thalamic inputs (White, 1978). Second, monosynaptically connected cortical cells with the characteristic fast spike thought to identify inhibitory neurons have been found by cross-correlation methods (Swadlow, 2003). Third, FSUs can show short-latency responses to whisker stimulation characteristic of monosynaptic thalamocortical input (Swadlow and Gusev, 2002; Wilent and Contreras, 2004). However, note that feedforward and feedback inhibition are not mutually exclusive mechanisms and the two may coexist.

The receptive fields of FSUs in barrels tend to be larger and less directionally selective than those of the RSUs (Simons and Carvell, 1989). If the FSUs project to the RSUs, the effect would be to limit the responses to whisker stimulation after a short delay through the extra synapse in the pathway compared with the monosynaptic excitatory input from the thalamus. If the weight of the transfer function for the inhibitory feedforward inhibition is set up to be greater at low intensities of whisker input than that for the excitatory drive, then the inhibition will tend to limit the receptive fields sizes of excitatory cells (see Figure 5.4) (Kyriazi and Simons, 1993; Pinto et al., 1996). The effect would be to tune the receptive field of the excitatory cells to a smaller number of whiskers and to limit the range of directions that excite the excitatory cells.

### 5.2.5    Lateral inhibition

Lateral inhibition was first described as a process for refining receptive field properties in the somatosensory system as far back as the 1950s (Mountcastle and Powell, 1959). The advantage conferred by lateral inhibition is that the level of acuity that can be achieved in the sensory system is related to the degree of overlap between receptive fields rather than the size of the individual receptive fields at the periphery and lateral inhibition can reduce that overlap. Multiwhisker receptive fields are common in the ascending whisker pathways providing scope for refinement of receptive field overlap. Lateral inhibition can be observed by stimulating a whisker adjacent to the principal whisker and noting the subsequent reduction in response to stimulation of the principal whisker. Lateral inhibition occurs to some degree in each of the nuclei in the ascending pathway from brainstem to cortex, but it tends to be rare in the principalis nucleus of the brainstem and consistently present in VPm (Minnery and Simons, 2003). In VPm, stimulation of an adjacent whisker before the principal whisker produces a reduction in the principal whisker response of about 40%. Lateral inhibition is maximal at approximately 10–20 ms and endures for approximately 100 ms (Figure 5.8) (Simons and Carvell, 1989). As noted above, thalamic inhibition is derived from the reticular nucleus and so this is an example of feedback lateral inhibition.

Lateral inhibition is somewhat greater in the cortex than in the thalamus, suggesting that cortical cells elaborate on the lateral inhibition that they passively acquire from their thalamic input. An adjacent whisker can reduce the principal whisker response an average of 70% if stimulated 20 ms before the principal whisker, though it endures for less time (approximately 50 ms) than does thalamic lateral inhibition.

The effect of lateral inhibition can be seen by trimming the whiskers and recording responses in an awake animal during a standardized whisking task (Kelly *et al.*, 1999). Under these conditions, responses to the principal whisker are increased in layer IV by approximately 20%. This effect is presumably because, during whisking, adjacent whiskers contact the object under interrogation by the animal within a few milliseconds of one another, which sets up a background of inhibition over several whisking cycles. Removing the immediately adjacent whiskers removes their lateral inhibitory effect and causes a net response disinhibition in the principal barrel for the spared whisker.

How is lateral inhibition produced within the cortex? As mentioned above, one possibility is that feedforward inhibitory neurons receive projections from thalamic cells that give them larger receptive fields than the cortical excitatory cells. There are two types of evidence that might support this idea: first, there should be some divergence of functional thalamic input to inhibitory cells over a wide area of cortex and, second, there should be convergence of whisker input on to individual inhibitory cells. Conceptually these are similar types of evidence, but experimentally they are tested in a different manner.

In the rabbit whisker representation, it has been shown that single thalamic neurons project to many inhibitory cortical cells. If a single thalamic cell is recorded over a period of four days, and several putative inhibitory neurons in the cortex are studied sequentially, it can be shown that a single thalamic neuron projects to several such cells (up to nine; Swadlow and Gusev, 2002). Similarly, using the 2-DG method, McCasland *et al.* (1997) have shown that stimulating a single whisker in awake hamsters leads to activation of inhibitory neurons in several barrels, not just those located in the principal barrel. These cells tend to be located at the bottom of the barrels at the interface between layers IV and V. The divergence of information necessary for feedforward lateral inhibition can, therefore, be seen in barrel cortex.

There is also evidence for convergence of whisker input on to inhibitory cells, as mentioned above. Extracellular studies show that FSUs tend to have multiwhisker receptive fields in layer IV (Simons and Carvell, 1989). Intracellular recordings have shown that receptive fields for identified chandelier cells comprise an average of 14 whiskers and those for other inhibitory cell types average 11 whiskers (Zhu *et al.*, 2004). Convergence of thalamic input on to putative inhibitory cells has also been reported for rabbit cortex, where cross-correlation is used to identify monosynaptic links (Swadlow and Gusev, 2002). The convergence of information necessary for feedforward lateral inhibition can also, therefore, be seen in the barrel cortex.

Lateral inhibition does not appear to be isotropic within the cortex or indeed within a receptive field. Cortical neurons show greater lateral inhibition if the neighboring caudal rather than rostral whisker is stimulated, and the ventral whisker is more effective than the dorsal whiskers (Brumberg *et al.*, 1996). Similarly, 2-DG studies show that stimulating the C-row of whiskers labels more glutamic acid decarboxylase-positive cells in dorsal barrel rows (row-B) than ventral (row-D) (McCasland and Hibbard, 1997). The anisotropy of lateral inhibition is thought to arise in the cortex as it is not found in the thalamus. The effect of asymmetrical inhibition is presumably important during active whisking. Inhibition within the row will be greater from the trailing whisker than the leading whisker in a whisker protraction movement and would, therefore, be expected to set up a different pattern of inhibition for several whiskers passing an object during protraction than during retraction. However, the consequences depend on the exact manner in which the whiskers are used, and there are several types of movement as discussed in Chapter 8.

## 5.3    Receptive field organization

### 5.3.1    *Receptive field size*

So far we have considered the effect of a single whisker on many neurons in the barrel cortex; the symmetrical concept is to consider the effect of many whiskers on a single neuron. Defining the subset of whiskers that drive a particular neuron and, in general, the best stimulus properties for driving the cell defines the receptive field for the neuron. Receptive field analysis can give an insight into the type of sensory processing that occurs in the barrel cortex as well as the way cortical circuits are composed (e.g. issues discussed in Section 5.2.4).

However, defining the receptive field is not a trivial exercise. Several factors influence the estimation of receptive field size, including the depth of anesthesia if used, the behavioral state of the animal if no anesthetic is used, the definition of a response, the means of detecting the response and the type of stimulus used. All these factors conspire to make the receptive field an elusive element, and it is useful, therefore, to consider methods of estimating receptive field size before embarking on a description of cortical receptive fields.

Broadly, there are two ways of choosing a stimulus to map the receptive field: by using a constant stimulus and measuring the response as it varies across different receptors, or by choosing a constant response level and measuring the stimulus intensity required to produce it as it varies across different receptors. The advantage of the constant stimulus method is that one can easily compare responses evoked in different cells. The advantage of the constant response method is that it avoids errors in measuring the relative levels of whisker response within a receptive field imposed by action potential threshold and response saturation. However, the former method is used more often. Occasionally, the threshold of the center receptive field response is measured and the stimulus intensity is set at a multiple of the threshold, which combines the advantages of both methods.

It is also known that anesthetic depth affects the receptive field size of thalamic (Friedberg *et al.*, 1999) and cortical (Armstrong-James and George, 1988) cells. Deep anesthesia, such as occurs with barbiturates, produces very small receptive field size estimates, while light anesthesia, such as can be achieved with urethane, produces larger receptive field size estimates. Anesthetic depths can be standardized at a particular level for comparisons by using a particular electroencephalographic state as a reference (Friedberg *et al.*, 1999). Alternatively, where no anesthetic is used, the behavioral state can be standardized by the same method in addition to behavioral metrics. Occasionally, the maximum receptive field size is measured under light anesthesia before deeply anesthetizing the animal to measure the minimum receptive field size (Favorov *et al.*, 1987). This method gives a sense of the center and the surround receptive field components.

Quantitative methods are usually used to measure the response of neurons to stimuli in the somatosensory system. Typically, poststimulus time histogram analysis is used, which allows detection of smaller responses than might be scored using audiovisual estimates of receptive field size (i.e. listening to the spike train on an audio speaker and watching the oscilloscope). This is particularly important for barrel cortex as the cells often produce responses of less than 1 spike/stimulus that are nevertheless accurately time locked to the stimulus.

Table 5.1 shows the various estimates made of receptive field size using these methods. Estimates are in reasonable agreement for cells located in extragranular layers but divergent for cells located in layer IV. This is surprising because whatever factors are likely to affect the receptive fields of layer IV cells might be expected to affect the receptive fields of cells in extragranular layers, to which layer IV projects strongly. Cells in layers II/III and V typically respond to an average of two to six whiskers (Armstrong-James and Fox, 1987), but layer V cells can respond to more than eight. Estimates of receptive field sizes for cells in layer IV range from 1.58 whiskers for RSUs under fentanyl sedation (Simons and Carvell, 1989) to eight for all classes of cell under barbiturate anesthesia (Waite and Taylor, 1978).

Table 5.1. *Variance in estimates of receptive field size for ventral posterior medial thalamic neurons and layer IV neurons in rat barrel cortex; estimates vary depending on anesthetic type, anesthetic depth and method of investigation, but in all cases, receptive fields of more than one whisker are reported and in most cases more than two*

| Average receptive field size | Anesthetic/conditions | Reference |
| --- | --- | --- |
| 1.58 | Regular spiking units; fentynal sedation | Simons and Carvell, 1989 |
| 1.4 | Center receptive field: light urethane | Armstrong-James and Fox, 1987 |
| 4.0 | Center and surround receptive fields | Armstrong-James and Fox, 1987 |
| 2.2 | VPm: halothane stage III-3 | Friedberg et al., 1999 |
| 5 | VPm: halothane stage III-2 | Friedberg et al., 1999 |
| 3.2 | Urethane | Ito, 1985 |
| 8 | Barbituate | Waite and Taylor, 1978 |

VPm, ventral posterior medial thalamic nucleus.

### 5.3.2    Dynamic receptive field analysis

The static count of whiskers included in the receptive field gives a slightly false impression of the cortical circuit unless timing is also taken into account. Although many cells respond to several whiskers, they do so at distinctly different times in almost all cases. Neurons involved in columnar processing respond far more quickly to stimulation of the principal whisker than the surround receptive field whiskers. For example, 40% of layer IV cells respond to principal whiskers within 5–10 ms of stimulation while only 2% respond to neighboring whiskers within the same interval (Armstrong-James and Fox, 1987). Conversely, 73% of layer IV cells respond to principal whisker stimulation before 15 ms, while 70% show their first response to surround whisker stimulation after 15 ms. This has led to the idea of a dynamic receptive field where the early responses can condition responses to input arriving late from surround whiskers (Armstrong-James and Fox, 1987). The same issue was considered in a different guise in Section 5.2 in discussion of intracortical processing. Looked at from the cellular viewpoint rather than the circuit viewpoint, the receptive field appears to evolve in time from a single whisker to several.

### 5.3.3    Cortical and subcortical receptive field components

One of the enduring challenges in this field is to determine the origin of different components of the receptive field. The first-order distinction is to determine the origin of the center receptive field and surround receptive field components. Are surround receptive fields generated intracortically, subcortically or both? The fact that responses to stimulation of surround receptive field whiskers occur at a greater latency than principal whisker responses suggests that surround receptive fields arise from intracortical relay and that relay takes more time the further away the barrel providing the excitatory source. However, it could be argued that surround responses are mixed with similar delays subcortically and then passed on to the cortex, which merely mirrors the responses subcortically.

There are certainly subcortical nuclei that have large multiwhisker receptive fields compared, for example, with cells in layer IV barrels. Among these are the neurons located in the interpolaris nucleus of the trigeminal nuclei and the POm. Interpolaris neurons appear to converge directly (Friedberg *et al.*, 2004) and indirectly via principalis nucleus (Timofeeva *et al.*, 2003) on to thalamic neurons and could be responsible for generating some of the surround receptive field in VPm for relay to the cortex. The POm cells tend to project outside the barrels but could be responsible for surround receptive fields in septum and extragranular layer cells. In addition, convergence from thalamocortical axons could also create surround receptive field components in cortical layer IV.

In order to address this question, Armstrong-James *et al.* (1991) ablated particular barrels in the rat barrel field to see whether this had any effect on the representation of the corresponding whisker in neighboring barrels. It was found that D2 barrel lesions almost completely abolished responses to D2 whisker in barrels surrounding D2 without affecting responses to other whiskers. Other laboratories have repeated this experiment and found similar results for the extragranular layer though a lack of effect for surround receptive fields in layer IV (Goldreich *et al.*, 1999). Using a different technique to achieve the same end, Fox *et al.* (2003) iontophoresed GABA agonists into a single barrel, which resulted in loss of the inactivated barrel's corresponding whisker responses in the neighboring barrels for all layers of cortex including layer IV. The response to the inhibited barrel's whisker returned once the inhibition was removed and this supports the original observation by Armstrong-James *et al.* (1991) made using irreversible lesions (Figure 5.9).

These studies suggest that the surround receptive field is generated intracortically rather than being passed on from a subcortical locus. This implies that individual barrels act like central hubs that disseminate excitation relating to a single whisker within the cortex. If this is true, then individual barrels should only respond to single whisker input from the thalamus, and all other responses would be derived from intracortical relay. This model is supported by experiments in which intracortical transmission is blocked by superfusing the cortex

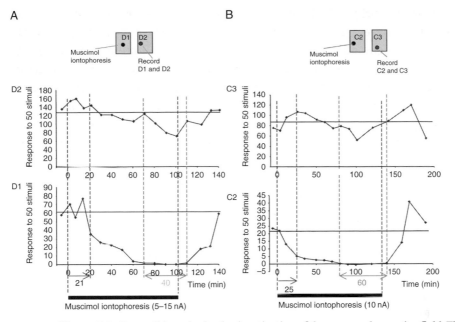

**Figure 5.9.** Reversible and selective inactivation of the surround receptive field. The graphs show the timecourse and effect of muscimol inhibition of the barrel adjacent to the barrel in which the cell is recorded (see insets). The principal whisker response is shown at the top and is relatively unaffected during muscimol application compared with the surround whisker response, which corresponds to the inhibited barrel (bottom). A. Inhibition of the D1 barrel with muscimol released iontophoretically at the time shown by the black bar at the bottom of the graphs affects the D1 whisker response in the D2 barrel. B. Iontophoresis of muscimol in C2 affects the C2 whisker response in C3 barrel. (Reproduced from Fox *et al.* [2003], with kind permission of the Society for Neuroscience.)

with a GABA agonist and local cells within a single barrel are relieved of inhibition locally by iontophoresis of a GABA antagonist. Under these conditions, the layer IV cortical cells exhibit single whisker receptive fields, implying that their surround receptive fields are generated intracortically (Fox *et al.*, 2003). Given that neurons in thalamic nuclei do not have single whisker receptive fields, this means that layer IV neurons must select thalamic input and refine thalamic receptive fields. The mechanisms for selection most likely depends on the sensitivity of those cells to the temporal synchrony of thalamic input (Section 5.2.1). Whether they do this entirely by excitatory mechanisms or whether inhibition is involved is not clear at present, as discussed below.

It has been suggested that inhibitory cells have relatively large receptive fields and by projecting to excitatory cells limit their receptive field size. As discussed above, the evidence in favor of this model comes from recordings made in cortex of the different cell subtypes. The responses of excitatory and inhibitory cells to whisker stimulation can be distinguished on the basis of the duration of their action potentials, which are faster in inhibitory cells than in excitatory cells (Simons, 1978). Using this method of classification, the inhibitory FSUs have larger surround receptive fields than the RSUs and so, provided the one projects to the other, would tend to limit the receptive field size of RSUs.

However, it is not clear at the time of writing that this mechanism is correct. The theory would predict that if the local inhibitory cell was disinhibited the thalamic surround receptive field would be revealed in the cortical cell. However, under conditions where local inhibition is blocked by a locally applied GABA antagonist and intracortically generated surround receptive fields are blocked globally by a GABA agonist, layer IV barrel cells exhibit single whisker receptive fields (Fox *et al.*, 2003). This does not argue completely against the role of local inhibition in restricting layer IV cells receptive field size because intra-cortical transmission is blocked in this experiment. It is possible that horizontal cells could activate local inhibitory cells and thereby generate lateral inhibition. However, it does imply that local inhibition driven by thalamic neurons does not limit the surround receptive field (Figure 5.4) and that excitatory mechanisms are sufficient to select the principal whisker from the surround receptive field. As far as the thalamocortical response transformation is concerned, this stems from the relatively weak input of individual thalamic synapses on to cortical neurons and the need for considerable synchrony and hence temporal summation to drive the excitatory cells (Bruno and Sakmann, 2006; see Section 5.2.1).

### 5.3.4    *Velocity sensitivity*

Neurons in the barrel cortex respond to deflection of the whiskers, but which aspect of the stimulus are they really sensitive to? Is it the amplitude of the displacement or one of the time derivatives of the displacement such as velocity or acceleration? Where these components of the stimulus have been varied independently, it has been found that barrel neurons are sensitive to amplitude and velocity (Wilent and Contreras, 2004). In other words, barrel neurons exhibit responses that increase monotically with amplitude and increasing stimulus velocity (Figure 5.10). This property originates in the primary afferents, which also show monotonic increases in number of spikes per stimulus to both increasing stimulus amplitude and increasing stimulus velocity (Shoykhet *et al.*, 2000). Whether barrel cells respond primarily to amplitude or velocity of the stimulus is not clear. It would seem that the early component of the response (i.e. the first 25–30 ms) is velocity dependent,

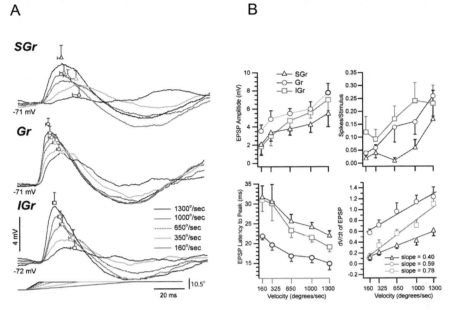

**Figure 5.10.** Sensitivity of barrel cortex neurons to velocity and amplitude. A. Population averages of synaptic responses to a range of whisker velocities in supragranular layer (SGr), granular (Gr) and infragranular (IGr) layers. B. The excitatory postsynaptic potential (EPSP) amplitude increases and latency to peak decreases with increasing velocity. (Reproduced from Wilent and Contreras [2004], with kind permission of the Society for Neuroscience and the authors.)

while amplitude is the most pertinent factor if a period of 600 ms is considered (Ito and Kato, 2002).

### 5.3.5    Directional organization

A small but important subset of the neurons in layer IV of the barrel cortex are sensitive to direction of whisker deflection (Simons and Carvell, 1989). The origin of direction selectivity lies in the organization of the afferents innervating the follicle. Afferents are located around the circumference of the follicle, which means that a specific subset will tend to be stimulated depending on the direction of the vibrissa movement. Approximately 80% of the whisker primary afferents in the trigeminal ganglion show a directional bias. The degree of selectivity varies from cell to cell, but 80% are tuned within 135 degrees and 30% within 45 degrees. Tuning properties differ between SA and RA fibers. The SA afferents show good angular tuning and as a population respond to a variety of directions. The RA afferents are not as directionally selective but, as a population, over-represent the vertical direction. Approximately 35% of cells prefer a vertical upward movement, whereas 9% prefer downwards and 12% prefer horizontal deflections in either direction.

The origin of the difference in SA and RA responses is thought to lie in the location of the receptors in the follicle. The RA receptors are thought to be lanceolate endings located around the follicle. They are all activated to some extent by the stretch of the follicle when the vibrissa moves, all, that is, except those that relax because they lie in the opposite direction to the deflection. The arrangement of RA fibers would be expected to convey some directional information but to respond to many directions to a lesser extent. The SA receptors are thought to be Merkel's discs and are located near the top of the follicle (Section 2.1). They respond to compression, which only occurs for one direction near where the whisker pivots at the top of the follicle (Rice *et al.*, 1986; Lichtenstein *et al.*, 1990). They should, therefore, convey the best directional information.

Most cortical neurons tend to show RA responses and, therefore, the directional SA information tends to be represented less well in the cortex than in the primary afferents. In fact, the proportion of direction-selective cells decreases as information ascends higher up the somatosensory pathway. The number of cells that show strong direction selectivity (within 135 degrees) decreases from 80% in the trigeminal ganglion to only 32% in thalamus and 15% in cortex (Simons and Carvell, 1989). If a less restrictive definition of direction selectivity is applied – the proportion of cells showing at least a 50% greater response to the preferred direction than to the response averaged over all directions – then the proportions of direction-selective cells are rather similar at 28% for thalamic cells and 27% for cortical cells (Bruno and Simons, 2002).

The exact estimate of the proportion of cortical cells selective for direction will depend on the proportion of FSUs and RSUs sampled. Whereas most FSUs are almost completely unresponsive to direction (79% show no bias) many RSUs show some directional bias (38%) (Bruno and Simons, 2002).

The mechanism underlying the direction tuning of the RSUs depends on several factors, and the relative contribution of each factor has not yet been conclusively ascertained. Treatment with bicuculline renders the cortical cell responsive to all directions of whisker stimulation (Kyriazi *et al.*, 1996b) suggesting a role for inhibition. However, cortical direction tuning depends partly on the tuning of the thalamic cells projecting to them, as well as on inhibition within the cortex. The EPSPs are weakly tuned to direction by comparison with the spike output of the RSUs (Figure 5.11). Three factors contribute to the non-linearity that sharpens the spike output to a particular direction. First, the synchrony of the thalamic input is greater for optimal than suboptimal

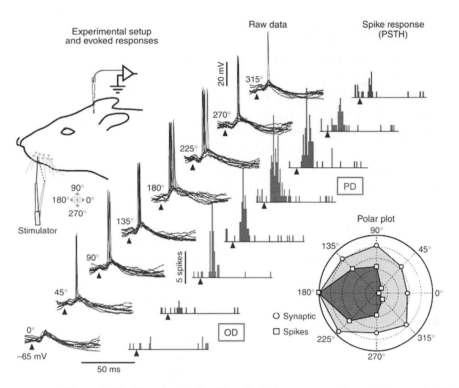

**Figure 5.11.** Directional selectivity of whisker responses in cortical receptive fields. Poststimulus time histograms (PSTHs) are recorded and compared with the intracellular recordings they correspond to for different directions of stimulation (PD, principal direction; OD, orthogonal direction). Note that the excitatory postsynaptic (EPSP) stimuli (raw data) are not tuned as strongly as the PSTHs. The normalized polar plot of the peak EPSP amplitude and the spike count is shown for the case illustrated. (Reproduced from Wilent and Contreras [2005], with kind permission of *Nature* publishing group and the authors.)

directions. It has been shown that direction-selective cells tend to receive input from thalamic cells of similar directional bias and, as described above (Section 5.3.3), synchronous activation is important for driving the thalamic recipient cell in the cortex with relatively weak and sparse thalamic connections (Bruno and Sakmann, 2006). Second, the spike threshold itself will naturally filter out smaller EPSPs and only produce spikes for the larger EPSPs at near the optimal direction. Third, inhibition will act in two ways to affect direction selectivity: (a) inhibition will control the spike threshold and (b) the relative timing, or phase, of the disynaptic IPSP to the monosynaptic EPSP rise time will determine whether a neuron reaches threshold (Wilent and Contreras, 2005). At the optimal direction, excitation is able to overcome the inhibition produced within the cortex, but at directions away from optimal the omnidirectional

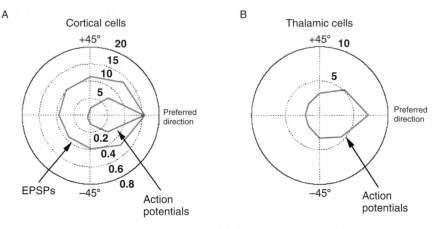

**Figure 5.12.** Directional tuning of thalamic versus cortical neurons. Polar plots illustrating the average normalized direction tuning of thalamic and cortical neurons to different angles of stimulation. Note that the thalamic cells (B) are tuned less than the cortical cells (A) (EPSPs, excitatory postsynaptic potentials). (Adapted from Bruno and Sakmann [2006].)

inhibitory cells (Lee and Simons, 2004) will respond better than the excitatory cells, which will tend to suppress the excitatory responses. Further, at the optimal direction, the shorter latency and faster rise time of the EPSPs are able to overcome the slower disynaptic EPSPs, but the situation is reversed at orthogonal and opposite directions because the EPSPs at these angles have a slower rise time that is slightly later than the IPSP (Wilent and Contreras, 2005). The net effect is that the proportion of cortical cells that do exhibit directional tuning actually recover a higher level of tuning than the average seen in the primary afferents, despite the information having travelled through several relays within which the tuning is worse (Figure 5.12).

### 5.3.6    Multiwhisker integration

How is information from several whiskers integrated in the barrel cortex? So far, we have considered neuronal responses to stimulation of a single whisker, but clearly a rodent uses all or several of its whiskers in combination to explore an object. So what is the effect of stimuli arriving in the barrel cortex from several whiskers? If an object moves across the whiskers, or the whiskers move across an object, the way the cortex processes the information will depend on temporal integration of sequential whisker stimulation and the direction tuning of individual neurons (Section 5.3.5). Both these factors will evoke facilitatory and suppressive effects in different cells in the cortex.

The neurons that are affected most by interwhisker facilitation are located in layers II/III. Deflecting an adjacent whisker approximately 3–5 ms before the principal whisker produces a supralinear summation of the response to the whisker activated second (Shimegi *et al.*, 1999). In other words, the whisker in the surround receptive field can facilitate the principal whisker response to produce a greater response than simply the sum of the individual responses from each whisker.

A response facilitation is shown by approximately 61% of neurons in layers II/III but only 24% in layers V/VI and 10% in layer IV. Neurons that show interwhisker facilitation tend to be located preferentially between two adjacent barrels within a row. The location of the cells is probably related to the need to sum rapidly excitation originating in neighboring columns. Because it takes 4.5–5 ms (on average) for excitation to travel from the principal barrel to the near side of the neighboring barrel-column's layer II/III cells, and only 2–3 ms to propagate within the column, there is only a narrow window for EPSP summation (Section 5.2). This probably explains why average facilitation curves show a half-height width of just 7 ms (Shimegi *et al.*, 1999).

It is possible that interwhisker facilitation is useful for decoding particular directions of stimulus movement across the whiskers. Both order of whisker activation and directional tuning are useful in this regard. Facilitation is sensitive to the order of whisker stimulation for most cortical neurons. Stimulating the rostral whisker of two first may produce facilitation while stimulating the caudal whisker first may not. More than half the neurons in layers II/III that show facilitation to stimulating the whiskers in a particular order also show a directional component (57%) (Shimegi *et al.*, 2000). The direction tuning and sequence preference often complement one another. Figure 5.13 shows an example where facilitation only occurs if the stimulus is swept in the caudal direction and the rostral whisker is deflected before the caudal whisker; both factors would serve to emphasize a stimulus moving from rostral to caudal across the whisker pad.

Interwhisker suppression also affects integration within the cortex, as discussed in Section 5.2.5, but it has mainly been studied in layer IV barrel locations where facilitation is rarely observed. Lateral inhibition occurs much later than interwhisker facilitation, which explains why it does not prevent it from occurring. While facilitation occurs for whisker stimuli paired up to 3 ms apart, lateral inhibition is maximal for intervals of 20 ms. Like facilitation, inhibition is also directionally tuned for many cells (Simons and Carvell, 1989). Using the same metric as above for direction tuning, 33% of RSUs will be inhibited by an adjacent whisker with a tuning of 135 degrees or less. The question arises of how lateral inhibition can be produced given that we have so far emphasized the lack

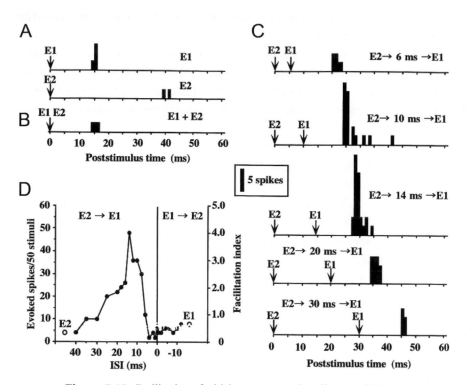

**Figure 5.13.** Facilitation of whisker responses by adjacent whiskers. Poststimulus time histograms are shown for stimulating whiskers alone (A), together at the same time (B) or in combination at various short intervals (C). Note the facilitation of the response when E2 stimulation precedes E1 whisker stimulation. D. Graphical representation of the response versus the interstimulus interval (ISI) for the example shown in A–C. (Reproduced from Shimegi *et al.* [1999], with kind permission of the Society for Neuroscience and the authors.)

of direction tuning in the inhibitory cell population. Broadly, there are two solutions involving inhibition: either the omnidirectional inhibitory cells are engaged by directionally tuned excitatory cells, or a separate population of directionally tuned inhibitory cells are involved. In favor of the hypothesis that a separate population of inhibitory cells is involved, approximately 21% of the FSUs studied in the cortex do show some directional selectivity (Bruno and Simons, 2002). In either case, the tuned excitation for the neighboring whisker must come from cortical rather than thalamic cells because the thalamic cells are less well tuned (Figure 5.12). The best tuned inhibitory or excitatory cells have relatively low levels of thalamic input, as assessed by spike-triggered averaging of cortical responses (Bruno and Simons, 2002). Given that the tuned cells are tuned to the adjacent not the principal whisker, the excitatory drive for direction-selective lateral inhibition is most likely to come from the neighboring barrel-column.

The third possibility is that suppression is a withdrawal of excitation (Higley and Contreras, 2003). This is not inconsistent with the inhibitory mechanisms described above provided that the inhibition acts on excitatory interneurons and causes them to decrease excitatory drive in response to stimulation of the adjacent whiskers.

In conclusion, receptive field analysis shows that rather specific information from different whiskers is integrated using facilitation, inhibition, velocity, directionality and whisker sequence in different combinations in different cells. One of the challenges for the future will be to determine how these elementary properties might be used as feature detectors. In addition, it will be important to relate them to their use in active touch, which is the topic of the next and final section on sensory processing.

## 5.4 Dynamic sensory processing

In the preceding sections, we have considered the passive response of the barrel cortex to touch. We now consider the modification of these basic circuit properties during active tactile exploration. Briefly, exploration involves three factors: moving the whiskers back and forward rhythmically, moving the head and generally adjusting posture accordingly, and moving the whole body through the environment. Because all three factors affect whisker position during exploration, determining the location of an object contacted by the whiskers requires a complex integration of information from tactile, proprioceptive and vestibular sources. However, if we simplify the problem for the moment to one of where the object is located relative to the head, the main question becomes where is the object relative to the whiskers? We can simplify the question further if we restrict our analysis to a single forward and backward whisking movement: that is, a whisk cycle. Under this scheme, where the object is located corresponds to when the object is contacted during the whisk cycle.

There are two basic forms of whisking pattern. One form is known as twitching, which is low amplitude 7–11 Hz movements and can be related to a synchronized electroencephalographic trace. The other form is the better known whisking movement referred to above, which involves whisker movements of larger amplitude but similar frequency to twitching; this can also vary in amplitude in a slow cycle of 1 Hz or so. The latter is associated with exploratory behavior.

There appear to be several advantages to moving the whiskers actively. First, the receptors in the follicle transmit information from RA receptors, which would be activated more strongly by rapid onset of the stimulus. Second, VPm neurons are activated more synchronously by rapid velocity whisker displacements and, as we have discussed, this is important for activating cortical layer IV cells. When the animal is whisking, the velocity of whisker deflection can be controlled to optimize this parameter, and there is evidence that the whisk velocity is appropriate to the preferred range for synchronous VPm activation (Pinto *et al.*, 2000). Third, and rather obviously, the animal samples a greater volume of space by moving its whiskers and, therefore, has a better chance of encountering the object. Finally, whisking ensures that the stimulus is repeated several times. Repeating the stimulus is known to improve discrimination for humans in tactile tasks (Sinclair and Burton, 1991).

Does whisking demonstrably help the animal to sense an object? There is certainly evidence that when rats were asked to distinguish between a rough and a smooth surface the ones better able to perform the task whisked more in the 7–12 Hz range (Carvell and Simons, 1995). It is possible, then, that the rate at which the whiskers interact with the object optimizes repetitive timing within the vibrissae system. There is also evidence that two whiskers are better than one in discriminating between two very similar rough surfaces (Carvell and Simons, 1995). This suggests that low spatial frequency discrimination requires multiwhisker integration. Finally, rats trained to detect differences in horizontal position using their whiskers can perform the task at higher resolution ($< 1.5$ mm) than the spacing between the whiskers at contact (approximately 4.8 mm), but only if they are able to whisk (Knutsen *et al.*, 2006). Paralysis of the whisker pad leads to performance at chance levels.

Given that whisking is an advantage for the animal, it comes at a price, which is that decoding spatial information requires decoding temporal information. The animal has to know where its whisker is relative to the whisk cycle in order to interpret where the object is located. The effect of whisking on the temporal properties of neurons in the barrel cortex is considered in the following section, together with a possible scheme for decoding position from timing.

### 5.4.1    *Whisking and active touch*

So far we have mainly considered the response of the barrel cortex to a discrete deflection of one or two whiskers. However, rodents usually use their whiskers by rhythmically moving them back and forth at whisking frequencies of 5–15 Hz. Whisking imposes a cyclic timing pattern on processing within the barrel cortex, with a set period between repetitions of the same stimulus. For a mid-range whisking frequency of approximately 10 Hz, the period would be 100 ms. As we have seen above, many of the responses of cortical cells to individual whisker stimulation and the radiation of excitation into neighboring

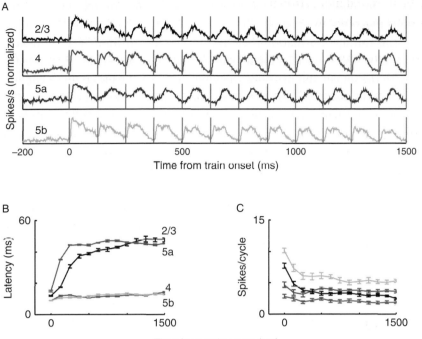

**Figure 5.14.** Phase sensitivity of neurons to repeated whisk-cycle stimuli. A. Average responses to 8 Hz whisker stimulation from each layer. Stimuli were air puffs aimed at moving several whiskers in synchrony (vertical lines indicate the stimulus onset). B. Evolution of response latency during the stimulus train. C. Change in spikes per stimulus during the stimulus train (bars indicate standard errors). (From Ahissar *et al.* [2001], with kind permission of the American Physiological Society and the authors.)

cortical columns last only about 20–50 ms at most, which means that the excitatory responses alone are unlikely to interact purely as a consequence of the stimulus repetition. However, other factors come into play, including longer loop feedback pathways to the thalamus and brainstem from the cortex (Section 5.4.2), local cortical inhibition, which can last for up to 100 ms (Section 5.2.4), and synaptic dynamics of individual excitatory pathways within the cortex. The result is that responses to, stimulation evolve to a steady state over several whisking cycles for some cells in the barrel cortex. Figure 5.14 shows an example of responses of cells in four layers of cortex to a number of whisking cycles. The responses at layer IV and Vb cells are relatively stable from the start to the end of the cycles, whereas the cells in layers II/III and Va begin at shorter latencies, similar to those seen in response to single stimuli, and rapidly evolve into responses of longer duration and longer latency (Ahissar *et al.*, 2001).

For example, layer II/III responses increase in latency by approximately 40 ms over four or five whisking cycles.

How is this timing information used to compute the position of the whiskers relative to the object? One idea is that the system must have cells that code for contact with the object and phase of the whisk cycle. Let us take these each in turn. First, cells in the trigeminal ganglion code for contact during whisking. The RA receptors are sensitive to initial contact and detachment of whiskers from an object surface, while the SA receptors are sensitive to the pressure that can occur during sustained contact. Therefore, the passive properties of "on," "off" and "sustained" response described in Section 5.3.5 correspond, respectively, to the active properties of "contact," "detachment" and "pressure" during a whisk cycle. Of these, the RA responses are relayed to the cortex more effectively. Second, 50% of SA and RA primary afferents respond to whisking (Zucker and Welker, 1969; Szwed et al., 2003), which results in a proportion of trigeminal nucleus neurons firing in phase with the whisk cycle (Nicolelis et al., 1995). This information is also relayed to the cortex. The electromyograph trace for the whisker pad, which correlates well with whisker position, is correlated with spiking of cells in barrel cortex (Fee et al., 1997). The fact that it is possible to predict the whisker pad electromyograph from the cortical spike train over a period of a whisk cycle serves to illustrate how good the correlation is between the two. During whisking without contacting an object, cortical cells tend to fire during the protraction phase and their firing is more highly correlated during large-amplitude whisk cycles. Overall, most phases of the whisk cycle are represented by one or other cortical cells (Fee et al., 1997) with approximately 50% of the cortical neurons showing at least 2% modulation of their firing rate within the whisk cycle (for review see Kleinfeld et al. [2006]).

What is the effect of superimposing the response from contact with an object on to the firing pattern of the cortical cell? For any given cell, contact will produce a change in the relative phase of spiking, which would otherwise be at the steady-state level determined by the whisking pattern (Figure 5.14). Given that cells tend to fire across the range of phases of the whisk cycle, different phase changes will occur for each cell. In principle, the location of the object is then computed from the difference in time (or phase) between the in-phase firing and the object-contact firing. The means by which this type of signal can be decoded to produce a picture of where the object is located is the subject of a good deal of research and has not been resolved at the time of writing. Broadly, this type of signal can be decoded in two ways. In one scheme, the reference signal modulates the sensitivity of the cortical neurons to the contact signal. Contact is registered as a facilitation of the response of a subset of neurons. In the second scheme, the reference and contact signals combine so that they produce a minimal response in the cell when they occur at the same time and a response that is proportional to the difference in phase (viz. timing) at phases away from this null point (Kleinfeld *et al.*, 1999).

There is some evidence that the latter system occurs in barrel cortex. The latency of many cell responses in layers II/III and Va change with whisk frequency. For example, a layer Va cell with a latency of 15 ms at 2 Hz will change to one closer to 60 ms at 11 Hz and behave in a relatively linear fashion at frequencies between these (Ahissar *et al.*, 2001). This has led to the idea that some components of the vibrissae system act like a phase-locked loop (Ahissar *et al.*, 2000). A phase-locked loop is a device used to decode frequency-modulated information in conventional radios. It works by having a phase comparator, which keeps the phase relationship between the input and output constant for a constant frequency. Any change in the frequency alters the phase angle proportionally. For a rodent whisking at a constant frequency, the phase angle would be constant until the whiskers came into contact with an object. Touching an object would introduce extra frequency components, which would be represented by changes in relative phase (or latency) of the response. The anatomical basis of such a system is explored in the next section. At present, this idea is formative and requires more evidence to substantiate it. For example, it is not clear where the phase comparator part of the circuit would be located. Further, there would presumably be many phase comparators given that different cells tend to fire at many phases of the whisk cycle. However, one key aspect, that frequency is proportional to latency, does hold for several cell populations in the cortex (Ahissar *et al.*, 2000, 2001) and one would imagine this unusual property is used somehow by the system.

### 5.4.2    *Cortical feedback*

Feedback loops become particularly important for information processing when the process is cyclical, as it is during whisking. If the feedback is rapid enough and long lasting enough it will affect processing during the second and subsequent phases of the cycle. There are two types of cortical feedback loop to consider in this context. One is the anatomical feedback loop created by pathways that send projections back to their source of afference. One such anatomical loop is made by the cortical back projections to the interpolaris nucleus of the trigeminal nucleus, which of course sends forward projections to the thalamus and hence to the cortex. The other type of feedback loop is formed if the whiskers are included as an element in the feedback pathway. The whiskers can be considered as an active part of the loop when the animal whisks, because the neuronal signal that drives the mechanical movement of the whiskers thereby also drives the sensory receptors from which it receives input (Figure 5.15B).

A

B

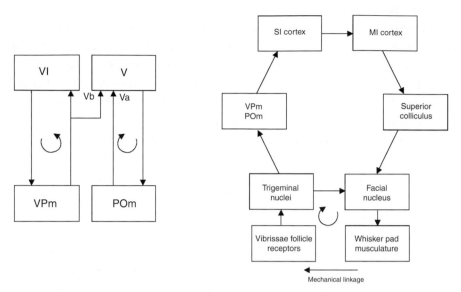

**Figure 5.15.** Sensory and sensory–motor feedback loops. A. Sensory feedback loops are made between barrel cortex and somatosensory thalamic nuclei. Cortical layer VI forms reciprocal excitatory connections with the ventral posterior medial thalamic nucleus (VPm) while layer V cells project to the posterior medial thalamic nucleus (POm). B. Two sensory–motor loops are illustrated: a short loop involving the trigeminal nucleus and the facial nucleus and a longer loop involving somatosensory area I (SI) (barrel cortex) and motor cortex area I (MI).

Before considering this sensory motor loop, we first explore the effect of the sensory feedback loops within the whisker–barrel pathway.

### 5.4.2.1   Sensory loops

Cortical feedback to subcortical sensory nuclei is derived from layer V and VI cells. Feedback to VPm comes from cells located in layer VI while feedback to POm comes from cells in layer V (Hoogland *et al.*, 1987; Figure 5.15). The feedback to VPm is a relatively minor component of the excitatory drive to this nucleus compared with the effectiveness of excitatory drive delivered to POm from the cortex. The functional consequences of cortical feedback have been assessed by experiments where cortical neurons have been inhibited while recording responses in the thalamus. Cortical inhibition practically abolishes responses in POm whereas it has relatively little effect on VPm (Diamond *et al.*, 1992b; Wallace *et al.*, 2001). One study has reported that inhibition of cortex decreased long-latency components of whisker responses in VPm (Ghazanfar *et al.*, 2001). The longer latency response was observed at a latency centered around 30 ms and was abolished by inhibition of the cortex, suggesting that the cortex is the source of the late response.

In contrast to the small effect of thalamic feedback on VPm responses, the entire response to whisker stimulation in POm can be abolished by blocking cortical activity (Diamond *et al.*, 1992b). Feedback to POm is derived from cortical layer V cells. As mentioned in Section 5.4.1, a subset of layer V cells in layer Va show a frequency-dependent phase shift characteristic of a phase-locked loop system (Ahissar *et al.*, 2001). Furthermore, POm neurons preferentially project to layer Va cells within the cortex. In concert with these findings, POm neurons also show frequency-dependent phase shifts similar to layer Va cells. It is likely that this behavior arises from a local thalamocortical loop rather than a loop including brainstem nuclei because neither the principalis nucleus nor the interpolaris nucleus of the trigeminal nuclei show frequency-dependent phase shifts (Ahissar *et al.*, 2000).

Cortical layer V neurons also make one other sensory loop where they project back to neurons of the interpolaris nucleus (Jacquin *et al.*, 1990). These neurons characteristically show larger receptive fields than cells in the principalis nucleus and it is conceivable that part of the reason for this is feedback from cortical layer V cells, which have large receptive fields themselves, although studies to date are inconclusive on this subject (Jacquin *et al.*, 1990).

### 5.4.2.2    Sensory–motor loops

The second class of feedback loop we need to consider is the sensory–motor loop that is formed during whisking, where the motor pathways are driven to stimulate the sensory receptors in the follicles. There are a large number of these loops: too many to detail here (for reviews see Kleinfeld *et al.* [1999, 2006]). Instead, we will consider two sensory–motor loops, one that might be considered as a low level loop, involving brainstem nuclei, and the other, which we might consider a long loop, that includes the cortex. First, one low level or short loop is formed by the projections from the trigeminal nuclei to the facial motor nucleus of the brainstem (Figure 5.15B). The facial motor nucleus, or at least its lateral subnucleus, provides the motor afferents that drive the musculature of the whisker pad and thereby control whisking. The facial nucleus mainly receives sensory input from the interpolaris and caudalis subdivisions of the trigeminal nuclei. One might assume from their anatomical location that this loop is intimately involved with controlling the basic mechanical parameters of the whisk cycle. Unlike many muscles, muscles in the whisker pad do not contain muscle spindles, presumably because the forces under control are too small to demand them. However, this does mean that the only feedback to the motor system about where the whiskers are located within the whisk cycle comes from the tactile sensory receptors, and this information is relayed to the facial nucleus from the trigeminal nucleus. The sensory feedback pathway is not necessary for whisking, however. Animals with sensory nerve block are able to whisk (Welker, 1964) and so the importance of these short-loop pathways remain to be determined.

As an example of a longer loop system, there is one formed by projections to the cortex from the ascending lemniscal system (trigeminal nuclei and thalamic nuclei) and descending projections from the barrel cortex and motor cortex to the superior colliculus, which then projects to the facial motor nucleus (Figure 5.15B). It is known that the very cells that project from the superior colliculus to the facial nucleus receive input from the vibrissae component of the motor cortex (Kleinfeld *et al.*, 1999). The role of barrel cortex in control of this pathway comes not from its role in producing the whisk cycle itself, although it has been shown that stimulating motor cortex can initiate a whisk cycle (Brecht *et al.*, 2004). Rather the barrel cortex seems to be involved in controlling the amplitude of the whisk cycle. Unilateral lesion of the barrel cortex results in bilateral whisking that is asymmetrical in amplitude (Harvey *et al.*, 2001). Normally, the whiskers move in phase and show a gradual increase and then a decrease in their amplitude during an exploratory whisking episode at a low frequency of approximately 0.1–1 Hz (Fee *et al.*, 1997; Kleinfeld *et al.*, 1999; Harvey *et al.*, 2001). The fact that the barrel cortex is necessary for this modulation suggests that it modulates the whisk cycle in concert with the motor cortex via the control it exerts on the superior colliculus. The slow-amplitude modulations are known to be important for sensory responses in the barrel cortex. Neurons in barrel cortex tend to fire preferentially during the larger amplitude components of the whisk and on the protraction phase (Fee *et al.*, 1997), presumably owing to the velocity sensitivity of the cortical responses and the greater whisker velocity during the larger amplitude component of the overall whisking episode.

One might ask what the purpose of modulating the whisk cycle could be? One possibility is related to the fact that it takes several cycles to stabilize the frequency-dependent phase system described above for POm and layer Va cells (Figure 5.14). Therefore, the early few whisk cycles, which are low amplitude, may only be intended to set up and stabilize the phase lock rather than to investigate objects. Once the phase lock is stable, the animal increases the amplitude of the whisk cycle to try and contact objects and hence locate them in space.

## 5.5    Conclusions

The barrel cortex processes sensory information through sensory channels that are kept relatively, though not entirely, separate at the level of layer IV but then merge in extragranular layers to integrate information from neighboring whiskers. Integration involves facilitation of correlated information over a period of a few milliseconds and suppression over periods of tens of milliseconds. A great deal of effort is expended in the way the cortical circuit is constructed to make sure that the relative timing of information from each whisker is preserved at a cortical level. In particular, it is noteworthy that layer IV cells will fire better to strongly correlated thalamocortical input and that the positive feedback within layer IV produces a highly synchronized output only if there is a highly synchronized input.

Timing of inputs is critical to the performance of the barrel cortex because the time at which an input occurs signals where the object is located within the whisk cycle. During active exploration, the whiskers are made to scan an object so that the same stimulus features are played through parallel sensory channels sequentially. The process can be repeated on several whisk cycles, which presumably helps in the interpretation of the sensory information.

One of the challenges for the future will be to determine how the relative phase of response to contact with the object is related to a knowledge of where the whisker is within the whisk cycle. There are a number of intriguing studies into whether the phase-locked loop can decode this information. Another challenge will be to determine how information being processed by the barrel cortex is read by other areas to which it projects. For example, how do SII, MI, pons and striatum use the output from the SI cortical neurons? It is likely that the same features of the barrel system that have made it useful for studying primary cortical processing will also be useful for studying the outputs of the system, in particular the ability to trace outputs corresponding to individual whiskers in a topographic form from one area to another.

Finally, passive touch methods are being used to understand how information between neighboring whiskers is integrated. Future studies will need to discover how multiwhisker information is used during active touch. In particular, how are the multiplicity of properties exhibited by single cells such as facilitation, suppression, directionality and sequence sensitivity used to advantage in active touch?

# 6

## Synaptic plasticity of barrel cortex

Chapters 6 and 7 describe the mechanisms underlying induction and expression of plasticity in the barrel cortex. In using the term plasticity, synaptic plasticity is meant implicitly, including not only the second-to-second changes that ensue during in vitro forms of plasticity such as LTP and long-term depression (LTD) but also the growth of pre- and postsynaptic elements of the synapse that occur over longer time scales. This chapter deals with the cellular evidence on the nature of synaptic plasticity mechanisms, while Chapter 7 deals with the systems level evidence for plasticity induced in the whole animal. The extent to which all plasticity mechanisms in the cortex are underpinned by synaptic plasticity is, of course, a subject of much debate and an issue we take up in the following pages.

Historically, synaptic plasticity has been studied extensively in hippocampus, visual cortex and barrel cortex. In some respects, plasticity studies in barrel cortex have caught up with those parallel investigations in the visual system and in some areas overtaken them. There are a number of reasons why this has happened, including the ease of manipulation of the peripheral receptors in the whisker system, the introduction of transgenics and knockouts in rodents and the invention of the thalamocortical slice preparation (Agmon and Connors, 1991). Although synaptic plasticity is not as well understood in the barrel cortex as in the hippocampus, even at this early stage it is clear that some differences exist between the two systems. This makes it important to study neocortical plasticity in its own right rather than to expect hippocampal mechanisms to be duplicated in neocortex. Conversely, the insights gained into plasticity mechanisms in the barrel cortex are likely to inform the field at large on general principles of neocortical plasticity and may show commonalities with plasticity mechanisms in the visual cortex. In the following sections we begin by comparing LTP and LTD in barrel cortex with LTP and LTD in other cortical areas.

## 6.1    Long-term potentiation

### 6.1.1    *Historical context and significance*

Long-term potentiation was discovered in the hippocampus in the late 1960s and reported in the early 1970s (Bliss and Lomo, 1970, 1973), but it was not confirmed as a synaptic mechanism in the neocortex for almost a further 20 years (Artola and Singer, 1987). The delay can partly be attributed to two technical issues that make LTP more difficult to study in the neocortex compared with the hippocampus. First, the lack of simple geometric alignment of most pyramidal cells in the neocortex reduces spatial summation of EPSPs. Although the cortex contains layers of cells, the pyramidal cell bodies are not closely aligned in the same plane as they are in the hippocampus (Chapter 2). The misalignment of cell bodies and dendrites results in less spatial summation of dendritic field potentials in the neocortex and makes the field potentials relatively small and difficult to interpret (Figure 6.1D,E). Second, the fact that axonal pathways are generally aligned parallel with the main dendritic axis, principally a result of the columnar arrangement of many cortical pathways, makes it difficult to stimulate axonal inputs to cells without producing antidromic activation at the same time. Both technical problems can be overcome by intracellular recording and by stimulating horizontal or off-axis pathways (Figure 6.1).

By using intracellular recording, first in the visual cortex (Artola and Singer, 1987) and then in the somatosensory cortex (Bindman *et al.*, 1988), experimenters were able to observe long-lasting increases in excitatory transmission following short periods of tetanic stimulation. A variety of methods can be used to induce LTP, including 100 Hz stimulation delivered in a single train or in packets of four stimuli per burst repeated at 5 Hz (theta-burst stimulation), or by pairing pre- and postsynaptic spikes (Figure 6.1). In individual cases, EPSP amplitude can increase by two- to four-fold following induction, but a relatively low probability of LTP induction (approximately 35% in adults) reduces the average level of increase to 20% (Hardingham *et al.*, 2007).

Early studies reported that induction of LTP in neocortex required special conditions such as low magnesium (Lee *et al.*, 1991) or inhibition of GABAergic pathways (Artola and Singer, 1987) for reliable induction of LTP. The need for concurrent disinhibition during induction of LTP may be a consequence of the pathway stimulated. Stimulation of the white matter can evoke indirect

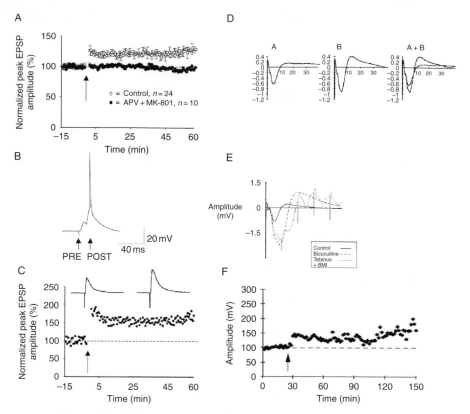

**Figure 6.1.** Different methods of inducing long-term potentiation (LTP) in layers II/III of the rodent barrel cortex. A. Spike pairing-induced LTP. Average LTP levels for excitatory postsynaptic potentials (EPSPs) evoked in layers II/III by stimulating layer IV in the side wall of the barrel. The layers II/III cells are recorded on the near side of the neighboring barrel-column and LTP is blocked by applying NMDA receptor antagonists (black circles). B. In this pathway, LTP is induced by timing a postsynaptic spike (POST) to occur 10 ms after a presynaptic stimulus (PRE). C. An example of LTP in an individual layer II/III cell. The inset waveforms are 10 min average EPSPs for baseline (left) and 50–60 min after pairing (right). (Adapted from Hardingham and Fox [2006] with permission of the Society for Neuroscience.) D. Extracellular field potentials before (A) and after (B) inducing LTP in layers II/III of rat barrel cortex with theta-burst stimulation in vivo. E. The effect of a single theta burst (four stimuli delivered at 100 Hz) on extracellular field potentials in the presence of bicuculline methiodide (BMI) to inhibit GABAergic transmission (tetanus + BMI). F. Increase in the peak amplitude of the field potential in rat barrel cortex in vivo following theta-burst stimulation at the point indicated by the arrow. The stimulation site was located in the layer IV septum and the recording site directly superficial to it in layer II/III. (Adapted from Glazewski *et al.* [1998a] with permission of Elsevier.)

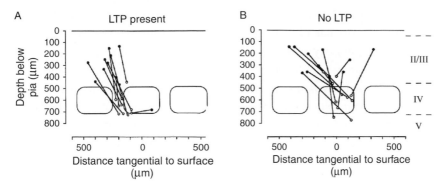

**Figure 6.2.** Optimal sites for inducing long-term potentiation (LTP) in rat barrel cortex. The stimulation sites are indicated by open circles and recording sites with solid circles and the pair of sites connected with a line. A. LTP is successfully induced in layers II/III of the near-side barrel-column if the stimulation site is in the septum or barrel wall of layer IV. B. LTP was induced less frequently, if at all, from sites located in the barrel, or in the wall of the barrel on the opposite side to the recording site (far-neighbor). (Adapted from Glazewski *et al.* [1998a] with permission of Elsevier.)

depolarization in layer II/III neurons via layer IV. Because excitation in layer IV is strongly controlled by inhibition (Chapter 3), it is difficult to transmit the higher frequency tetanic signals necessary for induction of LTP through layer IV to layers II/III (Rozas *et al.*, 2001). The problem is overcome by stimulating layer IV directly in order to activate layer II/III cells (Castro-Alamancos *et al.*, 1995). In the barrel cortex, the edges of the barrels provide the best sites for inducing LTP in layers II/III (Glazewski *et al.*, 1998a) (Figure 6.2). Alternatively, in order to study LTP in layer IV, it is preferable to use low-frequency stimuli coupled with direct depolarization of the postsynaptic cell (Crair and Malenka, 1995).

The significance of LTP in the barrel cortex is two-fold. First, experience-dependent and lesion-induced plasticity has been demonstrated in developing and adult barrel cortex, and one of the major hypotheses for how it is generated depends on the existence of synaptic plasticity in the excitatory connections of the barrel cortex circuitry. Other theories on how experience-dependent plasticity might work include changes in the inhibitory circuitry (Hensch *et al.*, 1998a) and growth of new pathways (Trachtenberg *et al.*, 2002). These are not mutually exclusive with, but rather compatible with, the mechanism of potentiation at excitatory pathways. Second, if barrel cortex can provide a model system for how columnar circuits operate in the cortex in general, then understanding LTP in the neocortex could help to explain the mechanisms underlying long-term memory formation. Long-term memory, lasting weeks and years, is thought to depend on neocortical plasticity (Lavenex and Amaral, 2000; Frankland *et al.*, 2004) and this suggests some specialization in cortical synaptic plasticity mechanisms compared with the shorter-term memory systems involved in hippocampal function. Barrel cortex has also been implicated in working memory during somatosensory tasks (Harris *et al.*, 2002), which operates over a shorter timescale than long-term or remote memory. It is conceivable that more than one type of synaptic mechanism is present in barrel cortex. In this chapter, we are primarily concerned with the role of synaptic plasticity in developmental and experience-dependent forms of barrel cortex plasticity as they have been studied most to date. Specifically, the following sections address developmental plasticity in the thalamocortical synapse on to layer IV cells and adult plasticity at intracortical inputs to layer II/III cells.

### 6.1.2    *Long-term potentiation at the thalamocortical synapse*

Plasticity is greatest in layer IV during development of the barrels (Chapter 4). The barrels show a critical period for both lesion-induced plasticity (Van der Loos and Woolsey, 1973) and experience-dependent plasticity (Fox, 1992), corresponding to barrel formation between P0 and P4. The thalamocortical slice preparation (Agmon and Connors, 1991) can be used to study plasticity of the thalamocortical inputs to the developing layer IV barrels during this period, and indeed it was found that thalamocortical synapses show a distinct critical period – the first postnatal week – for long-term synaptic plasticity (Crair and Malenka, 1995), roughly similar in timecourse to the macroscopic critical periods for sensory deprivation (see Fox [1995]). In the thalamocortical synapse, LTD can be induced by low-frequency pairing of presynaptic stimulation of the axons where they arise in the thalamus with postsynaptic depolarization of the postsynaptic layer IV cells to approximately 0 mV (Crair and Malenka, 1995). The probability of inducing LTP and the magnitude of the LTP induced both decrease between P3 and P7 in rat barrel cortex (Figure 6.3).

The mechanism underlying induction of LTP at the developing thalamocortical synapse appears to be insertion of AMPA receptors into the postsynaptic membrane. The first clue that this might be the case came from the observation that LTP causes unsilencing of silent synapses at the developing thalamocortical synapses (Isaac *et al.*, 1997), a process that requires NMDA receptor activation and BDNF (Itami *et al.*, 2003). Given that inducing LTP can convert silent synapses into active synapses in the barrel cortex (Isaac *et al.*, 1997; Lu *et al.*, 2003) and that unsilencing silent synapses is accomplished by insertion of AMPA channels into the postsynaptic membrane in the hippocampus (Malinow, 2003), this suggests that thalamocortical LTP during development involves insertion of AMPA receptors at a synapse that initially contains just NMDA receptors.

Contemporaneous with the increase in AMPA receptor function at thalamocortical synapses is a second process of kainate receptor decrease, which, while

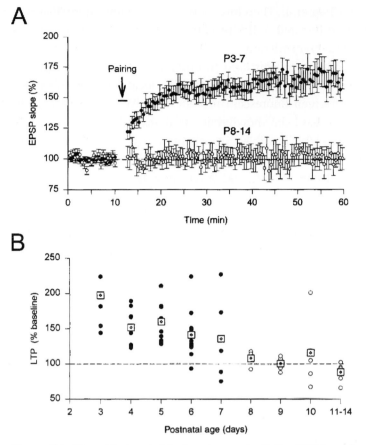

**Figure 6.3.** The critical period for long-term potentiation (LTP) in rat barrel cortex. A. LTP is induced in layer IV cells at postnatal days three to seven (P3–7) by stimulation of the thalamocortical afferents at 1 Hz while the postsynaptic cell is paired with depolarization (−10 to 0 mV; $n = 43$). The same protocol does not induce LTP at postnatal days 8–14 (P8–14) ($n = 20$). B. Individual cases (black circles) and average levels (squares) of LTP as a function of postnatal age. Note that LTP decreases to zero by eight days of age. (Reproduced from Crair and Malenka [1995] with kind permission of the authors and the *Nature* Publishing Group.)

not strictly an LTP process, helps to explain the development of early connections in this system. Kainate receptors have EPSPs of particularly long duration in the developing thalamocortical synapse and occur in separate synaptic locations to the silent synapse that gains AMPA receptor function with LTP and development (Bannister *et al.*, 2005). Protocols that cause LTP simultaneously reduce the kainate receptor components (Kidd and Isaac, 1999). Kainate receptors are also strongly downregulated during early development, suggesting that this is an endogenous process that can be mimicked by LTP in the slice preparation (Chapter 4). Therefore, both development and LTP at this synapse see an increase in rapid AMPA receptor transmission and a decrease in slow kainate receptor transmission.

Two methods have been used to observe insertion of AMPA receptors at synaptic sites. First, it is possible to view the location of the GluR1 subunit by tagging it with green fluorescent protein (GFP). Where this has been done in hippocampus, it has been shown that tetanic stimulation can drive GluR1–GFP into spines. It is also possible to track the entry of AMPA channels into the postsynaptic membrane by expressing homomeric GluR1 receptors in hippocampal slice cultures. Because AMPA receptors lacking the GluR2 subunit have rectifying I–V curves, insertion of the introduced GluR1 homomers can be measured as an increase in rectification of the synaptic EPSPs. This has been done in cell cultures and showed that AMPA channels were inserted in response to stimuli that induce LTP (i.e. coincident pre- and postsynaptic depolarization) (Hayashi *et al.*, 2000). Insertion can also be activated by autonomous $Ca^{2+}$-calmodulin-dependent protein kinase II (CaMKII) (Hayashi *et al.*, 2000), although this is not the only kinase involved (see below).

Further insight into the condition of thalamocortical synapses has come from studying the *barrelless* mouse, which has an impairment in AMPA receptor insertion owing to loss of ACI function (Abdel-Majid *et al.*, 1998). Thalamocortical synapses are rarely found in a completely silent state where no AMPA receptors are expressed at all, but rather contain NMDA receptors and few AMPA receptors (Lu *et al.*, 2003). In this sense, they are quiet synapses rather than silent synapses. This suggests that ACI probably acting via PKA is involved in insertion of AMPA receptors during development and LTP at this synapse (Lu *et al.*, 2003). The system of AMPA receptor insertion and regulation at this synapse also requires PKC during the first postnatal week, suggesting a complex interdependence of factors (Scott *et al.*, 2007). The GluR1 subunit of the AMPA channel has a PKC phosphorylation site located on its cytoplasmic tail that is important for LTP and AMPA receptor insertion in neonatal hippocampus, which could explain the finding at thalamocortical synapses (Boehm *et al.*, 2006).

The developmental mechanism of receptor insertion occurs in neonatal hippocampus and neonatal cortex, but it is not established at the time of writing that it occurs in adult animals. Insertion mechanisms for AMPA receptors are important for development but decrease or may even cease in adult hippocampus (Grosshans *et al.*, 2002), barrel cortex (Hardingham and Fox, 2006) and visual cortex (Rumpel *et al.*, 2004). Although thalamocortical LTP only occurs in barrel cortex during the first postnatal week, it continues in other layers of the cortex later in life including in layers II/III, which is the subject of the next section.

### 6.1.3    *Long-term potentiation at the layer IV to layers II/III synapse*

As mentioned above, the other major avenue of investigation for LTP in the barrel cortex so far has been to understand what underlies plasticity in the adult brain. The obvious site for study is the layer II/III cells of the cortex, as experience-dependent plasticity is present in these layers throughout life (Fox, 1992) and these layers exhibit prominent expression of NMDA receptors (Monaghan *et al.*, 1988; Fox *et al.*, 1989), which are known to be involved in LTP induction. In adult animals, LTP can be demonstrated in layer II/III cells by stimulating columnar, horizontal or diagonal pathways from adjacent columns (Aroniadou-Anderjaska and Keller, 1995; Castro-Alamancos *et al.*, 1995; Glazewski *et al.*, 1998a; Hardingham *et al.*, 2003). Potentiation in the barrel cortex shows a number of properties in common with that in the CA1 region of the hippocampus in that it is NMDA dependent (Castro-Alamancos *et al.*, 1995) and CaMKII dependent (Hardingham *et al.*, 2003). An example of the NMDA receptor dependence of cortical LTP in layers II/III is shown in Figure 6.1, and an example of CaMKII dependence is shown in Figure 6.6 (below).

Potentiation of synaptic transmission can be reversed by LTD induction protocols (Section 6.2) or potentiated following LTD, again a property that it shares with hippocampal synapses and which is known as bidirectionality (Feldman, 2000; Urban *et al.*, 2002). However, at least one aspect of barrel cortex LTP may not be shared with the hippocampus: while conventional thinking maintains that expression of LTP is postsynaptic in the CA1 region of the hippocampus, there is evidence for a large presynaptic component to plasticity in the neocortex. The postsynaptic component of LTP requires GluR1 in barrel cortex of animals older than 6 weeks of age (Hardingham and Fox, 2006). Quantal analysis and paired pulse analysis suggest that GluR1 knockouts lack any postsynaptic component to LTP. Nevertheless, both GluR1 knockouts and wild-type animals exhibit presynaptic LTP. Therefore, before discussing the nature of layer II/III plasticity further, it will be useful to review the evidence for presynaptic LTP, and this is done in the next section.

### 6.1.4    *Presynaptic long-term potentiation*

Markram and Tsodyks (1996) were the first to show that spike pairing could produce LTP and that the potentiation was frequency dependent. These pioneering studies were performed on layer V cells in developing somatosensory cortex and suggested a presynaptic component to plasticity. Spike pairing is a protocol for producing potentiation where a presynaptic action potential or spike is produced in the presynaptic axon to occur a few milliseconds before a spike in the postsynaptic neuron (Markram *et al.*, 1997). The presynaptic spike

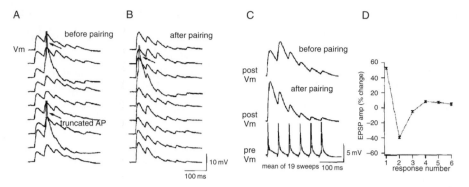

**Figure 6.4** Effect of long-term potentiation (LTP) on short-term dynamics in layer V to V synapses in neonatal rat somatosensory cortex. A. Sequential examples of excitatory postsynaptic potentials (EPSPs) evoked in response to a 23 Hz stimulus train of six presynaptic action potentials. B. The same cell after pairing to evoke LTP. Note that the synapse changes to a depressing synapse and only the response to the first stimulus is potentiated. C. The same data averaged for control (top) and after pairing (middle) periods. The stimulus train is shown (bottom). D. The change in response for each EPSP in the train. The first response is potentiated, the second depressed and the third to sixth marginally increased. (Reproduced from Markram and Tsodyks [1996] with kind permission of the authors and Elsevier.)

can be produced by an extracellular stimulating electrode and the postsynaptic spike by an intracellular somatic current pulse. The result is a form of LTP that shows potentiation when tested with low-frequency stimuli (say 0.1 Hz) but depression when tested with stimulation of higher frequencys (20 Hz) (Figure 6.4). In practice, both frequencies are delivered in a single stimulus by repeating a 20 Hz burst of five or six stimuli every second. The first response in the train occurs after a preceding interval of 10 s and in a depressing synapse has a greater amplitude than the subsequent responses to the shorter intervals (50 ms). Following potentiation, only the first pulse in the train is substantially potentiated (Figure 6.4D). These results are consistent with a presynaptic locus for LTP because if release probability is increased by LTP at a synapse with a low number of release sites per synaptic bouton, it increases the postsynaptic response by releasing more vesicles; however, it also thereby reduces the vesicles available for subsequent release within a short time period (see Section 3.4.3, which discusses short-term dynamics). This is particularly evident in intracortical synapses, which tend to have a small number of release sites per bouton, for example one per bouton in layer IV to II/III synapses (Silver *et al.*, 2003).

Further evidence for a presynaptic component to neocortical LTP comes from studies where quantal analysis has been used to probe the locus of LTP. In wild-type mouse barrel cortex, LTP exhibits both a pre- and a postsynaptic component to LTP and the presynaptic components generally develop more slowly (over 20–30 min) than the postsynaptic components, which occur almost immediately after pairing pre- and postsynaptic spikes (Hardingham and Fox, 2006). In GluR1 knockout mice, the only form of LTP at the layer IV to II/III synapse is pre-synaptic in origin, implying that the postsynaptic component is GluR1 dependent and normally occurs in addition to a presynaptic component (Hardingham and Fox, 2006).

As shown in Figure 6.4, the consequences of purely presynaptic LTP for a cell responding to a train of pulses at around 20 Hz or more are that only the first pulse in the train of EPSPs is actually potentiated, while the subsequent pulses are either mildly increased or strongly depressed. A number of models have been formulated that capture the properties of dynamic synapses and shown how such dynamics are useful for emphasizing changes in firing rate rather than absolute rate (Abbott *et al.*, 1997). Furthermore, such networks can retain memories and are capable of several real-time computing tasks (Carpenter and Milenova, 2002; Maass *et al.*, 2002, 2004; Abbott and Regehr, 2004). One yardstick by which to measure the relevance of pre- and postsynaptic components of plasticity is to test whether they occur in vivo, and this subject is addressed in the next section.

### 6.1.5    *Mechanisms of long-term potentiation and relationship to experience-dependent plasticity*

One of the studies that first gave a clue to the importance of an LTP-type mechanism of the type described by Tsodyks and Markram (1997) for experience-dependent plasticity in the barrel cortex was performed by Finnerty *et al.* (1999), who showed that whisker deprivation can affect the short-term dynamics of cortical neurons in a manner that is closely related to the changes observed in vivo in particular pathways between spared and deprived barrels. Removing all the whiskers except those in a single row led to an increase in transmission between the spared whisker barrels and the cells located in neighboring barrels deprived of their principal whisker input (Section 7.2.1). If slices of barrel cortex were prepared from rats that had undergone a period of whisker deprivation, then the pathways running between layers II/III in a spared barrel and layers II/III in a deprived barrel were found to be altered in a fashion consistent with pot-entiation (Figure 6.5). Specifically, the short-term dynamics of the synapse change such that the frequency response is decreased compared with that found in a normal undeprived pathway or in the reverse pathways between deprived and spared barrels (Finnerty *et al.*, 1999). In other words, the response to the first pulse is potentiated rather than responses to subsequent pulses in a high-frequency train. This mirrors the changes that occur in the short-term dynamics

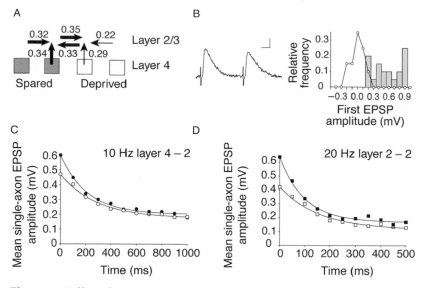

**Figure 6.5** Effect of sensory deprivation on electrically evoked responses in barrel cortical pathways. A. Summary of the changes in synaptic strength in various intracortical pathways between spared (grey) and deprived (white) barrel-columns. The numbers represent a conditional probability of vesicular release and are similar to synaptic strength (Tsodyks and Markram, 1997). Values for undeprived vertical pathways are 0.28 and for horizontal 0.27. (See Finnerty *et al.* [1999] for details.) B. Minimal stimulation in the IV to II pathway evoked excitatory postsynaptic potentials (EPSPs) with amplitudes as shown (first EPSP grey; open circles noise). Scale bars = 20 ms and 0.2 mV. C. Mean EPSP amplitude in response to 10 Hz stimulation in deprived (open circles) and spared (filled circles) columns. Note that the first response is smaller for deprived cases. D. Amplitude of EPSP for stimulation of the deprived to deprived pathway in layers II/III (open circles) compared with the spared to deprived pathway (filled circles). Note that the first response is greater in the spared to deprived column pathway. (Reproduced from Finnerty *et al.* [1999] with kind permission of the authors and *Nature* Publishing Group.)

of a synapse when it potentiates (Figure 6.4). Therefore, the effect of sensory deprivation is to leave behind the signature of a potentiated pathway leading from the spared to the deprived barrel.

Experiments on the probability of inducing LTP in layers II/III of deprived barrel cortex provide further evidence of the role of LTP in cortical experience-dependent plasticity. In animals with all their whiskers intact, the incidence of LTP induction is relatively low, at approximately 35%. However, this value rises to 70% following whisker deprivation, suggesting that many of the synapses are already saturated in normal barrel cortex and cannot be potentiated further (Hardingham and Fox, 2007). Whisker deprivation has been shown to produce

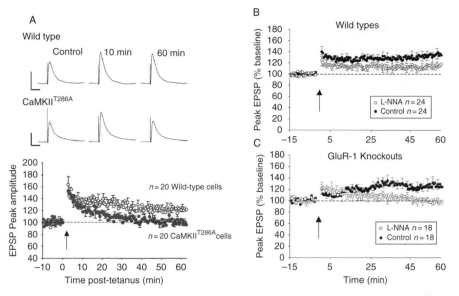

**Figure 6.6.** Factors involved in production of long-term potentiation (LTP) in layers II/III of the mouse barrel cortex. A. A point mutation of calcium-calmodulin-dependent protein kinase II (CaMKII) at the T286 site prevented autophosphorylation of CaMKII and LTP in layers II/III cells. Waveforms above the graph are average excitatory postsynaptic potentials (EPSPs) before (−15 min) immediately after (0–10 min) and an hour following pairing (50–60 min). (Reproduced from Hardingham *et al.* [2003] with permission of the Society for Neuroscience.) B. Application of a nitric oxide synthase antagonist (L-NNA) reduced but did not eliminate LTP in wild types. C. Application of L-NNA in knockouts for glutamate receptor subunit 1 completely abolished LTP. (Adapted from Hardingham and Fox [2006] with permission of the Society for Neuroscience.)

similar effects to LTD (Section 6.2) and, therefore, depriving the whiskers appears to reset the synapses to a state where they can undergo LTP, thereby increasing the probability of LTP induction. There is an argument for considering this extra LTP to be more properly described as de-depression rather than LTP, as will be discussed in Section 6.2.

One further piece of evidence linking LTP to the type of plasticity induced by whisker deprivation comes from studies where the molecular mechanisms underlying cortical plasticity have been studied. Both LTP and experience-dependent potentiation depends on CaMKII and autophosphorylation of CaMKII (Glazewski *et al.*, 2000; Hardingham *et al.*, 2003). The role of CaMKII in barrel cortex plasticity appears to be to control AMPA receptor phosphorylation via the GluR1 subunit and also to play a role in release of nitric oxide (Figure 6.6), which affects presynaptic function. The GluR1 subunit of the AMPA channel has a CaMKII phosphorylation site, which, once phosphorylated, produces an increase in conductance through the channel. This component of LTP is missing in barrel cortex of GluR1 knockouts, resulting in a loss of the postsynaptic component of LTP (Hardingham and Fox, 2006). If, however, nitric oxide synthase activity is blocked within the cell, there is a selective loss of the presynaptic component of LTP. Blocking either CaMKII autophosphorylation or inhibiting nitric oxide synthase in GluR1 knockouts completely blocks residual LTP (Figure 6.6).

In developing animals, the insertion of AMPA receptors also plays an important role in strengthening synapses, and this mechanism is also involved in LTP (Section 6.1.2). The AMPA-controlled channels have also been shown to insert in the developing barrel cortex (Takahashi *et al.*, 2003; Clem and Barth, 2006) and this process requires the postsynaptic density protein 95 (Ehrlich and Malinow, 2004), which is a scaffolding protein that is required to localize AMPA receptors at synapses.

One of the questions surrounding cortical plasticity has been whether the underlying mechanisms rely on inhibition. For example, it is possible that a selective loss of inhibition in a deprived sensory pathway could produce potentiation of the spared sensory pathways by disinhibition. This idea gains some support from the studies of Calford and Tweedale (1991a, b) showing immediate disinhibition in cortex following digit amputation or destruction of peripheral C-fires (Calford and Tweedale, 1991a–c). However, the fact that CaMKII is essential for cortical plasticity and that it is not present in cortical inhibitory cells (Liu and Jones, 1996) suggests that this is not the same mechanism as that involved in whisker-deprivation plasticity (Section 7.2). Similarly, the fact that LTP and experience-dependent plasticity rely on the same mechanisms and affect the incidence of one another implies a role for excitatory pathways in experience-dependent plasticity. This is not to say that inhibition does not play a role in induction of experience-dependent plasticity, however (as discussed in Section 7.2), but rather it places some bounds on its role in expression of plasticity.

## 6.2    Long-term depression

### 6.2.1    *Historical context and significance*

It was not clear when LTP was discovered that there would necessarily be an activity-dependent process capable of decreasing synaptic gain. Conceivably, decreases in synaptic gain could be autonomous. Synapses might turn over and be replaced by new synapses, thereby renewing the substrate for LTP, or synaptic gain at existing synapses could be predisposed to decay with time in the absence of a continuous LTP process. In the event, a heterosynaptic depression mechanism that could decrease synaptic gain was discovered first in the hippocampus (Barrionuevo *et al.*, 1980) and shortly after in the cerebellum (Ito and Kano, 1982; Ekerot and Kano, 1985). Heterosynaptic processes are defined as those where the synapses undergoing plasticity are different from those instigating the plasticity. For example, stimulation of climbing fibers gives rise to LTD at parallel fiber inputs on to Purkinje cells. Shortly after these findings, homosynaptic plasticity was discovered in the hippocampus (Bramham and Srebro, 1987; Stanton and Sejnowski, 1989). With homosynaptic processes, a pattern of activation carried by the same inputs cause their own depression of synaptic gain. The discovery of homosynaptic LTD meant that LTD was a process that could reverse the effect of homosynaptic LTP. It also meant that synaptic gain could be controlled by active down regulation rather than passive decay with time; in other words, synapses are likely to be relatively stable unless they are depressed by signals from their inputs.

Synaptic depression mechanisms have always been likely candidates for explaining plasticity in the visual cortex during ocular dominance plasticity. Closing one eye during the critical period early in life causes cortical neurons to lose responsiveness to that eye (Hubel and Wiesel, 1977), and while structural changes clearly result from monocular deprivation (Antonini and Stryker, 1993), it is at least likely that structural changes are preceded by earlier synaptic changes that either cause them or run in parallel with them. In favor of this theory, LTD was discovered in the visual cortex a few years after it was established as a synaptic mechanism in the hippocampus (Artola *et al.*, 1990; Dudek and Bear, 1992). The evidence linking the actual mechanism of LTD to the experience-dependent process has been rather long and complicated, because there actually appear to be several different synaptic mechanisms that can result in the same outcome of depressed transmission (Malenka and Bear, 2004). This is taken up in Section 6.2.5. However, initially it was the link between LTD and development that led to the first demonstration of LTD in layer IV of the barrel cortex (Feldman *et al.*, 1998). Using the thalamocortical slice, it was shown that thalamocortical afferents on to layer IV cells were capable of LTD when low-frequency stimulation was presented while holding the cell at a negative potential ($-50\,\mathrm{mV}$; Figure 6.7).

### 6.2.2    *Properties and methods of induction*

There are three main methods for inducing LTD in cortex low-frequency stimulation (typically 1 Hz for 900 pulses), anti-hebbian spike pairing, where the presynaptic spike occurs after the postsynaptic spike (typically by 50 ms), and chemical LTD where NMDA is applied to a cortical slice for a period of time. It is not clear at the time of writing whether any of these three methods leads to equivalent molecular changes at the synapse. However they do all produce a decrease in synaptic gain.

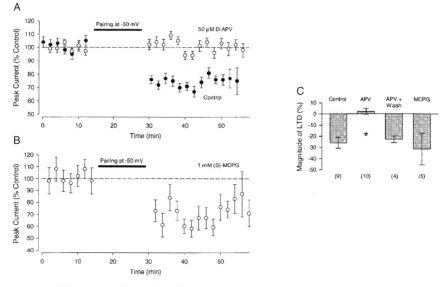

**Figure 6.7.** Induction of long-term depression (LTD) in the rat barrel cortex depends on NMDA receptors but not metabotropic glutamate receptors (mGluR) in neonates. A. Pairing stimuli delivered at low frequency (0.1–0.33 Hz) with depolarization to −50 mV induced LTD (black circles) unless an NMDA receptor antagonist (APV) was applied (white circles). B. An mGluR antagonist (MCPG) did not prevent induction of LTD. C. Average values of LTD in the presence of the antagonists shown. Animals were four to five days of age. (Reproduced from Feldman *et al.* [1998], with kind permission of the authors and Elsevier.)

Low-frequency stimulation has mainly been used in the visual cortex to induce depression (Dudek and Bear, 1992). Chemical LTD has mainly been used in slice cultures, or in cases where the experiment requires that a large number of cells be affected at the same time (Kamal *et al.*, 1999; Huber *et al.*, 2001). In barrel cortex, spike timing is the most commonly used induction method and probably the most physiologically justifiable given that induction of experience-dependent plasticity alters spike-timing contingencies in the barrel cortex (Celikel *et al.*, 2004). Spike-timing LTD is induced by recording intracellularly and generating a postsynaptic spike by injecting current into the postsynaptic cell and timing stimulation of the presynaptic pathway to lag the postsynaptic spike typically by 10–50 ms (Figure 6.8). The exact timing window is relatively broad for LTD compared with LTP. With LTP, the timing window is approximately 10–20 ms whereas for LTD it can be up to 100 ms (Figure 6.8) at some ages (Allen *et al.*, 2003). In layer IV, the timing window for LTD decreases with age and, therefore, progressively greater precision of timing amongst thalamocortical inputs on to layer IV cells is required in order to induce

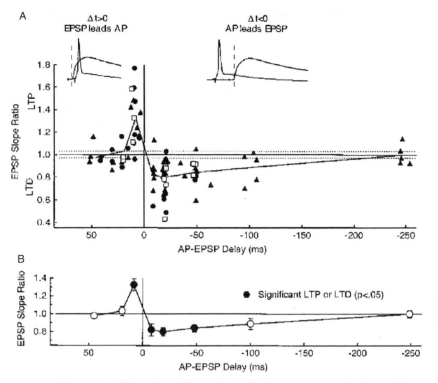

**Figure 6.8.** The spike timing window for long-term potentiation and depression (LTP and LTD, respectively) in adolescent rat barrel cortex. A. Relative phase of the pre- and postsynaptic spike is shown versus the change in synaptic gain it produces. Individual cases are plotted for room temperature (black circles) and at 32 °C (open squares). Insets show examples of pairing pre- before postsynaptic action potential (left), representing positive intervals, and pairing post- before presynaptic action potentials (right), representing negative intervals. B. Averages of the data in A showing the asymmetric time window for LTP (10ms) compared with LTD (at least 100ms). (Reproduced from Feldman [2000] with kind permission of Elsevier and the author.)

LTD as development proceeds. If LTD is a precursor to removal of synapses during development, then synapses firing later than the postsynaptic cell would gradually be pruned, while those firing before would be retained and potentiated. The wider LTD timing window occurs at the stage of development when LTD is most required; that is, the period when synaptic connection errors are made but then eliminated (Section 4.2.4).

### 6.2.3    Long-term depression at the thalamocortical synapse

The mechanism of synaptic depression has been studied during development at the thalamocortical synapse. Using the thalamocortical slice preparation, it is possible to record from layer IV cells and stimulate an isolated thalamic input from VPm. Pairing low-frequency stimulation with a mild depolarization to −50 mV causes LTD of approximately 25% at the barrel cortex in P4–P5 rats. This form of LTD is NMDA receptor dependent in layer IV and shows a critical period ending at the end of the first postnatal week (Feldman *et al.*, 1998). Since LTP at this age is partly attributable to unsilencing silent synapses (Section 6.1.2), the possibility exists that LTD reverses this process and creates silent synapses. However, the present evidence indicates that LTD acts by decreasing the quantal amplitude of synaptic transmission rather than by silencing synapses (Feldman *et al.*, 1998). The occurrence of LTD appears to involves a change in postsynaptic gain, perhaps by altering the transmission characteristics of AMPA channels. In support of this idea, it has been found that postsynaptic PKA is required for reversal of LTD in the barrel cortex (Hardingham and Fox, 2007). This is consistent with the hypothesis that LTD involves dephosphorylation of the GluR1 subunit Ser-845 site (Section 6.2.4) and explains why mice lacking elements of the PKA activation pathway exhibit reduced levels of GluR1 Ser-845 phosphorylation in barrel cortex (Inan *et al.*, 2006). Alternatively, phosphorylation of the Ser-880 site on the GluR2 subunit of the AMPA receptor may play a role in depression of synaptic transmission by decreasing AMPA receptor recycling at the postsynaptic density (Kim *et al.*, 2001; Seidenman *et al.*, 2003).

### 6.2.4    *Long-term depression at the layer IV to II/III pathway*

Whisker deprivation can depress responses of cortical layer II/III neurons while leaving responses of layer IV cells in the same barrel-column unaffected (Fox, 1992; Glazewski and Fox, 1996). These findings predict that a depression mechanism exists between layer IV and layer II/III cells in the barrel cortex, and subsequent studies showed that spike timing-dependent LTD could indeed occur in this pathway (Allen *et al.*, 2003). Similar to layer IV thalamocortical afferent plasticity, LTD at this synapse can be induced by pairing a postsynaptic spike to occur 50–100 ms before the presynaptic spike (Figure 6.9). The mechanisms underlying LTD at the layer II/III synapse are more complicated than might have been predicted and have pre- and postsynaptic components in different measure. The complexity of LTD mechanisms in general has been commented on by Malenka and Bear (2004) and continues to challenge the Ockham's razor approach to science. Here we discuss the evidence for two mechanisms bearing in mind that others may come to light in the future.

First of all, it is thought that NMDA receptors are involved in induction of at least some forms of LTD (Lee *et al.*, 1998; Malenka and Bear, 2004). It might seem curious that LTP and LTD can have opposite effects but be initiated by activation of the same receptor. Theories have been put forward for how this might work,

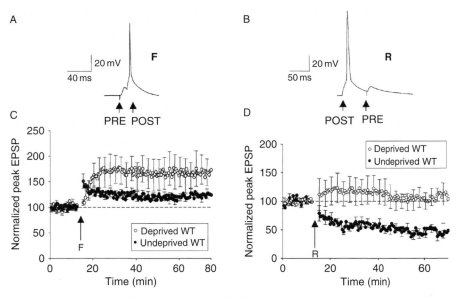

**Figure 6.9.** Effect of whisker deprivation on long-term potentiation and depression (LTP and LTD, respectively) in layers II/III of the mouse barrel cortex. A. Example of the timing of a presynaptic (PRE) and postsynaptic (POST) action potential for forward pairing (PRE before POST) used to induce LTP. B. Example of the timing of a presynaptic and postsynaptic action potential for reverse pairing (POST before PRE) used to induce LTD C. Following bilateral whisker deprivation for seven days, the average level of LTP increases, induced by forward pairing (F) in barrel cortex mainly owing to an increase, in probability of evoking LTP. D. Conversely, the same deprivation abolishes LTD cause by reverse pairing (R) (WT, wild type). (Data from Hardingham and Fox, 2007.)

including the idea that smaller increases in postsynaptic calcium are required for LTD to be expressed while higher levels result in LTP. This idea is consistent with the notion that LTP requires phosphorylation processes to be activated while LTD requires dephosphorylation and the fact that phosphatases are more sensitive to calcium than the kinases in the postsynaptic density (Cho *et al.*, 2001; D'Alcantara *et al.*, 2003). There is some evidence that the direction of synaptic plasticity can be predicted by the timecourse of calcium entry into the dendrites during spike pairing, with a faster rise predicting LTP and a slower rise LTD (Ismailov *et al.*, 2004). The resolution of this issue may come from studies examining the sub-synaptic locations of phosphatases and kinases with particular receptor subunits (Blackstone and Sheng, 1999; Kennedy, 2000). In addition, there is also evidence that the presynaptic component to LTD may require presynaptic NMDA receptors in young (P16–P23) animals (Bender *et al.*, 2006).

To consider the postsynaptic component first, one important factor involved in LTD in the layer IV to layers II/III pathway is the GluR1 subunit of the AMPA channel. Without it, LTD is almost completely abolished in this pathway (Hardingham *et al.*, 2006): interestingly, so too is experience-dependent depression (Hardingham *et al.*, 2006). Since AMPA channels are located postsynaptically, this could explain the postsynaptic component of LTD. The reason GluR1 is important for LTD is that the channel conductance is controlled by phosphorylation of the cytoplasmic tail of GluR1 at its CaMKII site (Derkach *et al.*, 1999) and surface expression and/or channel open probability at its PKA site (Banke *et al.*, 2000). The dephosphorylation of a PKA site occurs during LTD in the barrel cortex (Hardingham and Fox, 2007). This is similar to findings in the visual cortex where monocular deprivation causes a depression of cortical responses to the reopened, previously deprived eye and occludes a form of LTD induced by low-frequency stimulation (Heynen *et al.*, 2003). Both LTD and monocular deprivation cause dephosphorylation of the Ser-845 PKA phosphorylation site of the GluR1 subunit. Therefore dephosphorylation of the PKA site on the GluR1 subunit is important for LTD in the layer IV to layers II/III pathway in visual and barrel cortex.

What of the presynaptic component of LTD seen in some studies? There is some evidence that the presynaptic component results from a decrease in presynaptic release caused by postsynaptic release of cannabinoids (Bender *et al.*, 2006). The cannabinoid receptor CB1 is expressed in barrel cortex, particularly in layer II (Bodor *et al.*, 2005). It has previously been shown to be located on presynaptic GABAergic terminals where it controls GABA release (Bodor *et al.*, 2005). Neurons that are excitable and fire postsynaptic spikes at a high rate release cannabinoids, which increase the rate of GABA release at presynaptic neurons and hence homeostatically decrease the neuron's firing rate (Chapter 3). However, studies in the barrel cortex have shown that excitatory synapses can also be affected by cannabinoid release. Excitatory connections between layer V cells and between layer IV and layers II/III cells show depression following spike pairing, which is dependent upon both cannabinoids and presynaptic NMDA receptors (Sjostrom *et al.*, 2004; Bender *et al.*, 2006).

### 6.2.5    *Mechanisms of long-term depression and relationship to experience-dependent depression*

As mentioned above, synaptic depression can occur in the layer IV to layers II/III pathway following whisker deprivation. A period of single whisker experience of seven days will produce a depression of the sensory responses of cells located in layers II/III to stimulation of the principal whisker, once it has been allowed to regrow for seven days to enable sensory stimulation (Glazewski and Fox, 1996). However, layer IV cells show very similar levels of sensory response to the same stimulus and seem unaffected by the whisker deprivation. Layer IV cells have a strong projection to cells in layers II/III radially superficial to them in the same barrel-column (Lubke *et al.*, 2000). The two facts suggests that the link in the pathway of excitation occurs somewhere between layer IV and layers II/III, most likely including the layer IV to layers II/III pathway itself.

There is reasonable evidence that some form of LTD process is involved in barrel cortex plasticity. Not only is LTD occluded in the barrel cortex in response to whisker deprivation (Figure 6.9), specifically in the pathways that show depression in vivo (Glazewski and Fox, 1996; Allen *et al.*, 2003), but also the same molecular mechanisms, such as GluR1 and dephosphorylation of PKA sites, appear to be involved. Furthermore, the circuit conditions set up by whisker deprivation cause a situation that would be expected to drive a spike timing-dependent depression mechanism. Celikel et al (2004) have used in vivo recording to show that when recordings are made from layers II/III of a barrel that has been deprived of its principal whisker, layer II/III cells tend to fire before cells located in layer IV. Because the principal whisker is absent, cells of both layers II/III and layer IV only fire in response to surround receptive field inputs, which are transmitted faster to layer II/III cells than to layer IV cells from neighboring barrels (Section 5.2.2). Since layer II/III cells receive a substantial projection from layer IV, this means that the layer IV to layers II/III connection will fire after the layer II/III cells have discharged, a condition, which if replicated in vitro, would lead to LTD for a time lag of around 50 ms between pre- and postsynaptic discharge (Section 6.2.2). This situation is different of course from that prevailing in normal animals with all their whiskers intact because, with the principal whisker intact, the layer IV cells tend to precede firing of the layer II/III cells by a period of 2–3 ms or so (Section 5.2.2).

The idea that synaptic depression could be produced by a decreased firing rate seems less likely because average firing rate is not changed by whisker deprivation (Celikel *et al.*, 2004). This throws into question the utility of studying LTD induced in vivo by a low-frequency stimulation at 1 Hz, because the natural firing rates in the system are (a) rarely at this level and (b) do not differ significantly between conditions that cause depression of sensory responses and conditions that do not. However, it is possible that low-frequency stimulation leads to activation of the same types of plasticity involved in spike-timing processes, though this has yet to be determined.

## 6.3    Conclusions

The field of synaptic plasticity is complex, which is a reflection of the complexity of the synapse and the emphasis placed on regulating synaptic transmission by evolutionary processes. As a consequence, despite the rapid progress made in understanding LTP and LTD in recent years, reviewing studies on cortical plasticity gives one a sense that we have only so far scratched the surface and there is much more to come. Plasticity studies in the barrel cortex have the advantage that it is possible to check the relevance of many of the mechanisms discovered in vitro at the cellular level with the whole animal in vivo. This is especially important given that mechanisms activated in vitro may not be engaged by the normal activity of the cortex during sensory tasks. A second advantage that has become clear, and may become more important with time, is that in order to understand neocortical plasticity in general it is important to understand the circuitry of the cortex, because it is likely that plasticity will differ at synapses between different cell types. This has already become apparent when considering the three major types of synapse in the hippocampus. For example, plasticity at the CA1 synapse is NMDA receptor dependent while that at the mossy fiber CA3 synapse is not. Similarly, in neocortex, plasticity at the thalamocortical synapse is different from that at the layer IV to layers II/III synapse. Therefore, the advantage of studying synaptic plasticity in the barrel cortex is that an understanding of the circuitry involved is already well advanced (Chapter 3) and likely to advance more rapidly in this area than others because the barrel structure provides reference points for the columnar organization of the system. Given that cortical plasticity needs to be understood in some area of the cortex, it may as well be barrel cortex, which should then provide insight to plasticity in other cortical areas.

# 7

# Experience-dependent plasticity

Plasticity is an important topic in neuroscience, both from a philosophical and a practical viewpoint. Plasticity is involved in development, learning and memory and in shaping the nervous system's response to injury and disease. With regard to development, some topics have been covered in Chapter 4, but here we concentrate in more detail on the mechanisms of plasticity rather than their developmental sequence and consequences for development. On the question of learning and memory, in Section 7.2 we look at the extent to which synaptic plasticity mechanisms are activated by changes in sensory experience. This issue relates in a general way to the means by which experience creates memories. Sensory experience can induce lasting memories and memory is thought to depend on synaptic plasticity. Therefore, understanding how sensory experience induces synaptic plasticity is germane to understanding learning and memory. In both cases, experience changes synaptic function. On the question of the nervous system's response to injury, we treat this topic separately from the general treatment of experience-dependent plasticity because even though it may involve components of the latter it certainly involves other factors too (Section 7.5). In many ways, this may be the more urgent category of plasticity to tackle because a full understanding of injury-induced plasticity may lead to therapies for the consequences of damage to peripheral or central structures.

The early studies on somatosensory cortical plasticity were concerned with the cortical response to peripheral injury. In the early 1980s, the pioneering studies of Merzenich, Kaas and colleagues, established that the somatosensory cortex shows significant plasticity of the hand representation (Merzenich *et al.*, 1983a, b). Nerve injury caused the somatotopic maps of the affected digits to rearrange in the cortex such that cortical neurons that used to respond to the de-nervated digit changed to respond to the adjacent intact digits. Similarly, studies by Kossut and

Hand (1984) showed that ablation of all but a single whisker follicle led to an expanded cortical column in the barrel cortex. Plasticity was functional in the sense that areas of cortex altered the degree to which they responded to different whiskers. Individual cells within the cortical maps were, therefore, essentially functionally rewired by whisker follicle ablation. Unlike plasticity in the visual cortex, the plasticity of somatosensory cortex did not appear to show a clear critical period. Whisker follicle ablation had a similar effect in adult as in developing animals (Kossut et al., 1988). Several questions arose at this point. First, could experience alone rather than nerve lesions alter functional maps? Second, could the lack of critical period be attributed to inducing the plasticity by peripheral injury rather than experience? Third, was the plasticity cortical in origin or passively transmitted from subcortical structures? These questions have been addressed in the barrel cortex by looking at functional maps of the whisker representations and their response to whisker deprivations. The following sections deal with the nature of plasticity in the cortex (Section 7.1) and the evidence that plasticity is cortical in origin (Section 7.2), including the current understanding of the anatomical pathways that might be involved (Section 7.2.2), before going on to explore the molecular (Section 7.3) and structural (Section 7.4) mechanisms that underlie map plasticity. The final section considers the issue of lesion-induced plasticity and its similarities to and differences from experience-dependent plasticity (Section 7.5).

## 7.1    Map plasticity in barrel cortex

### 7.1.1    *The effect of altered tactile experience*

Can the somatosensory system change in response to something as subtle as altered tactile experience? This question has been addressed in several studies. Hand (1982) and Simons and Land (1987) showed that trimming the whiskers could be sufficient to alter receptive fields and cortical vibrissae domains. Similarly, Clark et al. (1988) showed that syndactyly, where two fingers are surgically joined together, led to altered receptive fields in the mature monkey cortex. Subsequent studies in barrel cortex confirmed and extended these early findings by showing that whisker deprivation produced plasticity that decreased in layer IV with age but remained high in layers II/III into adulthood (Fox, 1992).

The form of experience-dependent plasticity seen in the cortex depends on the nature of the deprivation or altered experience. In early studies, Kossut and Hand (1984) created a simple but clever whisker deprivation condition where a single whisker follicle was spared on one side of the face and the surrounding

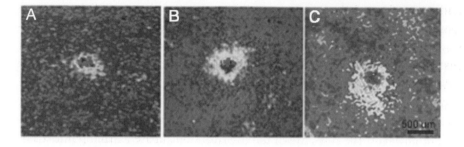

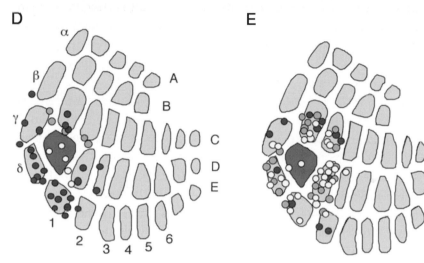

**Figure 7.1.** Whisker deprivation causes expansion of the spared whisker's domain. A–C. Autoradiograms using 2-deoxyglucose to identify the area of cortex in layer IV activated by single whisker (C3) stimulation in an adult mouse. A. Control condition showing C3 domain centered on the C3 barrel. B. The C3 domain two months after vibrissectomy of all but the C3 whisker. C. The C3 domain following two months of whisker deprivation sparing just the C3 whisker. (A, B Adapted from Kossut *et al.* [1988]; C adapted from Hand [1982].) D, E. Activation domains for the D1 whisker. Composite of penetrations made through layers II/III of barrel cortex in wild-type mice. Each circle represents the average response in layers II/III sampled from at least four different cells per penetration. D. Control from an undeprived animal. Note the domain is largely restricted to the D1 barrel. E. After 18 days of single whisker experience, the domain expands to the neighboring barrels. Responses indicated as <0.5 spikes/stimulus (black circles), 0.5–1.0 spikes/stimulus (grey circles) and ≥1.0 spikes/stimulus (white circles). (Adapted from Glazewski *et al.* 1996, 2000.)

follicles lesioned, which led to an expansion of the area of cortex activated by that single whisker (C3 in this case) beyond the boundaries normally seen in an animal with all its vibrissae intact. Similarly, depriving the whiskers in a manner that does not damage the follicle innervation also led to expansion of the area of cortex sensitive to the spared whisker (Figure 7.1).

Other studies have used more complex deprivation patterns, including sparing two whiskers (Diamond *et al.*, 1993), sparing a row (Simons and Land, 1994), removing a single row (Shepherd *et al.*, 2003) and chessboard pattern deprivation (Wallace and Fox, 1999a) where every other whisker is deprived (Figure 7.2). In each case, the effects that occur can be summarized as an increase in the response to the spared whiskers and a decrease in the response to the deprived whiskers. Measuring the response of the spared whisker is, of course, straightforward; however, the response of the deprived whisker are usually measured after the whiskers have been allowed to regrow for a short period of time (six to eight days). This potentially compromises the measure to some extent because it could allow some recovery of function. Therefore, the responses of the deprived vibrissae referred to in the following pages might be considered as an underestimate of the degree of depression caused by deprivation.

The magnitude of potentiation for a surround receptive field whisker response is typically two- to four-fold for mouse and rat barrel cortex and the magnitude of depression is typically about 50% for a principal whisker in a deprived barrel, again for both mouse and rat barrel cortex (Glazewski and Fox, 1996; Glazewski *et al.*, 2000). The change in response brought about by altered experience is, therefore, opposite in direction for the spared and deprived whiskers and approximately reciprocally equivalent to one another.

The timecourse of depression and potentiation are not the same, however, and depression occurs over a shorter time period than potentiation. In rats deprived of all but the D1 whisker, potentiation takes at least 18 days to develop, while depression is present after just seven days (Glazewski and Fox, 1996). Where experiments have been conducted in animals deprived in a chessboard pattern, potentiation can be accelerated somewhat so that the effects can be seen within seven days for the spared-whisker response in the deprived barrels. However, depression can be observed in animals deprived in a chessboard pattern after just four days of deprivation. To conduct the latter experiment, the whiskers need to be trimmed for four days and reglued at the time of recording because the whiskers do not regrow sufficiently to test responses in less than seven days. These observations relate to plasticity outside the spared barrels. Earlier plasticity events can be seen inside the spared barrel in layers II/III as early as 24 hours after deprivation has been initiated (Barth *et al.*, 2000) or, in whisker-paired animals, after 15 hours if the animal experiences an enriched environment (Rema *et al.*, 2006).

The location of the potentiation depends on the type of deprivation pattern adopted. When two adjacent whiskers are spared, the spared-whisker responses increase in the adjacent spared barrels (Diamond *et al.*, 1993). When a single whisker is spared, the spared-whisker responses increase in the

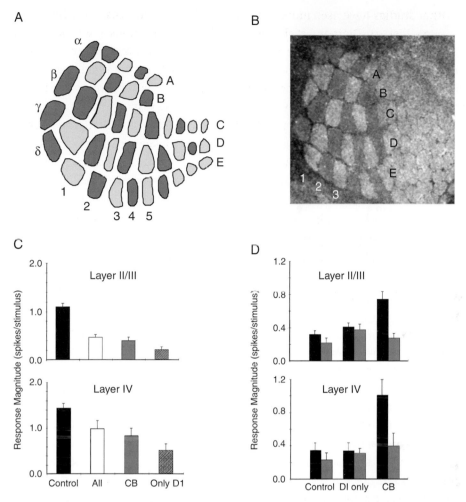

**Figure 7.2.** Chessboard deprivation pattern and effect. A. The chessboard pattern of whisker deprivation causes every other barrel to be deprived in the cortex. B. Zinc staining following chessboard pattern deprivation for 12 hours shows up the pattern of deprived barrels (grey, increased zinc) and spared barrels (white, lower zinc) in layer IV of the barrel cortex. Note the posterior barrels are affected and the anterior barrels have not undergone deprivation. (Adapted from www.neurobio.pitt.edu/ barrels/ figure7.html after Brown and Dyck [2003].) C. Depression of the deprived whisker occurs to a greater extent in animals with some spared whiskers in adolescent animals. Depression is approximately equal when all whiskers are deprived (All) to that in chessboard deprived (CB) cases but greater when only one whisker is deprived (only D1). Recordings taken from the deprived barrel principal whisker in each case. D. Potentiation is faster in animals undergoing chessboard deprivation than in animals where only a single whisker is spared (D1 only spared). After 7 days of deprivation, potentiation occurs where the deprivation is in the chessboard pattern (but not in the D1 spared case) and is most pronounced on the near side of the barrel (black) rather than the far side (grey). (Adapted from Wallace and Fox. [1999a].)

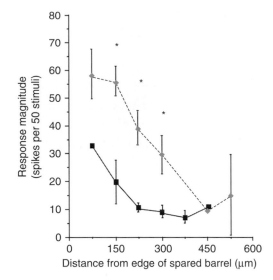

**Figure 7.3.** Fall off in response to the D1 whisker at distances away from the edge of the D1 barrel. The normal rate of fall with distance in a mouse with all whiskers intact is shown as the continuous line. The greater response levels to D1 whisker stimulation in barrels surrounding the D1 barrel following whisker deprivation sparing D1 for 18 days is shown by the dotted line. The asterisks mark statistically significant differences at three distances (100–300 μm). (Adapted from Glazewski *et al.* [2000].)

adjacent deprived barrels (Fox, 1992; Glazewski and Fox, 1996; Shepherd *et al.*, 2003). It is not clear how far out into the neighboring barrel field the potentiation of the response of the spared whiskers can range. Estimates based on extracellular spike recording suggest it ranges over at least a neighboring single barrel in mouse and rat, but the responses are potentiated far more on the near side of the barrel than the far side (Glazewski and Fox, 1996). Figure 7.3 shows the fall off in the size of potentiated response with radial distance away from the spared-whisker's barrel in the mouse barrel cortex estimated using extracellular spike recording. Subthreshold EPSPs may potentiate over a greater distance than this, given that even the unpotentiated responses range over several barrels (Petersen *et al.*, 2003; see also Figure 5.2).

There is some evidence that the spread of spared-whisker responses can reach further within the septal regions than within the barrel-columns themselves (Shepherd *et al.*, 2003) presumably because of the relatively long-range septal connections within layer IV (Hoeflinger *et al.*, 1995).

Depression of the deprived-whisker response also ranges over the neighboring barrels, causing a loss of deprived-whisker responses in the principal barrel-column and surrounding barrel-columns. It is perhaps not surprising that a loss, or decrease, of response in the principal barrel entails loss of response in surrounding barrels, given that responses to a particular whisker in non-principal barrel-columns depend on the responses to that whisker in the principal barrel-column (Section 5.3.3).

### 7.1.2    The effect of local cortical interactions on plasticity

One of the advantages of studying the barrel system is that the peripheral sensory input can be readily manipulated in a variety of ways to clarify different aspects of experience-dependent plasticity. Through using a variety of whisker-deprivation patterns, four main aspects of plasticity have been discovered:

- homosynaptic depression
- heterosynaptic depression
- cross-whisker potentiation
- potentiation within a deprived barrel.

Two of these forms of plasticity do not overtly require interaction between neighboring sensory inputs (i.e. homosynaptic depression and potentiation within a deprive barrel), while the other two accentuate plasticity as a result of interactions either between two spared vibrissae domains (cross-whisker potentiation) or between a spared vibrissa domain and a deprived vibrissa domain (heterosynaptic depression). Before describing the evidence for this view, it is useful to consider the relationship between the whisker-deprivation pattern and the cortical activity domains the deprivation pattern produces.

Because the barrel cortex is an isomorphic map of discrete whisker inputs, the pattern of spared and missing whiskers on the face is mirrored by the same pattern of active and less-active barrels in the cortex. Experiments in the visual and barrel cortex suggest that the distance between the active and inactive cortical barrel-columns is important for determining the degree of plasticity induced (Wallace and Fox, 1999b). In the visual system, monocular deprivation sets up a pattern of cortical domains where each neuron in a deprived eye column is not more than 150–200 µm from the nearest open eye column: each closed eye ocular dominance column is surrounded by open eye ocular dominance columns and the columns themselves are approximately 300–500 µm wide (Hubel and Wiesel, 1977; Hubel *et al.*, 1978; Anderson *et al.*, 1988). In the barrel cortex, both potentiation of the spared-vibrissae responses and depression of the deprived-responses are known to decrease with distance from the spared barrel-column (Glazewski and Fox, 1996; Glazewski *et al.*, 1998a), which suggests that plasticity should be greater if every neuron in a deprived column is close to a spared or active input. Together these results suggest a mechanism for competition between sensory inputs. In the following sections, the evidence for

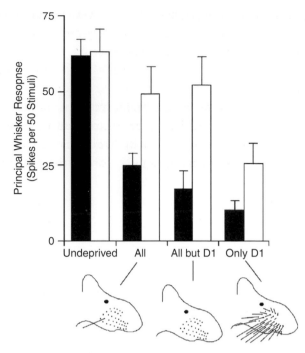

**Figure 7.4.** Evidence for heterosynaptic and homosynaptic depression mechanisms in layers II/III (black bars) and layer IV (white bars) of rat barrel cortex. Depression occurs when all the whiskers are removed (All) but greater depression occurs if only one is removed (Only D1). Chessboard deprivation (All but D1) achieves an intermediate level of depression for layers II/III. (Adapted from Fox *et al.* [1996b].)

local interactions affecting depression and potentiation of sensory responses is considered.

### 7.1.3    *Two components to depression of sensory responses*

Experiments where either all the whiskers are deprived simultaneously or just one single whisker is deprived have revealed two components to depression of sensory responses. Depriving all the whiskers simultaneously (or at least the major caudal ones on one side of the muzzle) causes depression of responses to the regrown whiskers, mainly in layers II/III (Glazewski *et al.*, 1998a). However, the depression is much greater if only one single whisker is deprived (Glazewski *et al.*, 1998a; Figure 7.4). This implies that simple inactivity (or at least decreased activity) is capable of depressing whisker responses, but that superimposed on this effect is the suppressive effect of the active whiskers. This result is conceptually similar to those obtained in the visual cortex, where binocular deprivation causes some depression of response to the deprived eyes (measured once the eyelids are reopened), but monocular deprivation causes far greater depression of the closed eye responses (Wiesel and Hubel, 1965). The general rule appears to be that depression occurs if all inputs are simultaneously removed but depression of deprived inputs is greater if other inputs remain.

Evidence that the proximity of spared and deprived cortical domains is a factor in active depression of deprived inputs by active inputs comes from experiments where a single whisker is spared and the others removed. In this case, the depression is greatest on the side of the barrel closer to the spared whisker's barrel-column (Glazewski and Fox, 1996). As discussed in Section 7.2, the interactions leading to depression are most likely cortical because plasticity is not expressed in the thalamus (Fox et al., 2002).

These results are corroborated by findings in animals deprived of whiskers in a chessboard pattern (Figure 7.2), where each deprived barrel is surrounded by a set of four active barrels. Again, no depression occurs in the thalamus, but the degree of depression in layer IV of the cortex is greater than would have been expected purely from removing all the whiskers (Wallace and Fox, 1999b). Confirmation of the cortical origin of the interactions leading to depression comes from studies where activity is blocked selectively in the cortex, which prevents cortical depression (Wallace et al., 2001). In conclusion, depression consists of two components; a component from the decreased activity in the pathway and a component from the activity contrasts between the deprived and spared inputs; both effects occur intracortically and both require cortical activity to occur.

### 7.1.4     Interactive and non-interactive potentiation of sensory responses

In the same way that it is possible to test whether active and inactive cortical domains interact by comparing the effect of different whisker deprivation patterns, so too can interactions between active domains be interrogated. At one extreme, just a single whisker is spared and all the others removed. This creates a single active domain in a "calm sea" of inactive barrels. Under these conditions, potentiation does occur in the surrounding deprived barrels after a period of approximately 18–20 days (Glazewski and Fox, 1996).

If several whiskers are spared, it opens up the possibility of interactions between neighboring active domains. In a chessboard pattern of deprivation, each deprived barrel-column is surrounded by four spared barrel-columns. The result is that potentiation in the deprived barrels occurs much faster than with a single spared whisker, occurring within seven days rather than 18 (Wallace and Fox, 1999a). Furthermore, potentiation occurs within layer IV as well as layers II/III in adolescent rats. This implies that there is a cooperative interaction between the spared vibrissae domains in the cortex which leads to increased potentiation. An interaction might occur through excitation, originating in the two or more spared columns, propagating to the deprived column, where it summates to produce a larger response than either input individually (Wallace and Fox, 1999a, b). Understanding whether this is feasible requires a closer look at the responses of cortical cells to whisker stimulation.

In a normal barrel cortex, cells respond in layer IV of the appropriate or principal barrel first, closely followed by cells in layer III then II of the same barrel-column 2–4 ms later. Excitation spreads to neighboring barrels, activating cells on the near side fully 7–10 ms earlier than cells on the far side (Armstrong-James *et al.*, 1992). In order for inputs originating in two active barrels to coincide in a deprived barrel, the stimuli would, therefore, need to be separated by 7–10 ms. This is feasible in an animal whisking at a rate of about 7 Hz and could be carried out by AMPA-mediated summation (Chapter 3). Facilitation of neighboring whisker responses occurs over periods of this order of magnitude (Shimegi *et al.*, 1999; Section 5.3.6). Integration over far longer time periods could be achieved by activation of NMDA receptor currents, which decay far more slowly (in the order of 100 ms).

If the active barrels are closer together, as they are in the undeprived animal, interactions can be very rapid as the difference in timing between activation of cells in layers II/III of the principal barrel (at 10.5–12.5 ms) and invasion of surround input on the near neighbor side of the barrel (at 13.0–13.5 ms) is only 0.5–3.5 ms (Armstrong-James *et al.*, 1992). This situation does not normally produce plasticity, of course, unless all but two whiskers are removed (Armstrong-James *et al.*, 1994). One possible reason for this is that lateral inhibition is able to suppress the cross-barrel excitation to a level that is not conducive to plasticity. The lateral inhibition can be alleviated, however, by whisker deprivation (Kelly *et al.*, 1999), and indeed where all but two whiskers have been deprived, potentiation of the spared-whisker response is seen in the neighboring spared barrel (Armstrong-James *et al.*, 1994).

### 7.1.5    Plasticity at different ages

Plasticity has been studied across a wider age range in barrel cortex than in other cortical areas. This enables an assessment of the similarities and differences between developmental plasticity mechanisms, on the one hand, and adult plasticity mechanisms, on the other, in the same animal. Three main periods of development have been studied in the barrel cortex: early postnatal, adolescent and adult.

#### 7.1.5.1    Early postnatal plasticity

The age at which an animal is born is somewhat arbitrary in relation to its development. Rodents are born relatively immature at a stage when the

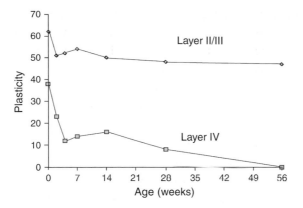

**Figure 7.5.** Critical period for layer IV plasticity in rat barrel cortex. Plasticity is measured as the percentage of cells in barrel-columns surrounding the D1 barrel-column that have greater responses to the spared D1 whisker than their own deprived principal whisker. Timepoints represent the start of a 60-day deprivation period. Layer II/III plasticity stays high throughout the first two months of life, while layer IV plasticity decreases rapidly during barrel formation (P0–P4) and gradually from P14 to P56. (Adapted from Fox [1992].)

cortex is incomplete and most cortical cells have not yet migrated to their final position (Chapter 4). The early postnatal period is the first postnatal week and for the rodent corresponds to a period of cortical development when many other mammals are still in utero. One of the consequences of this is that the brain is prone to the shaping influence of the external environment. Indeed, experiments have shown that experience does affect cortical development. During the first postnatal week, cortical plasticity is experience dependent and can be detected using physiological (Simons and Land, 1987; Fox, 1992), anatomical (Micheva and Beaulieu, 1995b) and behavioral (Carvell and Simons, 1996) methods. Chapter 4 and several reviews address this period of plasticity, which is, therefore, only dealt with briefly here (see also Fox [1995, 1996]).

The main thalamic input to layer IV develops into the characteristic barrel pattern over the first few postnatal days (Chapter 4). During this period, layer IV is at its most plastic. Lesion-induced plasticity in layer IV affects the disposition of presynaptic thalamocortical arbors and hence the barrel formation only if induced before P4 (Woolsey and Wann, 1976). Receptive field plasticity is greatest at P0 before the barrels are formed and decreases rapidly to a low level by P4 (Figure 7.5). During this period, thalamocortical afferents show a form of LTP, which involves conversion of silent synapses to active synapses (Crair and Malenka, 1995; Isaac et al., 1997; Chapter 4). The NMDA receptors appear to be involved in unmasking AMPA currents, perhaps by insertion of AMPA channels, and NMDA receptors are involved in lesion-induced plasticity as well as elimination of synaptic errors during development (Fox *et al.*, 1996a). Beyond that age, there is a progressive, decrease in the degree of plasticity observed in layer IV while plasticity in layers II/III is maintained almost at postnatal levels into adolescence (Fox, 1992).

### 7.1.5.2    *Plasticity in adolescents*

The adolescent period is a term used to describe a stage occurring approximately one or two months after birth in the rodent, when the major development of the cortex is complete, the animal's body is increasing rapidly in size and sexual maturity is reached. Not all aspects of neuronal development are complete, however, and some aspects of plasticity are present that will later disappear in older animals (Glazewski and Fox, 1996). The critical period for ocular dominance plasticity in the visual cortex occurs around this time (Fagiolini *et al.*, 1994). Because the visual system develops much later than the somatosensory system, and the critical period for the visual system occurs at approximately one month, it is reasonable to assume that barrel cortex plasticity at one to two months corresponds to a timepoint late in the critical period for the visual system (Fox, 1996).

Plasticity is less in all layers of the cortex at one to two months compared with the situation at birth (Fox, 1992), but layer IV plasticity decreases most and no longer shows anatomical plasticity, LTP, or experience-dependent plasticity with the single spared whisker paradigm at this age (Woolsey and Wann, 1976; Fox, 1992, 1996; Isaac *et al.*, 1997). The decrease in plasticity in layers II/III between birth and adolescence is small, however.

Adolescence is a useful age to study plasticity because the animals are still young enough to undergo substantial plasticity and, therefore, plasticity is relatively easy to measure, yet interventions do not evoke large-scale reorganization of connections. At this age, two different processes characterize plasticity, upregulation of the spared input (potentiation) and downregulation of the deprived input (depression). Depression of input from deprived whiskers appears to be restricted to the first two months of life and has not yet been detected in older animals (Glazewski and Fox, 1996). By comparison, potentiation of input from spared whiskers appears not to show a critical period in layers II/III of the barrel cortex and is present in adult animals (Glazewski and Fox, 1996; Glazewski *et al.*, 1998a).

### 7.1.5.3    *Plasticity in adulthood*

The beginning of the adult period has not been defined accurately in the rodent. In order to distinguish safely between adolescence and adulthood, a period around about 6 months of age has usually been taken as adult. This corresponds to an age at which 25% of the total lifespan has elapsed and is equivalent ratiometrically to about 20 years of age in a human or three or four years of age in a cat. The cortex is still plastic, up to about 15 months in a mouse, and it is not clear when plasticity really ends, if at all. At some point, senescence sets in, with the associated loss of function, but exactly when this occurs is not known. Researchers studying Alzheimer's disease and aging in rats and mice usually study animals not younger than 12–15 months (Chapman *et al.*, 1999).

The fact that experience-dependent plasticity is present in adult animals addresses one of the questions raised by the original work on lesion-induced plasticity, namely whether the lack of a critical period in somatosensory cortex in contrast with the clear critical period in visual cortex is a consequence of inducing the plasticity by injury rather than by experience. Clearly, somatosensory plasticity can occur through altered experience in the adult. The apparent difference between the two cortical systems can be attributed in part to the greater dependence of layer IV plasticity on age than is seen in layer II/III plasticity. Layer IV shows a critical period in both visual (Shatz and Stryker, 1978; LeVay *et al.*, 1980) and somatosensory (Fox, 1992) cortex, and recent work has shown that superficial layers of visual cortex show potentiation in mature animals (Sawtell *et al.*, 2003) in common with barrel cortex (Fox, 1992; Glazewski and Fox, 1996).

The most obvious difference between plasticity in adults and that in adolescents is that depression of deprived input is not present in adults. Depression, therefore, appears to show a late critical period ending somewhere between two and six months of age for the rodent (Glazewski and Fox, 1996). Potentiation is still present in layers II/III of the cortex, however, and plasticity is, therefore, a superimposition of the new representation on the old, rather than a replacement or realignment.

## 7.2 The locus of experience-dependent map plasticity

### 7.2.1 *Cortical versus subcortical locus*

In general, the critical period for subcortical plasticity tends to occur at younger ages than for cortical structures (Durham and Woolsey, 1984; Simons and Land, 1994), which means that age is a factor in defining the locus of plasticity. Here we begin by considering the adult case, which shows least subcortical experience-dependent plasticity if any at all.

There are four main arguments in favor of experience-dependent plasticity being cortical in origin, and these are based on the following observations: blocking cortical activity blocks cortical experience-dependent potentiation

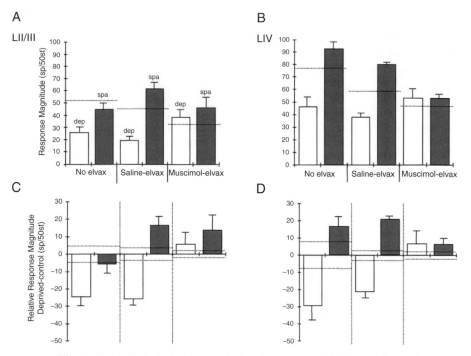

**Figure 7.6.** Effect of blocking cortical activity on potentiation and depression in rats deprived of whiskers in a chessboard pattern A, B. Average absolute response levels in three groups: animals without treatment of the cortex (no elvax); animals with elvax slow-release polymer implants containing saline (Saline-elvax) and animals with elvax doped with muscimol (GABA agonist; Muscimol-elvax). All animals receive chessboard deprivation for seven days. A. Layers II/III show significant differences between spared and deprived whiskers except for muscimol-treated animals. Dashed lines indicate baseline values of whisker response from undeprived animals for each group. B. Layer IV responses mainly show deprived-whisker depression and moderate potentiation. Depression and potentiation are prevented by muscimol treatment. C. Layers II/III: difference between control undeprived average responses and responses in treatment groups are shown. Dashed lines indicate standard errors for undeprived baseline condition. D. Muscimol treatment blocks depression in layer IV as with layers II/III. (Reproduced from Wallace *et al.* [2001] with permission of the Society for Neuroscience.)

and depression; paradigms that cause experience-dependent cortical plasticity do not cause subcortical plasticity; ablating specific cortical pathways prevents expression of experience-dependent plasticity; and whisker deprivation causes changes that can be observed directly in the cortex, such as changes in spine dynamics or changes in synaptic function.

The first argument and perhaps the strongest in favor of experience-dependent plasticity being cortical in origin is that if cortical activity is blocked by chronic muscimol application (Figure 7.6), neither potentiation nor depression occur

(Wallace *et al.*, 2001). Cortical activity blockade does not affect thalamic receptive fields either acutely or chronically, which could otherwise complicate interpretation. These result show that experience-dependent plasticity occurs in the cortex and that one need not postulate the existence of subcortical plasticity to explain the effects of whisker deprivation on cortical receptive fields. Nevertheless, it is conceivable that subcortical plasticity occurs but that the effect is not relayed on to the cortex. In order to test this idea, it is necessary to record sensory responses in the thalamus following whisker deprivation.

Studies that test for thalamic experience-dependent plasticity have shown that VPm neurons exhibit almost identical responses to spared and deprived whiskers following deprivation when compared with control and compared with each other (Armstrong-James and Callahan, 1991; Fox *et al.*, 1996b; Glazewski *et al.*, 1998a; Wallace *et al.*, 2001). With chessboard pattern deprivation (Figure 7.2), the differences between spared and deprived responses diverge as the responses are transmitted from thalamus to cortex. In the thalamus, the responses to the spared and deprived whisker are the same; at the next stage of relay in layer IV of the cortex, spared-whisker responses increase 17% while deprived-whiskers responses decrease 35%. At the next stage, in layers II/III outside the principal barrel in the near neighboring barrel, spared-whisker responses increase by 120% and responses to deprived principal whiskers decrease by 48% (Wallace and Fox, 1999a).

The fact that thalamic responses are not affected by deprivation while their target cells in layer IV are affected suggests that plasticity occurs at the cortical or thalamocortical level rather than within the thalamus. However, it is possible that, while individual thalamic cells show similar responses before and after deprivation, the number of cells responding to whisker stimulation within the thalamus changes. Therefore, a second measure of subcortical plasticity is to estimate the area over which responses to spared and deprived whiskers can be recorded in the thalamus. This can be achieved by measuring the distance between the spared-whisker representations and the distance between the deprived-whisker representations (i.e. the domains of each). Studies show that the distance between spared and deprived whisker domains within the thalamus are not affected by whisker deprivation (Fox *et al.*, 2002), ruling out thalamic domain changes as a possible source of thalamic plasticity.

The third piece of evidence in favor of plasticity being cortical in origin comes from studies where plasticity has been induced in the cortex and measured, then selectively abolished in a particular location in the cortex by a small lesion. If an animal has all but one whisker removed for a period of time, responses to the D1 whisker increase in all the barrels immediately surrounding the D1 barrel. However, any response to the spared D1 whisker can be abolished by ablating the D1 barrel (Fox, 1994), implying that the potentiated response is routed through the D1 barrel (Figure 7.7). An internal control is provided by the principal whisker response, which is unaffected by the lesion. That the potentiated response is transmitted radially from the spared barrel-column becomes clear from studies where lesions are made in a row along the septum between two neighboring barrels. In this case, the potentiated D1 response is lost in the barrel severed from the spared whisker's barrel, but not in an unsevered barrel (Figure 7.7). This approach serves as a useful internal control to check that the lesion does not prevent responses by causing non-specific damage. The principal whisker responses are unaffected in the same cases, again arguing for a specific effect on the D1 whisker response. If plasticity had been subcortical in origin (i.e. the D1 information had diverged subcortically), one would have expected some component of the D1 whisker response to have survived the cortical barrel lesion. The fact that it does not implies that plasticity occurs beyond the spared whisker's principal barrel in the cortex.

The fourth piece of evidence comes from studies which demonstrated that the function of particular pathways within the cortex is affected by whisker deprivation. These studies provided direct evidence of cortical components of plasticity rather than evidence against changes elsewhere. First, it has been shown that spines and filopodia protrude and retract during development, presumably sampling space to search for presynaptic terminals or perhaps in response to the proximity of a growing presynaptic growth cone. A proportion of synapses continue this process into adolescence and even at a lower rate in adulthood (Trachtenberg et al., 2002). However, in an animal undergoing chessboard pattern whisker deprivation, it has been shown that spines in superficial layers of the barrel cortex increase their rate of turnover even further. These spines may be on apical dendrites of layer V and layer II/III cells.

Finally, it is known that altering whisker patterns for a few days causes changes in the layer IV to layers II/III pathway in the cortex that can be seen in cortical slices prepared from the whisker-deprived animals. Depression of miniature EPSPs and evoked EPSPs, and decreases in the paired pulse ratio all occur in the responses of layer II/III cells in the deprived column (Finnerty et al., 1999; Allen et al., 2003; Celikel et al., 2004). Furthermore, changes in the ability to undergo LTP and LTD occur. Depriving all the whiskers causes an increase in the magnitude of LTP in the cortex and a reduction in the probability and magnitude of LTD (Figure 6.9).

In conclusion, there is substantial evidence that plasticity does occur in intracortical pathways and that it does not occur with the same manipulations in subcortical pathways. This is not to say, however, that plasticity cannot be produced in subcortical structures; this certainly occurs at younger ages

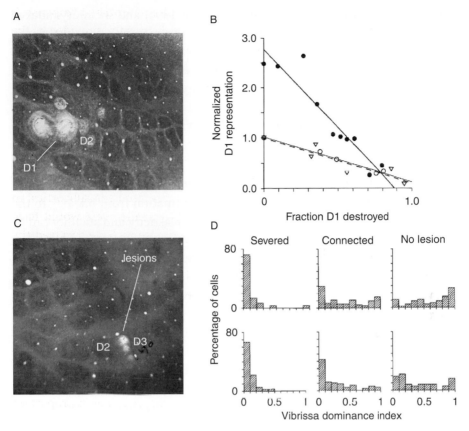

**Figure 7.7.** Effect of lesioning cortical pathways on expression of plasticity. A. Two large lesions destroy most of the D1 barrel. The small lesions correspond to marks made at the end of recording tracks around D1. B. The normalized response of cells in barrel-columns immediately surrounding D1 to stimulation of the D1 whisker as a function of the fraction of D1 destroyed by the lesion(s). Data on the effect of lesion size in normal undeprived animals from Fox (1994) (open circles, full line) and Armstrong-James *et al.* (1992) (open triangles, dashed line). Steep line filled circles: effect of D1 lesion size in animals reared with just D1 from birth to 60 days of age. Note that the response is approximately three times greater in unlesioned deprived animals (points at $x = 0$). Responses decrease to the same levels as undeprived animals when 80% of the barrel is ablated, indicating a cortical origin for plasticity. C. Septal lesions between the D2 and D3 barrel. Note that D2 and D3 are severed, but D2 and D1, for example, and many other pairs remain connected. D. Vibrissa dominance histograms for cells in barrel-columns severed from the spared column (Severed) or still connected (Connected) or in animals without lesions but with deprivation (No lesion). A value of 0 indicates the cells only respond to the principal whisker, a value of 1 only the D1 whisker and a value of 0.5 equally to both D1 and the principal whisker. Acute septal lesions shift the distribution away from the spared whisker to the principal whisker (shift left) for severed but not for connected barrels (recorded in the same animals). (A,B,D adapted from Fox [1994] with permission from the Society for Neuroscience.)

(Durham and Woolsey, 1984; Simons and Land, 1994) and in injury-induced plasticity (Section 7.5). Nevertheless, provided the manipulation just causes changes in experience, or in fact more directly activity in afferent pathways leading to the cortex, the cortex is sensitive to these alterations and responds by altering receptive field properties and plasticity properties accordingly. One question these studies raise is what pathways are responsible for experience-dependent plasticity, and this topic is addressed in the next section.

### 7.2.2    Pathways for plasticity

Plasticity is a useful property of a system, but clearly so too is stability, especially in a system that processes similar information from one day to the next like the barrel cortex. The balance between plasticity and stability can be achieved in a number of ways; for example, a subsystem of cells might form a scaffold of stable connections, with other pathways more specialized for plasticity. Alternatively, all cells could be plastic but the threshold for plasticity be set quite high in mature animals. Hybrids of these two strategies are also conceivable, and in fact there is some evidence for both ideas. In favor of specialized plastic connections, neurons in layer IV and in particular thalamocortical connections appear to be less plastic than layer II/III cells in adult animals (Glazewski and Fox, 1996). Conversely, in favor of high thresholds for plasticity, in adolescent rats, layer IV cells show little depression of principal whisker responses in deprived barrels with single-whisker experience, but significant depression in the deprived barrel with chessboard deprivation (Glazewski and Fox, 1996; Wallace and Fox, 1999a; Figure 7.4). In the following sections we consider the candidate pathways.

#### 7.2.2.1    Pathways for potentiation and horizontal spread

One of the salient features of experience-dependent plasticity is that the cortical domain occupied by the spared input spreads horizontally into neighboring columns (Figure 7.1). One way of determining which pathways are involved is to see whether lesions of particular horizontal pathways prevent expression of plasticity. Lesions of the septal region lying between the edges of two neighboring barrels have been found to be sufficient to prevent horizontal transmission of information between the two barrels (Fox, 1994). The specificity of this effect is clear from the finding that recordings made from the same animal in a neighboring barrel that had not been cut off by a septal region still received input from that barrel (Figure 7.7). In these examples, the animal has been reared with just the D1 vibrissa intact, which leads to potentiated responses in surrounding barrels (Fox, 1992). The septal lesions are, therefore, able to eliminate the potentiated responses in surrounding barrels and in fact reduce the D1 vibrissa representation to less than that found in a normally reared animal (Fox, 1994). These data suggest that a horizontal pathway exists between barrels that can, under certain rearing conditions, be potentiated.

Considerable evidence exists for horizontal pathways in the cortex. Bernardo *et al.*, (1990a,b) have shown that injections within barrels lead to a radiating pattern of horizontally projecting fibers in the cortex, which stretch furthest in extragranular layers. Other experiments in rats have shown that septal locations contain a pattern of linked horizontal pathways within layer IV (Hoeflinger *et al.*, 1995; Kim and Ebner, 1999). It is noticeable that there is little projection from the septal layer IV cells back into the neighboring barrel-column, however, which suggests horizontal spread via the septal regions probably links back into the neighboring barrels via their connections with supragranular layers. Given that several horizontal pathways exist for plasticity, one can ask whether they are all plastic or whether some specialized pathways are plastic.

Experiments examining LTP have shown that stimulating electrode locations are far more effective at evoking LTP in superficial layers if they are positioned in the septum/barrel wall of layer IV rather than in the center of the barrel (Glazewski *et al.*, 1998b). Furthermore, potentiation can be induced in a neighboring barrel on the near side but not the far side of the barrel. This suggests that diagonal pathways emanating from layer IV septum/barrel walls and reaching as far as the near side of the neighboring barrels are capable of potentiating, and, therefore, they are potentially involved in cortical plasticity. One complicating factor is that the targets of these layer IV cells (i.e. the layer II/III pyramidal neurons) have dendrites that reach more than 200 μm and hence stretch outside the limits of the barrel-column, at least in the mouse barrel cortex. This means that neurons of the supragranular layer can receive vertical input from their principal barrel and at least one adjacent barrel. In this sense, the diagonal pathways between layer IV and layers II/III referred to above, where it was envisaged that axons travel from one barrel to another, may be supplemented by vertical projections within the column on to distal dendrites of cells reaching over from adjacent barrels.

There are few studies detailing single cell pathways within barrel cortex. However, Lorente de Nó (1992) has shown a number of examples of pathways within barrel cortex using Golgi staining. Many cells drawn in that study projected to layer III from a horizontally displaced site within layers III, IV or V. Examples are picked out and simplified in Figure 7.8. Notice that the layer III projections are recurrent collaterals of axons projecting out of the barrel field; they branch within layer IV before making a diagonal track to layers II/III. Layer IV cells with dendrites within particular barrels also send a descending axon

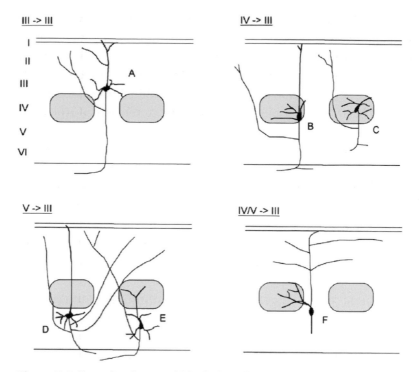

**Figure 7.8.** Lateral pathways within the barrel cortex for transmission between barrel-columns. A number of examples are redrawn in a simplified form from drawings of Golgi-stained sections of cortex by Lorente de Nó (1992) and the links to the original figure numbers in that paper are given. Top left. An example of a layer III pyramidal cell projection from the septal region into a neighboring barrel (similar to Figure 4 neurons B and C and Figure 5 neurons E and D). Top right. Two examples of layer IV projections, into a neighboring column (B) or septum (C) (B is similar to Figure 5 neuron A, and C to Figure 9 neuron A). Bottom left. Examples of two pyramidal cells projecting from layer V into neighboring columns (D is similar to Figure 14 neuron A and E to Figure 16 neuron C). Bottom right. Example of a cell located at the bottom of layer V with dendrites in a barrel and descending into layers V/VI and which projects to its own and neighboring barrel-column (similar to Figure 11, neuron A). (Reproduced from Fox [2002] with permission from Oxford University Press.)

that forms a collateral within layer V and projects to layers II/III. Several examples of inverted pyramidal cells at the bottom of layer IV are also shown where their main axonal projection is directed to superficial layers where it branches to send off horizontal fibers within layers II/III. Finally, layer V cells project axons out of the cortex but send diagonally oriented recurrent collaterals to neighboring columns in supragranular layers.

A septal lesion in layer IV could have severed each of the pathways represented by these examples (Figure 7.8). Similarly, they could all have been activated by the electrical stimulus that evoked LTP in neighboring layers II/III, either directly or via axons of passage. However, though these represent the most direct pathways, it should be borne in mind that other polysynaptic routes may also have been affected. It is also likely that other pathways exist which have yet to be catalogued.

Layer V cells themselves also show high levels of interconnectivity, which might account for horizontal spread. Layer V to V synapses can potentiate or depress when tested with spike pairing protocols (Markram and Tsodyks, 1996; Sjostrom et al., 2003). Layer V cells also show similar experience-dependent plasticity to the layer II/III cells in that they exhibit depression of their center receptive fields and potentiation of their surrounds. However, a difference exists between the IB and RS cells with only IB cells showing potentiation (Petreanu et al., 2007). Given that layer V cells are highly connected between columns, one pathway for lateral spread could be via multisynaptic layer V connections, and these may potentiate during experience-dependent plasticity. In conclusion, a number of pathways exist for horizontal spread of information between columns that are capable of synaptic plasticity. One challenge in the future will be to see which of these are involved in experience-dependent plasticity, bearing in mind of course that several may be.

### 7.2.2.2    *Pathways for depression and vertical spread*

The first clue about the natural sequence of information processing within the cortex came from studying the latency of response of neurons within the barrel field to a brief stimulus. A full account of latency analysis and the natural sequence of cortical activation can be found in Section 5.2.3. The earliest responses following whisker stimulation occur in the principal barrel itself within layer IV and layer Vb and responses then radiate out into the surrounding barrels over the next 20–30 ms or so. The first relay is within the column to layer II/III cells, and since the layer Vb recurrent collaterals' projection to layers II/III is not as strong or as focused within a column as that from layer IV, supragranular layer excitation at this early stage is likely to be from layer IV. This pathway is, therefore, highly likely to be the one responsible for depression during whisker deprivation since layer II/III cells show far more depression than layer IV cells if they show depression at all (Glazewski and Fox, 1996). This view is supported by studies that show that LTD can be produced quite readily in vertical connections from layer IV to layers II/III in normal animals, and yet LTD is occluded in the same pathway in whisker-deprived animals both in the rat and mouse (Allen et al., 2003; see also Chapter 6).

Layer V cells in deprived columns also show center receptive field (principal whisker) depression following whisker deprivation. Part of this depression may originate from depression of thalamocortical inputs on to the layer Vb cells. However, it has also been shown that a projection from layers II/III to layer Vb is also depressed after 10 days of whisker deprivation (Petreanu *et al.*, 2007). In conclusion, principal whisker pathways travel within the column and can depress in at least two locations, between layers IV and II/III and between layers II/III and Vb. Other pathways are likely to be involved but have not yet been studied at the cellular level.

### 7.2.3    *Traces of plasticity following deprivation*

Finally, one further type of study that has yielded information on the cortical origin of experience-dependent plasticity involves ex vivo investigations where the effect of deprivation on synaptic physiology and connectivity can be seen in a slice of barrel cortex maintained in a recording chamber. Whisker deprivation can be imposed at a certain age to alter the animal's experience and the effect of altered experience can then be observed in a slice preparation of the affected circuits in barrel cortex. Remarkably, the changes caused by experience are robust enough to survive the effect of preparing the slice. The fact that plasticity leaves a robust trace in the slice is more understandable where experiments have been performed on younger animals during development of intracortical circuits. In these cases, deprivation would be expected to cause a lasting structural change in the tissue. However, other experiments have been performed in older animals where the structural changes, though present, are more modest, and yet traces of plasticity can still be observed.

In developing animals (P11–P15), layer II/III to II/III horizontal pathways are altered by deprivation of two rows of whiskers (Finnerty *et al.*, 1999). Connections between pyramidal cells show increased depression of short-term dynamics (Section 6.1.4) when they link spared to deprived columns compared with those linking deprived to deprived columns. As discussed in Chapter 6, this could be indicative of a presynaptic LTP-type process occurring in the spared to deprived pathways during deprivation. Vertical pathways are also affected by deprivation, with the layer IV to II connections showing greater depression of EPSPs at 5–10 Hz than control in spared columns (Finnerty *et al.*, 1999). Again this could be indicative of presynaptic potentiation in the IV to II pathway. Curiously, signatures indicative of both potentiation and depression tend to occur in animals with all their whiskers deprived from P14 to P16 (Shepherd *et al.*, 2003). If photolytic release of caged glutamate is used to stimulate the presynaptic cells in layer IV, EPSPs in layer II/III cells in spared barrel-columns tend to be weaker than those in normally reared animals, while layer IV to layers II/III pathways are stronger in septal columns. The reduction in barrel-column transmission explains the reduction in principal whisker input seen in whole animal recordings in (Fox, 1992). The consequences of an increase in septal-column transmission are not known at present, but again, given that septal cells may link to surrounding barrels via their horizontal connections (Hoeflinger *et al.*, 1995), they could provide a substrate for horizontal expansion of spared-whisker domains.

In older animals, where the deprivation has been started beyond the critical period for layer IV (Van der Loos and Woolsey, 1973) or layer II/III (Woolsey and Wann, 1976; Stern *et al.*, 2001) development, traces of plasticity can still be seen in a slice preparation of barrel cortex. For example, depriving a single row of whiskers occludes LTD in the layer IV to layer II/III pathway of the rat cortex within the deprived column but not in the spared column (Allen *et al.*, 2003). The same effect can be seen in mouse barrel cortex, where total whisker deprivation from four weeks of age has the effect of reducing the probability of LTD induction from approximately 80% to less than 30%, and simultaneously increasing the probability of LTP from approximately 30% to 70% (Hardingham and Fox, 2007). These ex vivo experiments imply that the synapses have changed state in some sense as a result of the deprivation. One likely explanation is that whisker deprivation causes depression of the synapses (experience-dependent depression) and so they are unable to undergo any further depression (LTD) in the slice. Conversely, if the synapses are depressed by deprivation then they are more likely to repotentiate than before and the probability of LTP increases.

These studies provide further evidence that the layer IV to layers II/III pathway and the horizontal supragranular layer pathways are involved in cortical plasticity. One of the questions it will be important to address in the future is what other pathways show plasticity and how they interact as a circuit to produce the effect seen in whole animal recordings.

## 7.3    Early-phase molecular mechanisms of map plasticity

The concept of plasticity involves an implicit dualism; on the one hand, it obviously involves mechanisms that instigate and conduct change but it also implies the existence of mechanisms that resist change and confer some level of stability. In considering molecular mechanisms for plasticity, there is a need to explore mechanisms that instigate synaptic plasticity, but also to explore those that confer stability in all other circumstances. Stability in this sense is, of course, a relative term and might involve relatively short periods of absolute stability or a level of dynamic stability where the population remains constant while individual synapses change.

A good deal of progress has been made into the candidate plasticity mechanisms of LTP and LTD, which induce plasticity and express it during its early phases (Chapter 4). It is envisaged that these rapid processes allow synapses to be selected and altered in function over time spans of hours. Insertion and removal of AMPA receptors from the synaptic membrane, alterations in AMPA phosphorylation state and changes in presynaptic proteins associated with release are likely to be involved in these early stages of plasticity. However, to cause lasting changes in synaptic function, the mechanisms involved are likely to be different because phosphorylation events, for example, are too easily reversed by dephosphorylation to last very long. The issue of how molecules retain stable structure over months and years is of course the long-standing question in biology of how form is maintained despite continual molecular turnover. Given the far greater lifetime of larger-scale neuronal structures such as dendrites and synapses compared with those of proteins and phosphorylation states, it is likely that long-term plasticity will involve changes at the structural level. Nevertheless, rapid plasticity mechanisms still have essential features for the early stages of plasticity such as the ability to detect and change in response to correlated neuronal activity.

In the following sections, we begin by reviewing the evidence of whether early-phase plasticity factors, more often associated with LTP and LTD (Chapter 6), are involved in experience-dependent plasticity in vivo (Section 7.3.1). What is the evidence that NMDA receptors and calcium-dependent postsynaptic enzymes are involved in real experience-dependent plasticity? This leads on to the subject of Section 7.3.2, regarding late-phase plasticity, including anatomical plasticity, for which there are presently some clues about the molecular mechanism involved.

### 7.3.1    NMDA receptors

There are some limits to what can be determined in vivo about the role of postsynaptic NMDA receptors in cortical plasticity. While it is clear that cortical activity per se is important as the instigator of cortical plasticity, it is not easy to demonstrate that the usual pathway by which this is achieved in vitro (i.e. via the NMDA receptor; Chapter 6), is also the critical pathway in vivo. The problem arises because the postsynaptic NMDA receptors are involved in normal synaptic transmission in the neocortex. This means that blocking NMDA receptors with an NMDA antagonist can cause a decrease in sensory responses in the same way as, for example, a small dose of GABA agonist would also decrease sensory responses. This problem is avoided in vitro because NMDA receptors are not activated substantially under the condition in which cells in the slice operate, except during high-frequency stimulation. Therefore, blocking NMDA receptors does not affect the baseline synaptic responses. In vivo, baseline sensory responses are definitely reduced by NMDA receptor antagonist, and since any factor decreasing transmission of sensory information would be likely to affect plasticity, NMDA receptors are no exception; however, unfortunately, because of this, neither can they be shown to have a special role in plasticity by this method.

Ideally, there would be a way of distinguishing between the role of postsynaptic NMDA receptors as a non-specific cation channel allowing transmission of excitation, and their role in allowing calcium into the spine to trigger plasticity. In an attempt to avoid this problem, experimenters have tried to change activity minimally with NMDA receptor antagonists and see whether this affects plasticity substantially. In the barrel cortex, superfusing the cortex with 500 mmol/l APV reduced the long-latency components of sensory responses without acutely affecting the main short-latency response to stimulation (Rema et al., 1998). This procedure prevented plasticity of surround receptive fields in layer IV, but curiously not that in layer II/III cells, which is a major site for cortical plasticity (Rema et al., 1998). In the visual cortex, injection of a low dose of MK801 (glutamate receptor antagonist) caused a decrease in the amount of ocular dominance plasticity with a significant effect on a minority (23%) of cells' cortical visual responses to stimulation (Daw et al., 1999). While these studies provide some indication that NMDA receptors are doing more than just adding to depolarization of the cell, they are not conclusive. A different tactic is to look at the calcium-triggered pathways downstream of the NMDA receptor that are associated with the molecule on the cytoplasmic side (Husi et al., 2000). With the advent of knockout technology, it has become clear that calcium-sensitive enzymes are required for cortical experience-dependent plasticity (such as CaMKII and calcineurin). The calcium must come from somewhere – possibly from NMDA receptor activity (Glazewski et al., 1996; Yang et al., 2005). A few of these molecular pathways are explored in the following sections.

### 7.3.2    Calcium-calmodulin-dependent kinase type II

The first evidence that CaMKII might be involved in experience-dependent plasticity came from studies in the barrel cortex (Glazewski et al., 1996). The idea that CaMKII might be involved in plasticity has a long history. The "Lisman–Kennedy switch" hypothesis has been discussed in the literature for a number of years as a possible molecular mechanism for maintaining potentiation at synapses. The idea is that CAMKII forms a molecular switch, which is activated by postsynaptic calcium/calmodulin, autophosphorylates and becomes calcium independent and thereby functional for an extended period of time (Lisman, 1985; Miller and Kennedy, 1986; Lisman and Goldring, 1988). This allows the forward reaction of phosphorylation to outpace the reverse dephosphorylation reaction and could, in principle, create a switch to a stable autophosphorylation state maintaining LTP. In support of this idea, αCAMKII appears to be necessary for LTP in the hippocampus (Silva *et al.*, 1992) and neocortex (Kirkwood *et al.*, 1997), is able to phosphorylate AMPA receptors and is well situated to affect plasticity as it forms some 16% of the postsynaptic density (Miller and Kennedy, 1985; Barria *et al.*, 1997).

Experience-dependent plasticity in the barrel cortex has also been found to be dependent on αCAMKII, raising the possibility that experience-dependent potentiation mechanisms may be related to LTP mechanisms. Potentiation of spared-whisker responses occurs in neurons located in layers II/III of wild-type adult mice but not in null mutants lacking a functional gene for αCAMKII (Glazewski *et al.*, 1996).

As mentioned above, a key component of the Lisman hypothesis is that the molecule retains a "memory" of past synaptic activity by phosphorylating itself. The Thr-286 site is where autophosphorylation normally occurs. In order to test the Lisman switch hypothesis, it is necessary to see whether synaptic potentiation can be induced in an animal with normal levels of αCAMKII but lacking the autophosphorylation site in that enzyme. In this way, one can distinguish between the more general kinase function of the molecule and its specific postulated role in maintaining potentiation over an extended period of time at the synapse. Altering threonine to alanine at position 286 thereby preventing CAMKII autophosphorylation, also prevents the induction of LTP in CA1 and leads to severe impairments on behavioral tests that are sensitive to hippocampal lesions (Giese *et al.*, 1998). This evidence suggests that αCAMKII autophosphorylation is necessary for LTP and that LTP itself is required for hippocampus-dependent learning and memory. Results in the barrel cortex have shown that threonine at position 286 is also necessary for experience-dependent plasticity (Figure 7.9). Potentiation does not occur in animals with two copies of the mutated allele (Glazewski *et al.*, 2000).

The "Lisman switch" molecule may play an essential role in bridging the time between postsynaptic calcium entry and secondary changes required to maintain potentiation, but it is unlikely that a kinase could produce a change for longer than a matter of hours; phosphorylase activity would eventually dephosphorylate CAMKII, returning it to its original form. One idea is that in order for plasticity to last longer, de novo protein synthesis, of channels, enzymes or structural proteins, is required following induction of plasticity. The longer lifetime of these molecules would increase the lifetime of the plastic changes (Davis and Squire, 1984), as explored in Section 7.4.2.

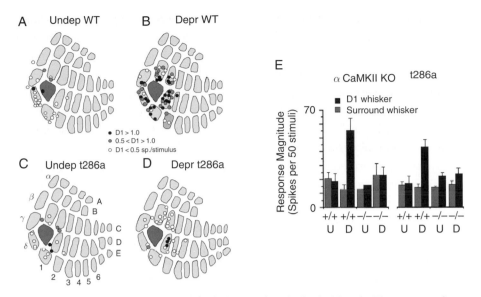

**Figure 7.9.** Lack of plasticity in layers II/III of mice lacking the Thr-286 autophos-phorylation site on calcium-calmodulin protein kinase II α-subunit (αCaMKII) in adolescent mice. A. Spared D1 whisker domain for an undeprived (Undep) wild-type animal. Each circle represents an average response to D1 for several cells located in a single penetration through layers II/III (see key). B. Cells respond more powerfully to D1 following 18 days of deprivation (Depr) of all but the D1 vibrissa. C. Undeprived mutants with altered Thr-286 (to Ala; t286a). D. There is no potentiation of the D1 responses in the point mutants. E. Average responses to D1 (black bars) and a surround receptive field whisker (grey bars) summed for layers II/III in two αCaMKII mutants. Left. In the αCaMKII knockouts (KO), potentiation does not occur in the null mutants (−/−) but does in the deprived wild-type (+/+) littermates (U, undeprived; D, deprived). Right. In the point mutants, again potentiation is prevented in the mutants but not in the wild-type littermates. (Adapted from Glazewski *et al.* [2000] with permission of the *Nature Publishing Group*.)

### 7.3.3    *Protein kinase A*

Protein kinase A is not involved in cortical LTP nor experience-dependent potentiation in the same way as CaMKII. Inhibition of PKA does not affect the magnitude of LTP in the IV to II/III pathway in mouse barrel cortex, whereas LTP is not possible in this pathway in the CaMKII Thr-286 mutants (Hardingham *et al.*, 2003; Hardingham and Fox, 2007). However, following whisker deprivation, LTP is larger in magnitude and sensitive to inhibition of PKA (see Figure 6.9). Because whisker deprivation causes depression of synapses, one explanation is that the extra ability to undergo LTP is created by depressing synapses that would otherwise be too potentiated to potentiate any further. In other words, whisker deprivation causes desaturation. Several other studies have found that it is difficult to obtain LTP in undeprived barrel cortex without having first produced LTD (Urban *et al.*, 2002; Froc and Racine, 2005). This implies that in normal barrel cortex many of the synapses are saturated with respect to LTP, having already undergone an LTP-like process previously. To produce potentiation from this condition requires that some or many of the synapses be first depressed to a lower state from which potentiation can occur. If this argument is correct, then the further inference is that potentiation from the depressed state requires PKA while potentiation from the basal state does not.

### 7.3.4    *Kinase substrates: glutamate receptor subunit 1*

The GluR1 subunit of the AMPA channel is an obvious substrate for CaMKII and PKA that might affect plasticity as it contains phosphorylation sites for both kinases and can directly control transmission at the glutamatergic synapse. The AMPA channel is able to affect plasticity either by insertion of new GluR1 subunits into the synaptic membrane (Hayashi *et al.*, 2000) or by changing the AMPA conduction state (Barria *et al.*, 1997); both processes are CaMKII dependent. Studies have shown that knocking out the GluR1 subunit of the AMPA channel reduces LTP during the first few minutes post-tetanus (Hoffman *et al.*, 2002; Hardingham and Fox, 2006). However, potentiation eventually reaches levels similar to that seen in wild types. Quantal analysis reveals that this is because GluR1 is responsible for the postsynaptic component of potentiation and does not affect a prominent presynaptic component present at the layer IV to layers II/III pathway in the barrel cortex (Hardingham and Fox, 2006).

The presynaptic element of LTP is mediated by activation of nitric oxide synthase, which is both a CaMKII substrate (Bredt *et al.*, 1992; Watanabe *et al.*, 2003) and the source of the retrograde messenger nitric oxide, which has been implicated in LTP by several studies (e.g. Son *et al.*, 1996). Blocking postsynaptic nitric oxide synthase prevents presynaptic potentiation in the wild-type animals while leaving the postsynaptic component intact. Blocking the enzyme in the GluR1 knockouts blocks all LTP by abolishing the only component of plasticity present in these animals: the presynaptic component of LTP (Chapter 6).

The mechanisms involved in PKA-dependent potentiation could also act via the GluR1 subunit of the AMPA channel. It is possible that such depression causes dephosphorylation of the AMPA channel subunit GluR1 at the Ser-845 site. Phosphorylation at the Ser-845 site then increases the open time through the AMPA channel (Banke *et al.*, 2000) and could this explain the LTP unmasked by whisker deprivation and LTD (Chapter 6). Correlates of this process can be found in the visual cortex where monocular deprivation decreases phosphorylation of the Ser-845 site. In visual cortex, PKA plays an important role in ocular dominance plasticity. Knocking out the regulatory subunit of PKA (RIIβ) abolishes LTD and almost all the ocular dominance plasticity in the visual cortex (Fischer *et al.*, 2004). Knocking out the RIIα or RIβ isoform of PKA (Hensch *et al.*, 1998b; Rao *et al.*, 2004) does not have the same effect, possibly because of the associations of the RIIβ isoform with the postsynaptic density protein Yotiao and hence NMDA receptors (Kurokawa *et al.*, 2004).

An alternative explanation is that deprivation causes the production of new immature synapses that require PKA for potentiation, unlike the more mature synapses. Certainly, whisker deprivation in a chessboard pattern has been shown to increase the number of new synapses, or at least filopodia, even in older animals (Trachtenberg *et al.*, 2002). A number of studies have shown that immature synapses potentiate via a PKA-dependent mechanism in hippocampus and a developmental switch to a more mature form occurs later in life (Yasuda *et al.*, 2003). Similarly, developing thalamocortical synapses require PKA to potentiate in young barrel cortex (Lu *et al.*, 2003). It is possible, therefore, that the PKA-dependent potentiation occurs at a subset of newly formed synapses generated during the deprivation period.

Reversal of phosphorylation of GluR1 (i.e. dephosphorylation at either the CaMKII or the PKA site) could also play a role in plasticity by depressing synaptic responses. There is some evidence for this in the visual cortex, where monocular deprivation leads to a lower level of GluR1 phosphorylation at the PKA site than normal (Heynen *et al.*, 2003). In the barrel cortex, it has been found that knockout of the GluR1 subunit of the AMPA channel prevents the depression of synaptic responses that normally accompanies whisker deprivation. Deprivation of all but a single spared whisker in an adolescent mouse leads to selective depression of layer II/III responses but not layer IV responses to whisker stimulation, which implicates the pathway from layer IV to layers II/III in depression (Section 7.2). However, depression does not occur in GluR1 knockout mice undergoing the same whisker deprivation, demonstrating that experience-dependent depression requires GluR1 (Figure 7.10). The GluR1 knockout does not affect potentiation as severely as depression however, presumably because the alternative mechanisms of potentiation via nitric oxide are still present to produce potentiation (Hardingham and Fox, 2006).

## 7.4    Late-phase plasticity: gene expression and structural changes

Late-phase plasticity is envisaged as a process that occurs after the initial plasticity events at the synapse and leads to longer-lasting structural

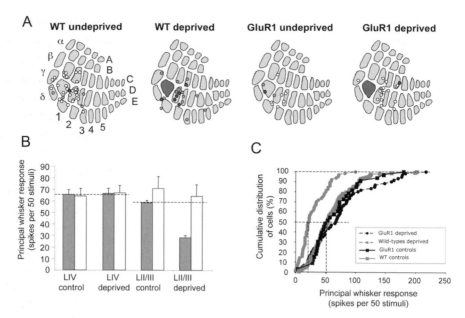

**Figure 7.10.** Lack of depression in knockout mutants for the glutamate receptor subunit 1 (GluR1). A. Penetration maps are shown as with Figures 7.1 and 7.9 except in this case for principal whisker responses. Penetrations are coded for strong responses in white and low responses in black (white, >1 spike/stimulus; grey, 0.5–1.0 spike/stimulus; black < 0.5 spikes/stimulus). Note that in wild types (WT), depression occurs in animals deprived of all but the D1 vibrissa (WT deprived). However, responses are at normal levels in GluR1 knockouts receiving the same treatment. B. Average principal whisker response levels for layer IV and layer II/III cells in deprived and undeprived animals. Dashed line indicates the responses in undeprived wild types (grey bars). Note that no depression occurs in layer IV at this age (one month) with a D1-spared deprivation pattern, but it does occur in layers II/III of wild types. No depression occurs in layers II/III of GluR1 knockouts (white bars). C. Cumulative distribution function for responses of all cells in layers II/III and IV of wild types and knockouts. Note that only the distribution for wild-type layer II/III cells shifts left with deprivation (lower responses levels) and is unaffected in GluR1 knockouts (see key). (Adapted from Wright *et al.* [2007].)

changes, which are less susceptible to the effects of molecular turnover and involve much larger assemblies of molecules than early-phase plasticity. De novo gene expression is one method by which the effects of molecular turnover can be overcome and indeed may be required to sustain structural scale changes in the synapses.

There are two broad categories of late-phase plasticity to consider. First is the case where synapses are relatively stable and changes in transmission endure for long periods after the initial plasticity events. In this situation, no structural plasticity is required for plasticity to endure. Second is the case where synapses are potentially short lived and early-phase plasticity serves to determine whether the synapse endures or is discarded. Most synapses are stable and only somewhere between 5 and 20% are short lived in the barrel cortex, meaning that they appear or disappear with 24 hours (Trachtenberg *et al.*, 2002; Zuo *et al.*, 2005a). Similar turnover rates have been observed in adult primate visual cortex (Stettler *et al.*, 2006). Short-lived and stable synapses are, therefore, sufficiently prevalent to require consideration of both in a theory that accounts for experience-dependent plasticity. At present, it is simply not known whether short-lived synapses are sufficient to account for experience-dependent plasticity in cortex, and it may be safer to assume that selection of the short-lived synapses and modulation of the stable synapses are both involved. If new synapses are formed, it is likely that gene expression and de novo protein synthesis are involved. Here we consider first the evidence for experience-dependent structural changes, mainly considering the mechanisms associated with dynamic synapses (Section 7.4.1), and, second, the evidence for experience-dependent gene expression associated with plasticity (Section 7.4.2).

### 7.4.1    Structural plasticity

During development, large-scale changes in the structure of dendrites and axons occur as neuronal processes grow into position. Cells initially carry few synapses but they develop rapidly during critical periods of synaptogenesis. For excitatory cortical pyramidal cells, synaptogenesis involves the generation of spines. Valverde (1967, 1971) described changes in spine numbers with development in the visual system and noted that sensory deprivation could change the innervation of spines during development. In the somatosensory system, Micheva and Beaulieu (1995a) found that whisker deprivation led to an increase in inhibitory innervation of spines in the deprived barrel. More recently, in vivo two-photon microscopy has increased the time resolution with which spines can be studied in vivo and led to the realization that spine structure can change within tens of minutes (Chen *et al.*, 2000; Trachtenberg *et al.*, 2002).

### 7.4.1.1    Effect of experience on cortical spines

Spines can broadly be divided into two classes on the basis of their shape and motility. In young adult mouse barrel cortex, the highly motile filopodia are long thin spines that tend to come and go within a 24 hour period and make up approximately 20% of the total population (Trachtenberg *et al.*, 2002). At the other end of the spectrum, about 60% tend to be bulbous-headed or mushroom spines that last at least eight days (Trachtenberg *et al.*, 2002) at P42–P70. In even more mature mice of three to six months of age, the stable population can constitute

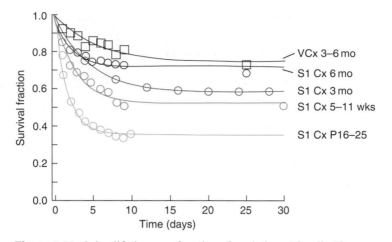

**Figure 7.11.** Spine lifetime as a function of age in layer Vb cells. The age range and cortical area are indicated on the right of the figure for each line on the graph. Squares (top line) are for visual cortex (VCx) as a comparison (three to six months of age). Other curves are for somatosensory cortex (S1) at the ages indicated (mo, months; wks, weeks). (Adapted from Holtmaat *et al.* [2005], with kind permission of the authors and Elsevier.)

approximately 75% of the total (Holtmaat *et al.*, 2005; Figure 7.11). These estimates of relative stability contrast with the situation in developing animals, where approximately 75% of the spines may turn over within four days at P8–P12 in layers II/III (Lendvai *et al.*, 2000), as described in Section 4.4.2.

Sensory experience can alter this background level of spontaneous change (Figure 7.12). Whisker deprivation in a chessboard pattern has been found to increase the rate of filopodia turnover and simultaneously increase the turnover of spines with a "stable" morphology. Spine turnover increases as a result of whisker deprivation, but obviously the degree of plasticity is partly a function of age because baseline levels of spine turnover are lower in older animals (Figure 7.11). At P11–P13, which is the height of the critical period for layers II/III forming connections, total whisker deprivation increases spine turnover by 37% (Lendvai *et al.*, 2000). Chessboard deprivation in animals imaged between P34 and P74 causes an increase in spine turnover of approximately 10% (daily turnover) in the same neurons (Trachtenberg *et al.*, 2002). This is what might be expected if cells were forming new synapses as a result of whisker deprivation. An alternative explanation might be that synapses are being formed and eliminated all the time and that whisker deprivation prevents the natural elimination that normally occurs. Deprivation at four to six weeks of age occurs during the period when spine dynamics are still naturally decreasing (Zuo *et al.*, 2005b). Therefore, deprivation at this time prevents 12% of the spine loss that would

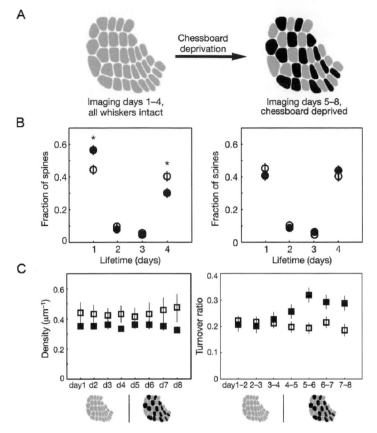

**Figure 7.12.** Effect of chessboard deprivation on spine turnover in barrel cortex. A. Neurons were imaged once per day for four days to establish a baseline before whisker deprivation in the pattern shown (dark barrels are deprived) and a further four days of imaging. B. Spine lifetime inside the barrel cortex (left) and outside the barrel cortex (right). Values are shown for baseline (open circles) and postdeprivation (closed circles). C. Spine density (left) and spine turnover (right) versus time (d, days) for spines inside (solid squares) and outside the barrel cortex (open squares). Note the increase in turnover for spines inside the barrel cortex following deprivation. (Reproduced from Trachtenberg *et al.* [2002], with kind permission of the authors and the *Nature* Publishing Group.)

normally occur in that period (Zuo *et al.*, 2005b). At present, this issue of whether deprivation increases spines or prevents a decrease in spines at these ages remains unresolved.

### 7.4.1.2    *Effect of experience on cortical presynaptic structure*

Changes in spines are presumed to occur in concert with changes in presynaptic terminals. It has been shown that newly formed spines make contact with presynaptic boutons and form terminals (Trachtenberg *et al.*, 2002). Therefore, one might expect axons to show plasticity as well as spines. In fact, similar to spines, axonal arbors are largely stable in barrel cortex over long periods of time, especially those corresponding to thalamic inputs to cortex (De Paola *et al.*, 2006). It has been estimated that 94% of the axonal arbor remains stable over a period of 24 days. However, some classes of axon reshape relatively often, and branches can elongate and retract by tens of micrometers over a period of one month. En-passant boutons seem to be more stable than terminal end branch boutons. For example, 60% of terminal boutons of layer VI recurrent projections to layer I are dynamic while only 15% of en-passant boutons show losses or gains in thalamic or intracortical connections over a period of one month (De Paola *et al.*, 2006). The most dynamic axons found to date are those of layer VI cells that project to layer I, and it would be of interest to know the function of this plasticity given the unique position of layer VI cells in controlling thalamic input to layer IV via projections to thalamus and layer IV inhibitory cells (Section 3.4.6)

Sensory experience is also known to affect the morphology of thalamocortical axons in developing animals. In the visual cortex, monocular deprivation leads to pruning of the geniculocortical afferents for cells responding to the deprived eye, and so their arbors become relatively sparse compared with those for cells responding to the open eye, or those seen in normal binocular animals (Antonini and Stryker, 1993). In barrel cortex, complete whisker trimming from birth does not affect thalamocortical afferents appreciably when judged by retrograde transport from injection sites to the corresponding barreloid in the thalamus (Keller and Carlson, 1999). However, depriving all but one whisker from birth does alter the distribution of short-latency responses corresponding to the spared whisker, which show up in inappropriate deprived whisker barrels (Fox, 1992), suggesting that thalamocortical segregation is incomplete and under the control of sensory input (Chapter 4). Whisker trimming from birth also affects the row orientation of intracortical axonal connections. Normally, intracortical connections are biased to project along the rows rather than along the arcs, but complete whisker trimming abolishes the row orientation and the connections become symmetrical around any single barrel (Keller and Carlson, 1999). A similar effect can be produced in developing barrel cortex by blocking cortical NMDA receptors (Dagnew *et al.*, 2003), suggesting that the connections require sensory experience acting via NMDA receptors to form correctly.

In adult barrel cortex, studies on inhibitory terminals have shown that increased sensory stimulation to a single whisker can lead to an increase in inhibitory presynaptic terminals in adult mouse barrel cortex (Knott *et al.*, 2002). Similarly, an increase in puncta positive for the glutamate decarboxylase 67 kDa isoform can be seen in the stimulated barrels of mice receiving single-row whisker stimulation paired with an aversive stimulus (Siucinska and Kossut, 2006). The functional consequence of increasing inhibition is to provide an element of long-term negative feedback to dampen the effect of a sustained increase in stimulus input. This suggests that anatomical plasticity can be employed to create a level of automatic gain control in the cortical circuit throughout life.

### 7.4.1.3    *Molecular mechanisms for structural change*

What guides the growth and retraction of spinous and axonal processes, and if synapse stabilization is related to early-phase plasticity mechanisms, how are they coupled at the molecular level? While the answers to these questions are not clear at present, some of the molecules involved have been identified. Dendritic spines move as a result of actin polymerization and depolymerization. Studies on cultured hippocampal cells show that spine heads are constantly making submicrometer changes in shape over periods of seconds and that inhibition of actin polymerization prevents this movement (Fischer *et al.*, 1998). Similarly, in cortical neurons, actin tends to be located at the tips of dendrites and spines and is, therefore, in the right location for exploratory movements by these processes into the surrounding extracellular space. In barrel cortex, it has been shown that filopodia often actually move toward existing synaptic terminals where they add to the synapses on a single spine (Knott *et al.*, 2006), implying that an attractant is sensed by the spine head and a signaling pathway translates this into actin-based movements.

Candidates for the signal that attracts the spine include glutamate, neurotrophins and extracellular matrix cues acting via integrins. It is beyond the scope of this chapter to explore all of these possibilities but for reviews see Luo, 2002) and Whitford *et al.* (2002). Instead, we sketch the evidence linking activation of the ionotropic glutamate receptors with spine motility, as synaptic activity is clearly involved in barrel cortex plasticity.

Activation of GluRs can influence retraction and protraction of dendritic spines. For example, NMDA receptor activation during LTP protocols causes de novo spine formation in hippocampal slice cultures (Engert and Bonhoeffer, 1999; Maletic-Savatic *et al.*, 1999). The direction of spine movement can be affected by the type of activity because theta-burst stimulation favors protraction and low-frequency stimulation favors retraction (Nagerl *et al.*, 2004). Conversely, stabilization of spines appears to require at least spontaneous release of glutamate on to AMPA receptors, which prevents spine retraction (McKinney *et al.*, 1999). Similarly, sustained levels of AMPA (1–2 µmol/l) causes a cessation of actin dynamics via depolarization of the cell (Fischer *et al.*, 2000).

These studies suggest that retraction, protraction, stop, and go signals are all influenced by GluR activation.

The GluRs are linked to actin remodeling via a class of molecules known as Rho-GTPases. In their active state they bind GTP and in their inactive state GDP. Coimmunoprecipitation studies have established that the Rho-GTPase RhoA associates with the GluR1 subunit of the AMPA channel and the NMDAR2a subunit of the NMDA channel when in its activated state (Schubert *et al.*, 2006a). The level of association of RhoA with AMPA and NMDA decreases with potassium-induced depolarization of the cell. Depolarization of hippocampal neurons by potassium, in turn, leads to active retraction of spines that requires RhoA (Schubert *et al.*, 2006a), suggesting that dissociation of RhoA leads to a reduction in its activity in changing the actin cytoskeleton beneath the spine head. The final link between GluR activation and actin is made via a kinase that is activated by RhoA (ROCK) and forms a complex known as ROCK–PIIa, which directly regulates actin polymerization (Schubert *et al.*, 2006a).

In conclusion, a number of molecular pathways have been identified that control actin-based spine and dendrite dynamics. So far it is not clear which pathways are important for the changes in experience-dependent spine dynamics observed in whisker-deprivation studies. One issue that will be important to resolve is the relative importance under different circumstances of the neurotrophin and extracellular matrix signaling pathways. For example NMDA receptors and integrins have convergent effects on spine plasticity in hippocampal neurons (Shi and Ethell, 2006) and might be expected to act similarly in barrel cortex.

### 7.4.2    *Changes in gene expression*

Changes in gene expression could potentially support late-phase plasticity in a number of ways. Gene expression could be activated to support growth and retraction of processes or new synaptic materials could be directed to the site of stable synapses in order to cement changes in synaptic gain. As mentioned above, it is probably safer to assume that both types of process occur in the cortex, as it is presently not known whether the population of 5–20% labile spines is sufficient on its own to account for experience-dependent plasticity.

A number of immediate early genes are activated by whisker-deprivation patterns that are known to result in plasticity (Figure 7.13). Notably, genes for c-Fos, inducable cAMP early repressor (ICER), Krox-24 and JunB are all activated in the spared barrel of a whisker-deprived animals exposed to an enriched environment (Bisler *et al.*, 2002). There is some temporal distinction between expression of the genes for these proteins, with genes for c-Fos and Krox-24 being earlier at 1–14 hours than, for example, ICER, which peaks at six hours but remains present up to five days later (Bisler *et al.*, 2002). This is similar

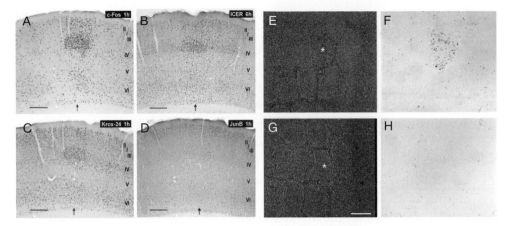

**Figure 7.13.** Expression of immediate early genes in barrel cortex following whisker deprivation. A–D. Coronal section immunohistochemistry in rat barrel cortex of c-Fos one hour after deprivation. (A), inducible cAMP early repressor (ICER) after six hours (B), Krox-24 after one hour (C) and JunB after one hour (D). Note the strong labeling in layer IV in the spared barrel in each case. Scale bars = 300 µm. (Reproduced from Bisler *et al.* [2002], with kind permission of the authors and Elsevier.) E–H. Horizontal sections showing expression in mouse barrel cortex of the CAMP-response element (CRE) and β-galactosidase in *Cre–LacZ* transgenic mice. E,G. The barrel field with DNA visualized with propidium iodide in the deprived condition (E) and on the control undeprived side (G). The asterix indicates the principal barrel for the spared whisker. F, H. Expression of *Cre–LacZ* as indicated by detection of beta-galatosidase after 24 hours of single-whisker experience (F). Note that the D1 (spared) barrel shows staining. The control undeprived side is also shown (H). (Reproduced from Barth *et al.* [2000] with permission of the Society for Neuroscience.)

to a related gene, that for the cAMP-response element-binding protein (CREB), which has an effect within 12 hours that is maintained for approximately seven days (Barth *et al.*, 2000). One issue is whether the genes are reacting to changes in activity in the pathways brought about by whisker deprivation, in other words are they involved in a homeostatic reaction to changes in activity, or whether they are actively involved in a plasticity process. One clue comes in noting where the genes are expressed. The genes for c-Fos, ICER, Krox-24 and JunB are all expressed in subcortical locations as well as barrel cortex and yet only barrel cortex shows plasticity at these ages. Therefore while these immediate early genes may or may not be involved in plasticity, they are certainly not sufficient for nor predictive of its expression. In contrast, *CREB* is not expressed in the thalamus in response to whisker deprivation but is in the cortex, suggesting that it could be involved in plasticity (Barth *et al.*, 2000).

The topic of gene expression and cortical plasticity is relatively new and unexplored and, therefore, here we just concentrate on two factors that might play a role: NeuroD2, which appears to be involved in transport of materials to new synapses, and CREB, which is important for long-term memory and plays some role in barrel cortex plasticity.

### 7.4.2.1   NeuroD2

The calcium-regulated transcription factor NeuroD2 is important for development of thalamocortical connections. One of the genes controlled by NeuroD2 codes for the growth-associated protein GAP43. Knockout mice for both NeuroD2 and GAP43 have deficits in barrel pattern formation as a result of incomplete segregation of axons in layer IV. The synapses formed by thalamo-cortical axons tend to be weak and layer IV in particular exhibits lower levels of GluR2/3 expression. The normal change from NMDA- to AMPA-dominated responses with development are, therefore, impaired by a loss of NeuroD2 (Ince-Dunn et al., 2006). Maturation of silent synapses involves rapid insertion of AMPA channels into the membrane and this process would appear to require support from NeuroD2-dependent gene expression. One aspect that remains to be determined is whether the calcium signal that induces NeuroD2 synthesis occurs at the same time as the signal to insert AMPA channels, which would argue for an instructive role in plasticity, or whether the calcium signal is normally generated by the general level of activity in the cell, which would argue for a permissive rather than an instructive role.

### 7.4.2.2   Cyclic AMP-response element-binding protein

Phosphorylation of CREB by PKA causes this cAMP-dependent transcription factor to dimerize, and it can then regulate transcription. Since PKA can be activated by calcium-dependent ACI, gene regulation can be activated by post-synaptic calcium (e.g. via NMDA receptor activation). The association of CREB with late-phase plasticity is suggested because it is generally implicated in the later stages of LTP and memory. It has been found that CREB is necessary for LTP to last longer than two hours in hippocampus (Bourtchuladze et al., 1994). It has also been found that it is necessary for long-term plasticity in aplysia (Alberini et al., 1994) and for long-term memory in flies and mice (Bourtchuladze et al., 1994; Yin et al., 1994). Whisker deprivation in barrel cortex certainly produces a form of plasticity that lasts longer than two hours. Changes in spines associated with whisker deprivation occur over periods of days (Trachtenberg et al., 2002). Similarly, changes in receptive fields tend to take several days to accumulate (Glazewski and Fox, 1996). Because changes cannot accumulate in this way if plasticity decays rapidly, plasticity must last at least several days in this system, which is consistent with the finding that vibrissae regrowth for a period of 8–10 days after deprivation does not negate the effect of the preceding deprivation.

These factors argue in favor of a role for CREB in barrel cortex plasticity, and indeed it has been found that *CREB* knockout mice show approximately half the potentiation of the spared whisker normally seen in wild-type littermates (Glazewski *et al.*, 1999). The fact that all plasticity is not abolished may be because the alpha–delta isoform knockout studied has a beta-isoform upregulated in the barrel cortex, which may cause a partial rescue of the mutation (Glazewski *et al.*, 1999).

Further evidence for the role of CREB in barrel cortex plasticity comes from studies using a CRE-reporter gene (*LacZ*) downstream of the CREB-activated promoter (Figure 7.13). In adult animals deprived of all but the D1 whisker, a strong (30-fold compared with the spared hemisphere) and highly place-specific upregulation of CRE-mediated gene transcription occurred in layer IV of the spared whisker barrel (Barth *et al.*, 2000). The difference between the spared and deprived barrels was so stark that the position of D1 could be seen in a whole mount brain. Reporter gene upregulation occurred within 16 hours and in some cases persisted for a week. The functionally related ICER is also upregulated in barrel cortex following whisker deprivation (Bisler *et al.*, 2002). The gene for ICER is a negative feedback gene that requires CREB for activation but then tends to repress further CREB production. The fact that both CREB and ICER are simultaneously synthesized suggests that they reach an equilibrium that maintains *CREB* expression, though presumably at a lower level than in the absence of ICER.

Expression of *LacZ* in layer IV is accompanied by an increase in responsiveness of a subpopulation of layer II/III cells to spared whisker stimulation, as determined by in vivo single-unit recording (Barth *et al.*, 2000). Therefore, CRE-mediated gene expression occurs presynaptically to the cells that exhibit changes in their receptive field properties.

Changes in CRE-mediated gene expression are specific to deprivation patterns that induce potentiation rather than simply change activity levels in the cortex. Sparing a single whisker in animals of this age causes potentiation of spared whisker responses without depression of deprived-whisker responses. However, no potentiation occurs if all the whiskers are deprived simultaneously (Glazewski *et al.*, 1998a). In concert with this observation, upregulation of reporter gene expression does not occur if all whiskers are deprived simultaneously (Barth *et al.*, 2000). Indeed, levels of CRE-mediated gene expression in both input-spared and input-deprived hemispheres are the same or lower than values from normal undeprived animals.

A number of genes associated with plasticity have CRE elements in their promoters including BDNF and CPG15 (also known as neuritin-1). The latter is a small membrane-bound protein that regulates growth of apposing axonal and dendritic arbors (Nedivi *et al.*, 1998; Cantallops *et al.*, 2000) and is upregulated in barrel cortex following single-whisker experience (Harwell *et al.*, 2005). The trophic factor BDNF has several effects on development of synapses (Sections 4.2.3, 4.4.1 and 6.1.2) and is upregulated in barrel cortex during increased whisker stimulation (Rocamora *et al.*, 1996). It is likely that these and other CRE-dependent genes play a role in plasticity, and the relative contribution of these factors to experience-dependent plasticity will need to be determined in the future.

In conclusion, while in its infancy, studies on barrel cortex plasticity in developing and adult animals do implicate gene expression in plasticity of the barrel cortex. One challenge for the future will be to determine the network of genes expressed during plasticity and how they are controlled.

## 7.5    Injury-induced plasticity

### 7.5.1    Developmental plasticity

In 1973, Van der Loos and Woolsey reported that ablating a row of follicles in neonatal mice and damaging the follicle innervation caused a loss of the corresponding barrels in the cortex when the animal had matured. Ablating a row of follicles led to fusion of the corresponding row of barrels in the cortex (Section 4.2.2) and the fused row occupied less space than the normal barrels or the surrounding rows that expanded into their territory (Van der Loos and Woolsey, 1973). Later studies showed that the effect had a distinct critical period between P1 and P5 in the mouse (Woolsey and Wann, 1976), peaking at P1 (Jeanmonod *et al.*, 1981). The brain is highly plastic during this period of development because the thalamocortical afferents grow into the cortex and segregate into barrels between birth and P5 and the cortical cells simultaneously form the cytoarchitectonic domains of the barrels (Section 4.2.2). The dendrites of layer IV neurons are also plastic during this period. Layer IV spiny stellate cells normally orient their dendrites in toward the center of the barrel (Figures 2.10 and 3.1), but follicle lesion causes the dendrites to loose their asymmetry and project dendrites equally in all directions (Harris and Woolsey, 1981). The dendrites show a slightly shorter critical period than the thalamocortical afferents between birth and P3.

Some of the effects of damage to the follicle innervation can be attributed to activity-dependent processes in the cortex itself. For example, blocking post-synaptic cortical activity at the same time as ablating the follicles during the first few postnatal days reduces cortical plasticity by about half (Schlaggar *et al.*, 1993). However, it is not possible to block fully the effects of lesion-induced plasticity by cortical treatments alone because some of the effects of the lesion are expressed subcortically. Peripheral lesions cause plasticity in VPm, brainstem nuclei and the primary afferents themselves. First in VPm, neurons in areas normally devoted to the whisker representation become responsive to input from the nose, cheek and lower jaw (Waite and Cragg, 1982). In the thalamus, the critical period closes earlier in the periphery (P3) than in the cortex (P5) (Durham and Woolsey, 1984). Second, lesion of the periphery also produces plasticity in the brainstem where the critical period occurs between P1 and P3 (Yamakado, 1995). The brainstem nuclei shrink following whisker ablation (Durham and Woolsey, 1984; Yamakado, 1995). Cutting the infraorbital nerve causes the interpolaris nucleus to shrink by as much as 33%, but the cell count is only reduced slightly (Hamori et al., 1986) and the loss of volume is mainly owing to loss of peripheral nerve innervation. Third, follicle lesions also induce plasticity in the primary afferents. Nerve lesions can lead to demyelination and degeneration of the affected axons, which probably undergo an apoptotic cell death following cautery (Waite and Cragg, 1982; Li et al., 1995). Nerve degeneration also shows a critical period. Cutting the nerve at P0 causes 62% of the axons to die but only 20% die if the cut is made at P10 (Waite and Cragg, 1979). The survival at earlier ages may be related to the ability of axons to regrow to the follicles (Waite and Cragg, 1982). However, cauterizing nerves even in relatively mature animals (P20) will cause expression of a range of neuropeptides in the ganglion such as neuropeptide Y and galanin (Li et al., 1995), showing that they still respond to lesions even though they do not degenerate fully at this age.

Some of the cortical plasticity effects at younger ages can, therefore, be explained by passive inheritance of plastic changes subcortically. Chief among these are the effects of neural degeneration at subcortical locations in neonates leading to reduced thalamocortical innervation. For example, cutting the infraorbital nerve at birth can increase the level of natural apoptosis in the thalamus (Waite et al., 1992). Cell loss in VPm reaches 24% of the total neurons following nerve section at P2 and continues to occur with lesions as late as P10. In a study using TUNEL (transferase-mediated deoxyuridine triphosphate–biotin end labeling) to judge apoptosis, section of the infraorbital nerve at birth was observed to cause apoptosis in VPm (Baldi et al., 2000). Apoptosis in VPm can also be induced by preventing axonal transport in the infraorbital nerve by vinblastine and can be rescued by BDNF and nerve growth factor applied to the infraorbital nerve. This suggests that infraorbital nerve section causes thalamic cell loss by limiting delivery of trophins to the thalamic cells rather than by reducing excitatory activity (Baldi et al., 2000). One further major effect of early deafferentation is to alter the proportion of synapses in VPm so that they mainly originate from cortex. Inhibitory synapses also increase as a proportion and they presumably originate from the thalamic reticular nucleus (Hamori et al., 1986). In conclusion, many of the effects of peripheral damage are far greater than can be accounted for purely by changes in synaptic activity.

### 7.5.2    Intracortical plasticity beyond the thalamocortical critical period

Some of the changes in thalamic innervation to barrel cortex caused by lesions between P1 and P3 can be explained by subcortical critical period changes in thalamus and brainstem. However, intracortical connections tend to have a longer critical period than thalamocortical connections and can be affected by peripheral lesions at later ages. Cutting the infraorbital nerve at P7 in the mouse prevents the proper maturation of horizontally directed transcolumnar projections from layer II/III and V cells (McCasland et al., 1992). Intracortical projections in layer IV are also affected by infraorbital nerve section but only up to P3 in the rat (Rhoades et al., 1997). Injection of tracer into the C3 barrel normally labels cells in septal areas more than barrel areas, giving a fenestrated pattern to the labeling, but infraorbital nerve section up to P3 changes the balance so that far fewer retrogradely labeled cells occur in the septa and most occur in the barrels or the fused barrel row (Rhoades et al., 1997).

Intracortical axons react to peripheral nerve lesion even in mature animals. If all innervation is cut save that to the C-row of vibrissae of young adult mice (P42), axons projecting horizontally from spared barrels do so over greater distances in all layers (except layer V) than either control axons or axons projecting from deprived barrel-columns (Kossut and Juliano, 1999). Furthermore, axonal density is 70% greater for the spared barrel-column projections, suggesting that the complexity of the projections also increased (Figure 7.14).

Lesion-induced plasticity also affects dendrites in layer IV of the cortex in adult animals. Denervation of the whisker follicles causes a reorientation of dendritic arbors in layer III and IV of adult rats (Tailby et al., 2005). Layer IV stellate cells normally have their dendrites oriented toward a particular barrel (Chapter 2), but after denervation they loose their orientation and grow into surrounding septal areas (Figure 7.15). This is similar to the rat forepaw representation of somatosensory cortex, where dendrites reorient relative to the boundary of the forepaw representation following denervation of the limb (Hickmott and Steen, 2005).

A similar conclusion is reached in considering cortical plasticity beyond the critical period for thalamocortical afferents as during the critical period: that plasticity is greater if caused by a peripheral lesion than if caused by whisker deprivation. Whisker trimming from birth has a far smaller effect on

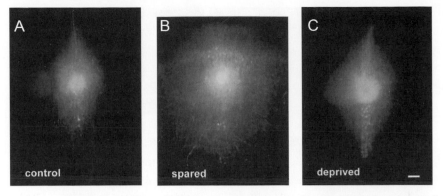

**Figure 7.14.** Effect of follicle ablation on intracortical axonal connections in barrel cortex demonstrated in coronal sections following injection of fluorescent dextrans into cortical barrels in layer IV. A. Control undeprived cortex. B. Labeling from injection of a spared barrel. All the whisker follicles were removed except the C-row in mice five to six weeks of age. The deprivation lasted 8–10 weeks. C. Labeling following injection in a deprived barrel. Scale bar = 100 μm. (Adapted from Kossut and Juliano [1999], with kind permission of the authors and Pergamon Press.)

thalamocortical afferent disposition than ablating the follicles (Killackey *et al.*, 1976; Fox, 1992; Keller and Carlson, 1999). Whisker trimming leaves most intracortical axonal arbors unaffected (De Paola *et al.*, 2006) but lesions can cause an increase in growth between barrels (Kossut and Juliano, 1999). Whisker trimming does not affect the dendritic structure in layer II/III cells beyond P15 (Maravall *et al.*, 2004) and yet follicle damage can induce new dendritic growth in layer IV in adults (Hickmott and Steen, 2005; Tailby *et al.*, 2005).

### 7.5.3    *Subcortical plasticity in adult animals*

In neonates, damage to the infraorbital nerve or individual whisker follicle innervation can cause plasticity at the level of the thalamus and brainstem as mentioned above (Waite and Cragg, 1982; Nicolelis *et al.*, 1991, 1997). In adult animals, subcortical plasticity is less pronounced because cell loss occurs to a far lesser degree. For example, after complete nerve transection, axons will still regenerate and grow back to the periphery. Nevertheless, plasticity can still occur at the subcortical level in the adult animal in response to peripheral nerve damage, which complicates interpretation of what might otherwise be considered as a cortical plasticity effect. One of the most remarkable examples of subcortical plasticity of this kind comes from the ability of adult axons in the infraorbital nerve to regrow to their distal targets. In adult animals, damage to follicle innervation results in reinnervation of adjacent follicles by the damaged nerves after 64 days of recovery. Plasticity appears to have occurred in the cortex

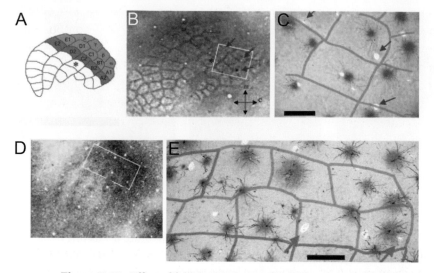

**Figure 7.15.** Effect of follicle ablation on dendritic orientation within layer IV. A.
The pattern of deprivation used. The posterior arcs of whisker follicles either A1–E1 *or*
A2–E2 were removed. Alpha, beta, gamma and delta were also removed. Rats were
more than eight weeks old at the start of deprivation and the deprivation period
lasted 8.5–11.5 weeks. B. Barrel field showing the cells filled with lucifer yellow made
permanent with immunohistochemistry. The area in the square is shown at higher
magnification in C. C. The basal dendrites of layer III pyramidal cells do not cross
barrel boundaries (grey lines) in undeprived animals. D. Barrel field showing the area
represented in E. E. In vibrissectomized rats, the dendrites of layer III cells cross
boundaries in deprived barrels (light grey boundaries, corresponding to the light grey
barrels in A) but not in undeprived barrels (dark grey boundaries, corresponding to
the dark grey barrels in A). The arrows show blood vessels used to align B with C and D
with E. (Adapted from Tailby *et al.* [2005], with kind permission of the authors and the
National Academy of Science.)

because cells in the deprived barrels show increased responses to adjacent
whiskers, but the effect can be explained by peripheral nerve regrowth (Melzer
and Smith, 1998). In this study the C1–C3 follicles were damaged in adult animals,
and the timecourse of the cortical plasticity was tracked in time using the 2-DG
technique (Section 7.1) together with histology of the whisker follicles. Increased
responses in the deprived barrels to surrounding whisker stimulation was not
seen before the first signs that follicles surrounding the damaged follicles were
reinnervated by the damaged nerves (Melzer and Smith, 1998).

The thalamus also shows plasticity effects in the adult, which do not fall
neatly under the heading of lesion-induced or experience-dependent plasticity.
For example, blocking activity in the peripheral nerve with lidocaine causes
rapid plasticity in the thalamus consisting of unmasking receptive field

components that are not normally seen (Krupa *et al.*, 1999). Overall, 60% of cells responding to the whiskers showed unmasked receptive field components, typically new whisker inputs, when lidocaine was applied to the nerve. This is similar to the observation by Calford and Tweedale (1991b) that local anesthetics applied to the digit caused rapid expansion of receptive fields in the cortex. The effect can partly be attributed to feedback projections from the cortex, because if the cortex is blocked with lidocaine during this manipulation fewer cells show unmasking (Krupa *et al.*, 1999).

The use of nerve blocks reveals aspects of circuit function that rely on spontaneous or tonic levels of activation. One of the explanations is that tonic inhibition is set up by spontaneous activity in the afferent nerve fibers that has a more diffuse projection pattern than the rapid Aβ-fiber input subserving the center receptive fields of cells in the somatosensory pathway. The surround tonic inhibition could be supplied by the C-fibers because they have more diffuse terminations in the spinal cord. Calford and Tweedale (1991a) tested this idea by applying capsaicin, which is a neurotoxin for C-fibers, to the peripheral nerve and found it could produce the same effect as local nerve blockade. Once again, cortical receptive fields expanded at their edges into areas somatotopically adjacent to the capsaicin-treated nerves (Calford and Tweedale, 1991a). The disinhibition is almost immediate (four minutes), implying that it is caused by a circuit effect. A similar result is obtained in the whisker pathway at the level of the thalamus. Capsaicin injection under the lip causes an increase in receptive field size in VPm within approximately 15 minutes of application (Katz *et al.*, 1999). Changes in barrel cortex are of the same order of magnitude and at the same period of time as those in VPm, suggesting that the cortical effects are the result of the subcortical consequences of capsaicin treatment. These studies throw light on an earlier finding that capsaicin treatment of the vibrissae nerves in neonates causes expansion of cortical receptive fields in adult animals (Wall *et al.*, 1982).

## 7.6    Conclusions

A number of themes have recurred in this chapter under different guises. First, there is the question of whether all cortical pathways are plastic or just some. From studies that have been conducted so far it would seem that most pathways are capable of plasticity under some circumstance or other, for example, most intracortical pathways show LTP or LTD when studied at the level of the single cell. A notable exception is the thalamocortical synapse on to layer IV cells, where LTP and LTD seem strongly developmentally regulated. This pathway is highly specialized within the cortex for transmitting accurate temporal information from the thalamus to the cortex (Chapter 5). Perhaps if plasticity were permitted in this pathway, it would fail in this primary function, resulting in loss of vital timing information to the barrel cortex; consequently, its plasticity is limited by developmental mechanisms. The structure of some pathways do seem more suited to expression of plasticity than others; for example, the septal pathways are ideally connected for horizontal spread of excitation between cortical columns.Where structural plasticity has been studied, it has been found that axons of layer VI cells are particular plastic. Furthermore layer Vb IB cells tend to show more potentiation following whisker deprivation than RS cells. So in conclusion, there is certainly evidence that some pathways are more plastic than others, but most can undergo plasticity.

The second issue that arises is the question of how stability is maintained in a structure where so much is plastic. Synapses continually turn over even in adult cortex. Could it be that despite making and breaking connections the synapses are in dynamic equilibrium, showing individual changes but no net change? Evidence from studies on spines suggest that a subset of spines actually turn over in cortex (5–20%) while the rest seem stable over a period of at least days in adult animals. The transient fraction could be in dynamic equilibrium while the rest are relatively stable.

The question of dynamic equilibrium recurs once more when considering how form is maintained despite continual molecular turnover. At the level of excitatory synapses, one can imagine AMPA receptors being recycled and maintained in the correct proportion by the correct number of slot proteins. But even the slot proteins would turn over at some finite rate. One possible solution to this dilemma is if the representation of what needs to be preserved involves not one synapse but many, and not one set of molecules at that synapse but many. In this case, the rate of turnover would become slow enough that recurring experience and use might be sufficient to maintain the synapses in their original condition. In this sense, the world becomes part of the stabilizing mechanism. This is not to trivialize the problem however, because in order to work, such a system still needs to organize and maintain a large complex of molecules in a given form, for example to organize the structure of a single synapse in all its detail. To understand this is, of course, the present challenge to those working on synaptic plasticity. The challenge in experience-dependent plasticity is to determine how synaptic plasticity is controlled by experience.

# 8

## New and emerging fields in barrel cortex research

This chapter differs from those preceding it in that it does not treat a single theme but several. Rather than concentrate on one particular field of barrel cortex research, this chapter explores research in several new and emerging fields. Each field is characterized by a strong continuing development of methodology. In each case, barrel cortex is either the central focus of the research or is particularly well suited to help to further research in an allied field. The area of cortical blood flow and stroke research is a good example of the latter category. Many of the common cortical strokes that lead to paralysis are caused by occlusions that involve or affect the middle cerebral artery, which supplies the somatosensory cortex in general and the barrel cortex in rats and mice. Stroke research is in many ways ideally suited to study in barrel cortex because the cortical tissue affected by the stroke can be readily defined from the barrel field histology and the clinically relevant artery can be occluded to observe its effect on barrel cortex blood flow, angiogenesis, cell death and recovery of function.

Arguably some of the topics treated in this section warrant chapters of their own or could add considerably to the previous chapters in this book. The reason they have been grouped together in one chapter stems from two main factors. First, it is too early to attempt a reasonable synthesis of research in each area at present, a circumstance that will no doubt change rapidly over the next few years. Second, the development of new technology and methods in each field is allowing new questions to be asked, often for the first time. In this sense, the research described in this chapter represents some of the pioneering work into new areas and outlines some of the future challenges in barrel cortex research. Section 8.1 describes how fundemental research into cortical blood flow in barrel cortex can help in the understanding of the clinical problem of cortical stroke and the associated recovery processes. Section 8.2 returns to a central question in barrel cortex research, which is somatosensory processing, but this time focusing on active touch and the ways in which the rodent actually uses its whiskers to sense. Section 8.3 on synaptic physiology revisits some of the themes touched on in Chapter 4, but this time concentrates on how extremely detailed knowledge of synaptic parameters are possible using the thalamocortical slice preparation. The section on computer modeling (8.4) describes one of the smaller subfields of barrel cortex research, but nevertheless one with great potential. The ability to model cortical function is of course limited at present by the lack of knowledge of various cellular and synaptic parameters, but given the advantages of studying these factors in barrel cortex, as described in Section 8.3, it is likely that great progress can be made in this area. Finally, the chapter ends on the genetic analysis of barrel cortex, a subject which deals on one level with the identity of the barrel cortex, and this is primarily a developmental question, but also with the ability to understand genetic make-up to the point where it can be manipulated to gain further understanding (Section 8.5). In this regard it is tantilizing to think that two transgenic strains have been produced that show restricted expression in barrel cortex and in specific layers of barrel cortex.

## 8.1    Cortical blood flow and stroke research

The same factors that have made barrel cortex such a useful tool for research in other fields has meant it also finds employment in cortical blood flow and stroke-related research: namely, that it is possible to link the function being studied to a defined cortical location. The location can be as specific as a single barrel-column if required because the barrel's blood supply is derived from relatively few arterioles. Endovascular casts made of the blood vessel pattern of the barrel field reveal that each barrel is supplied with a dense plexus of capillaries originating from one or two arterioles (Cox *et al.*, 1993; Woolsey *et al.*, 1996).

As with the other fields described in this chapter, cortical blood flow research has generated several methodological innovations in recent years. Early studies used a radiographic tracer such as iodo-[$^{14}$C]-antipyrene introduced via the femoral vein to measure blood flow. Whisker stimulation produces an increase in blood flow that can be seen in the developed autoradiograph of the sectioned barrel cortex postmortem (Sakurada *et al.*, 1978). The method has good spatial resolution but lacks any temporal resolution. Subsequently, the field has been characterized by a proliferation of methods for measuring blood volume, blood flow and blood oxygenation changes in the cortex in real time. In the following sections, we first consider the methodology involved (Section 8.1.1) before describing its application in the study of barrel cortex blood flow (Section 8.1.2), neuronal activity and haemodynamic coupling (Section 8.1.3), stroke research (Section 8.1.4) and angiogenesis (Section 8.1.5).

### 8.1.1    Imaging cortical blood flow and oxygenation levels

Before going on to consider the application of cortical blood flow and oxygenation measurements to biological and clinical questions, it may first be useful to review some of the methods being used in this field (although the expert may want to read ahead to Section 8.1.2).

Stimulation of the whiskers causes a measurable changes in local cerebral blood flow. There are three main methods for measuring blood flow: laser Doppler flow cytometry (Gerrits et al., 1998), fluorescence stroboscopic methods (Cox et al., 1993) and arterial spin magnetic resonance imaging (MRI) (Silva et al., 1995). By far the most common method is laser Doppler flow, which depends on the principle that illumination of the cortex at a single wavelength will be backscattered by the moving red blood cells and therefore undergo a Doppler shift proportional to the particles' average velocity (Riva et al., 1972; Stern et al., 1977). A receiver light guide is used to detect the backscattered light, which is demodulation to detect the Doppler shift. The advantages of the technique are that the time resolution is reasonably good (typically 100 ms) and the measurements can be made non-invasively by shining the light through the thinned skull overlying the cortex. The disadvantages are that the measurement is relative not absolute and the depth through which the measure is made is unknown. The separation of the probes affects depth of measurement and is typically 2 mm for laser Doppler flow fiber separations of 0.5 mm. Since rodent cortex is about 2 mm or less in vertical depth, this method is reasonably well suited to studying barrel field blood flow changes.

A second means of measuring blood flow involves fluorescence stroboscopic methods, where a marker is injected, typically isothyocyanated dextrans or fluorescent beads of 1–3 μm diameter, and then is bleached periodically as it flows through superficial blood vessels. The distance between the bleached bands and the repetition rate of the photobleaching then gives the velocity (Rovainen et al., 1993). This method allows accurate measurement of absolute flow rate, shear force at the vessel wall and the increase in flow as a function of vessel diameter. An alternative method is to measure the time it takes for a fluorescence marker to travel from one part of the blood vessel to another as the fluorescence wavefront moves through the arterial system for the first time.

Finally, a third and novel method for measuring flow also effectively involves stroboscopically magnetizing the arterial water in the bloodstream and measuring the resultant field at particular locations within the brain with MRI.

A magnetizing field at neck level continuously inverts the magnetization of the arterial water, which then perfuses the brain and is diluted by water of opposite magnetic polarity. The amount of longitudinal magnetization in the brain at any single location is then proportional to blood flow. Magnetization can be read using ultrafast MRI. Studies have shown that it is best to use a small magnetizing coil (Silva *et al.*, 1995). Changes in blood flow produced by whisker pad stimulation have been measured using arterial spin MRI in the rat barrel cortex (He *et al.*, 2007).

In addition to the three blood flow techniques, blood oxygenation level can be measured and this gives greater spatial resolution. Sensory stimulation causes deoxygenation of hemoglobin to fuel the increased neuronal and metabolic activity and an increase in local blood volume because of arterial dilatation. Measures of oxygenation level are, therefore, usually a combination of changes in blood volume and changes in blood oxygenation, although as we shall see the two can be separated to some extent.

Changes in blood oxygenation level can be detected using two main methods, spectroscopy and blood oxygenation level-dependent (BOLD) MRI. Spectroscopic methods rely on the different absorption spectra for oxy- and deoxyhemoglobin at wavelengths away from their isosbestic points. Useful peak absorption for oxyhemoglobin occurs at 577 nm and for reduced hemoglobin at 557 nm. Total hemoglobin can be measured at an isosbestic point where the absorption spectra coincide for the oxy- and deoxy-forms. This method is useful for measuring cortical blood flow spectroscopically. Variants on these techniques have been used by a number of laboratories to image visual and barrel cortex (Grinvald *et al.*, 1986; Masino *et al.*, 1993), quite often using higher wavelengths to avoid imaging blood vessels. However, more recently Sheth *et al.* (2004) have shown that the laser Doppler flow technique and intrinsic imaging at 570 nm can provide results with a good level of agreement and high spatial resolution if statistical methods are adopted for avoiding blood vessel artefacts. Using these methods it is possible, for example, to distinguish the C1 barrel from the C2 barrel in rat by stimulation of each barrel's principal whisker (Figure 8.1).

The BOLD functional MRI technique relies on the magnetic properties of hemoglobin itself. Oxyhemoglobin is diamagnetic while its deoxygenated form is paramagnetic. Changes in blood oxygenation can be detected by comparing the ratio of the two species. However, changes in activity cause changes in both blood volume and oxygenation, so to see changes in blood volume it is often preferable to use contrast agents with higher contrast than the hemoglobin oxygenation states (cerebral blood volume MRI). Comparing laser Doppler flow and functional fMRI during electrical stimulation of the whisker pad gives good correspondence between the two methods for superficial layers of cortex (Kennerley *et al.*, 2005).

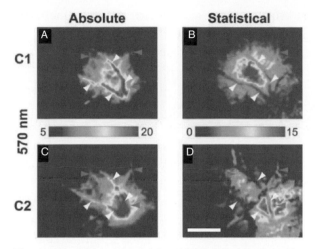

**Figure 8.1.** Imaging C1 and C2 whisker responses in rat barrel cortex using optical imaging at 570 nm. At this wavelength (approximately the isosbestic point for reduced and oxygenated hemoglobin), total hemoglobin (blood flow changes) can be measured and imaged with good spatial resolution. A, C. Using a simple threshold to view the changes in total blood flow for stimulation of the C1 (A) and C2 (C) whiskers accentuates the arterioles. B, D. Using a statistical method (Sheth *et al.*, 2004) relying instead on *P* values de-emphasizes major blood vessels and reveals total blood flow changes in the capillary bed for C1 (B) and C2 (D) whisker stimulation. Scales are fractional change ($\times 10^{-3}$; A, C) and negative $\log_{10}$ of the *P* value (B, D; medial is up and anterior is right). Scale bar = 1 mm (D). (Adapted from Sheth *et al.* [2004], with kind permission of the authors and the Society for Neuroscience.)

Having reviewed some of the main methods, the following sections describe their application to studying barrel cortex function.

### 8.1.2 Dynamic blood flow in the barrel cortex

Whisker stimulation produces a relatively rapid rise in local blood flow, which can be detected using optical imaging. The increase in flow peaks approximately 2.5–2.75 s after initiating whisker stimulation when measured using 570 nm illumination (Sheth *et al.*, 2004). The timecourse of the change in oxygenation is a little more complicated and involves an initial increase in deoxyhemoglobin, which peaks within 1 s of stimulus onset, and a later minimum, which occurs at approximately 4 s. The first peak is presumably caused by the oxygen demand in the tissue and the later minimum reflects increased perfusion of oxygenated blood through the increased flow (Figure 8.2). Similar observations have been made by other laboratories using 590 nm illumination to examine flow, or total hemoglobin, which peaks at about 2.2 s in an anesthetized animal (Berwick *et al.*, 2002).

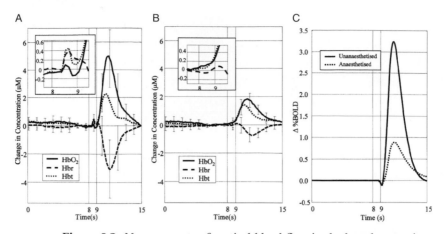

**Figure 8.2.** Measurements of cortical blood flow in the barrel cortex in response to whisker stimulation and the affect of anesthesia. A. The response to an air-puff stimulus to the whiskers delivered between timepoints 8 and 9 s in the unanesthetized rat results in an initial dip and then an increase in oxygenated hemoglobin (solid line, $HbO_2$) and an initial small increase followed by a large decrease in reduced hemoglobin (dashed line, Hbr). Total hemoglobin is shown as the dotted line (Hbt) and also increases. The inset panel shows the period during stimulation on an expanded timescale. B. Similar responses occur in anesthetized animals but at lower levels. C. The estimated effect of anesthesia on the BOLD signal that would be measured in an MRI scanner using the data in A and B and a model proposed in Davis *et al.* (1998). (Reproduced from Berwick *et al.* [2002], with kind permission of the authors and the International Society for Cerebral Blood Flow.)

Anesthesia can have a substantial effect on the magnitude if not the timing of cortical blood flow changes. For example, it has been found that urethane can reduce the peak blood flow measurements by more than 40% (Berwick *et al.*, 2002). Changes in oxygenation signal are affected even more, decreasing by about 65% with anesthesia, presumably owing to the far lower levels of neuronal activity in anesthetized animals (Table 8.1).

One further effect of anesthesia is to flatten the dynamic range of cortical blood flow response that is normally possible with increased whisker stimulation. Using laser Doppler flow cytometry, it has been observed that in unanesthetized animals blood flow increases relatively linearly with whisker stimuli up to 40 Hz, but in anesthetized animals the response curve saturates before 10 Hz (Martin *et al.*, 2006). This is presumably the effect of anesthesia on the following-frequency of the cortical neurons, and the blood flow parameters reflect their requirement for reoxygenation, which are of course similar at 10 and 40 Hz if the cells do not follow 40 Hz stimulation.

Table 8.1. *The effect of anesthesia on mean response magnitudes and latencies to peak for optical imaging spectroscopy of barrel cortex during whisker stimulation*

| Parameter (mean ± standard deviation) | Hemoglobin | | |
| --- | --- | --- | --- |
| | Total | Oxygenated | Reduced |
| Unanesthetized peak magnitude (μmol/l change) | 2.4 + 1.2 | 5.3 + 2.0 | −3.3 + 1.1 |
| Anesthetized peak magnitude (μmol/l change) | 1.4 + 0.4 | 1.9 + 0.6 | −0.8 + 0.4 |
| Unanesthetized latency (s) | 2.3 + 0.8 | 2.7 + 0.3 | 3.2 + 0.1 |
| Anesthetized latency (s) | 2.0 + 1.2 | 2.9 + 0.0 | 3.1 + 0.2 |

From Berwick *et al.*, 2002.

### 8.1.3    Metabolic coupling of neuronal activity and blood flow

Adenosine and nitric oxide are two of the molecules thought to be responsible for hemodynamic coupling, both of which have been studied in the barrel cortex. Adenosine is implicated because it increases both with metabolic rate and under conditions of hypoxia. Increased metabolism is powered by breakdown of ATP, and lack of ATP synthesis under conditions of low oxygenation will prevent ATP reforming; consequently, both factors conspire to create higher adenosine levels. Adenosine could, therefore, form the "error signal" in a negative feedback loop controlling local blood flow if it causes vasodilatation, and this has been studied in barrel cortex. Using laser Doppler flow, it was found that blood flow increases by about 17% in barrel cortex under chloralose anesthesia when the whiskers are stimulated manually for 1 min. Adenosine receptor blockade with theophylline (an antagonist for $A_1$ and $A_2$ receptors) superfused over the cortex reduced this increase by 40% without an effect on prior baseline levels of blood flow. These results suggests that basal levels of adenosine are low, that they increase during stimulation and that adenosine is indeed vasoactive (Dirnagl *et al.*, 1994).

There is some evidence that nitric oxide plays a role in metabolic coupling of blood flow over and above that provided by adenosine, although as we shall see a number of methodological issues make an absolute determination difficult at this stage. Dirnagl *et al.* (1994) found that nitric oxide synthase (NOS) inhibitors decreased stimulus-induced blood flow in the barrel cortex by approximately 20% over and above the 40% inhibition produced by adenosine antagonists. The degree of NOS antagonism tends to be variable from study to study; however, where it has been measured, the peak blood flow response to stimulation does show a linear relationship with NOS antagonism (Irikura *et al.*, 1994).

Studies in knockouts provide evidence that the neuronal NOS isoform (nNOS) couples blood flow to sensory stimulation. The NOS antagonist L-$N^\omega$-nitroarginine

(L-NNA) attenuates regional cerebral blood flow increases caused by whisker stimulation (Ayata *et al.*, 1996) and hypercapnia (Ma *et al.*, 1996) in wild-type animals and in the endothelial isoform (eNOS) knockouts, which suggests that nNOS is involved. However, interpretation is complicated by the fact that the eNOS knockouts are hypertensive and have more distensible blood vessels. Maximal dilatation of excised blood vessels with ethylenediaminetetraacetic acid (EDTA) causes greater dilatation in eNOS knockouts than in wild-type animals. For a reason that is not yet clear, the chronic lack of eNOS in the eNOS knockouts leads to wasting in the vessel wall that makes it more distensible. The eNOS knockouts are hypertensive but increased distension is not a result of chronic hypertension (Baumbach *et al.*, 2004). The combination of hypertension and more distensible blood vessels could potentially exaggerate the changes in blood flow seen in eNOS knockouts. Nevertheless, even when these factors are taken into account, these studies imply some role for nNOS in coupling blood flow.

Curiously, L-NNA does not have an effect on whisker stimulation-induced cerebral blood flow in nNOS knockouts (Ma *et al.*, 1996) despite the fact that eNOS is clearly present in blood vessels and certainly plays a role in vasodilatation in other parts of the body. It is conceivable that eNOS plays a role in the basal or tonic levels of cerebral blood flow; however, this is not currently known because the studies cited above have been conducted using laser Doppler flow, which cannot determine absolute levels of blood flow, only measuring changes in blood flow.

One further important methodological issue has been discovered and that is that prior treatment with halothane during surgery appears to increase the effect of another NOS antagonist (L-N$^{\omega}$-nitro-L-arginine methylester; L-NAME) on blood flow (Gerrits *et al.*, 2001). Both isoforms of NOS are blocked by L-NAME whereas 7-nitroindazole (7-NI) is more effective at blocking nNOS. Neither alters the total increase in blood flow measured with laser Doppler flow during automated stimulation of the whiskers unless the animals are pretreated with halothane earlier in the procedure. In fact, peak flow is actually slightly higher in the L-NAME-treated animals without prior halothane treatment. In these experiments, the halothane sensitization effect only lasted two to four hours unless urethane or another anesthetic was administered, in which case the effect endured (Gerrits *et al.*, 2001). Similarly, blood flow increases caused by whisker stimulation were only susceptible to inhibition with L-NAME if the animal was anesthetized and not if the measurement were made in awake animals (Nakao *et al.*, 2001). As a result of these methodological issues, the role of nitric oxide in cerebral blood flow remains to be resolved.

### 8.1.4    Models of cortical ischemia

The middle cerebral artery is often affected during stroke and is the major artery that supplies the barrel cortex and somatomotor cortex in general. Barrel cortex provides a useful model for stroke research because the area affected by the infarct can be defined quite accurately with reference to the barrels and because the ability to stimulate the whiskers provides an easy method for checking whether stimulus-induced increases in blood flow are affected by the stroke.

Thrombotic infarcts can be modeled by illuminating the cortex through the thinned skull using 560 nm light having first injected Bengal red dye into the blood stream 2–3 min beforehand (Ginsberg *et al.*, 1989; Hurwitz *et al.*, 1990; Jablonka and Kossut, 2006; Jablonka *et al.*, 2007). Alternatively, ministrokes can be created that affect quite local areas of the barrel field by selectively ligating branches of the middle cerebral artery using fine thread (Wei *et al.*, 1995).

In addition to enabling studies of blood flow and neuronal responses in and around the site of the infarct, creating a stroke in barrel cortex also allows the functional recovery time to be measured, either for specific behavioral tasks or for adaptive plasticity mechanisms. For example, in an active detection task, animals were initially trained to cross a gap using their whiskers to judge the distance, before one or both barrel cortices were compromised by a photo-thrombotic infarct. The animals that received a unilateral lesion recovered within two to three weeks while those that received bilateral lesions did not (Hurwitz *et al.*, 1990). Similarly in a passive detection task, animals were required to detect passive stimulation of the whiskers in order to know the correct location of a reward in a T-maze. Once more, animals with a bilateral stroke did not recover while those with a unilateral stroke recovered to within 10% of normal levels within about six weeks (Hurwitz *et al.*, 1990). These studies suggest that the surviving cortex, which lies ipsilateral to the whiskers, is used in the task and shows considerable plasticity despite the paucity of ipsilateral projections to the barrel cortex. Studies using 2-DG to measure activity levels in animals receiving unilateral photothrombotic infarcts do show increased levels of activation of the ipsilateral barrel cortex (Jablonka and Kossut, 2006), suggesting that ipsilateral cortex is indeed involved in the recovery process.

Higher spatial acuity strokes can be created (ministrokes) by vascular ligation and are useful for viewing the cortical response proximal to the infarct. Ligation of distal branches of the middle cerebral artery cause variable but quantifiable infarcts in the barrel cortex. After one week of recovery, injection of biotinyl-ated dextrans in the peri-infarct area reveal that the thalamic input to the cortex had decreased while the intracortical connections had increased. The

natural bias in intracortical connections within the barrel cortex tends to preferentially connect areas lateral and anterior to any given barrel, but following a
stroke located on the lateral side of the barrel cortex the bias in intracortical
connections reverses to become oriented predominantly posterior and medial
(Carmichael *et al.*, 2001).

Finally on this topic, it is also possible to look at the question the other way
around and to measure the effect of a lesion made outside the barrel cortex on
barrel cortex function (diaschisis). A photothrombotic infarct affecting frontal
cortex and part of MI cortex has been shown to cause a decrease in the whisker
stimulated 2-DG uptake and cortical blood flow (Ginsberg *et al.*, 1989).
Stimulation of the whiskers at a rate of 2–3 Hz normally causes an increase in
the 2-DG uptake of approximately 42%. However, a remote infarct reduces the
whisker-stimulated increase in blood flow by 20–30%. The mechanism is not
known at present but could involve a pathway traveling via the corticopontine
cerebellar route or, more directly, MI connections to SI (Ginsberg *et al.*, 1989).
Therefore, in contrast to the stimulative properties of a contralateral stroke on
the intact cortical hemisphere, an ipsilateral stroke outside the barrel cortex
impairs performance. This is also true of strokes occurring caudal to the barrel
field. In another study investigating photothrombotic infarcts, experience-
dependent plasticity induced by whisker trimming was abolished by a photothrombotic infarct located posterior to the barrel cortex (Jablonka *et al.*, 2007).
One of the questions for future study is what causes plasticity in ipsilateral
cortex following a contralateral infarct; for example, is it caused by altered
blood flow to the ipsilateral cortical area, by behavioral changes in the use of
the whiskers, by neuronal pathway changes, or a combinations of these factors?

### 8.1.5    Angiogenesis

Angiogenesis is an important topic in the field of cortical stroke because
it is likely to be key to reinstating function following an ischemic insult. Sensory
stimulation can increase angiogenesis, as discussed below, and barrel cortex is a
useful model system in which to study this effect. Intrinsic optical imaging can
be used to detect the barrel-columns of interest and measure their response to
whisker stimulation. Minstrokes can then be induced by vessel ligation in the
identified area. Ministrokes have been found to cause an increase in the collaterals of the preexisting blood vessels in the area immediately surrounding the
infarct (the ischemic border region) but not elsewhere (Wei *et al.*, 2001). The
increase is partly a result of an acute increase in existing vessel diameter but it
also involves active growth of the blood vessels, as judged by the appearance of
bromodeoxyuridine-labeled cells and increases in blood vessel length measured
at 30 days after the infarct.

Blood flow in the border of the ischemic area can be measured by injecting a fluorescent marker (Fluorescein isothiocyanate) into the bloodstream and measuring the time between the first appearance of fluorescence in the artery and the half maximal fluorescence in the area of interest. Immediately after the infarct, the peak blood flow produced in response to whisker stimulation is severely reduced in the border region, by approximately 50% (Wei *et al.*, 2001). After 30 days of recovery, the peak is still reduced but the time taken for the blood flow to increase following stimulation is much shorter, indicating a faster metabolic coupling between cortical activity and blood flow changes.

Studies on focal stroke have also recently been extended from rat to mouse, opening up the possibility of using transgenic and knockout approaches to understand and develop treatment for ischemic strokes (Whitaker *et al.*, 2007). There are a number of possible molecular targets to study in this field including various angiogenic factors such as vascular endothelial growth factor, fibroblast growth factor, angiopoietin 1 and 2 and their receptors Tie-1 and Tie-2, which are known to be important for angiogenesis (Eliceiri and Cheresh, 2001; Zhang and Chopp, 2002; North *et al.*, 2005; Scott *et al.*, 2005). In a study where mouse barrel cortex was infarcted by occlusion of the middle cerebral artery, it was found that increased whisker stimulation increased expression of a number of angiogenic factors. Increased whisker stimulation, therefore, ultimately resulted in increased blood flow to the affected barrel cortex 14 days following the stroke (Whitaker *et al.*, 2007). Recovery of blood flow measured with laser Doppler flow cytometry and angiogenesis were improved whether the whisker stimulation was delivered manually by the experimenter or whether the mouse was encouraged to use its whiskers more than usual by unilaterally trimming the whiskers projecting to the intact hemisphere (Whitaker *et al.*, 2007). Potentially, studies in barrel cortex can help in the understanding of the link between neuronal activity and angiogenesis. The judicious use of knockouts will allow molecular and behavioral therapies that can aid functional recovery to be tested.

## 8.2    Understanding active touch

The topic of whisking and active touch has already been introduced in Section 5.4.1, but this is an active area of research at present and several new methods have recently been applied to try to elucidate the mechanisms involved. The purpose of this section is, therefore, not so much to explain active touch, which is not presently possible, but more to describe some of the novel methods being applied to understand this process. Once again the barrel system is a good subject in which to tackle active touch because the anatomy of the various sensory–motor feedback loops are known and the active touch behavior itself is cyclic and stereotypic, which lends itself to averaging methods and relatively simple behavioral paradigms. Having said that, close observation of active sensing behavior in rats have revealed that the whiskers are not always used for whisking. Animals may use the whisker conventionally (as described in Section 5.4.1) by whisking them back and forth to palpate an object or, when faced with a texture discrimination task, may slide the whiskers across the surface causing stick and slip movements of the whisker bent against the surface. Because the whiskers tend to resonate during this process, the texture discrimination becomes a vibration frequency discrimination (Neimark *et al.*, 2003). As described below, the natural whisker resonances can also be used where the whisker is driven first into contact with and then past a vertical bar (Hartmann *et al.*, 2003).

Such observations have led to an interest in whisker mechanics and robotic whisking machines to try to discern what information is present in such a system, and this is addressed in Section 8.2.1. The other approach being pursued currently is to make the stimuli delivered to the animal more realistic or imitative of nature, either by recording in awake behaving animals performing a set whisking paradigm or by providing a complex stimulus using a multi-whisker stimulator. This is the topic of Section 8.2.2.

### 8.2.1    *Modeling whisker mechanics*

It is extremely difficult to understand the visual cortex without under-standing the retina and the lens. In the same way, it is difficult to understand the barrel cortex without understanding the follicle receptors and the whiskers. A number of advances have been made recently into understanding how the whiskers might be used in transducing tactile information during natural whisking tasks based on the observation that they resonate during natural exploratory tasks. For example, when whisking in space so as to encounter a vertical bar, the rat naturally drives the whisker past the vertical bar, causing the whisker first to be arrested and then to flick past the position it would normally occupy at that point in the whisk cycle (Figure 8.3). This sets up an oscillation in the whisker that is closely related to the mechanical resonance properties of the whisker (Hartmann *et al.*, 2003). Similarly, in a texture discrim-ination task, the tip of the whisker can be dragged past a rough surface causing irregular stick and slip movements that excite the resonance of the whisker (Neimark *et al.*, 2003). Conversely, the whiskers do not resonate when the animal is whisking in free air.

The natural resonance of the whisker is a function of its length, density and thickness, in the same way that a string on a stringed instrument depends on the

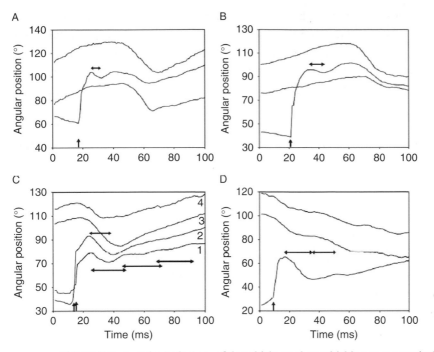

**Figure 8.3.** Angular trajectory of the whiskers when whisking past a vertical bar. The low-frequency oscillation (approximately 100 ms periodicity) is the whisk frequency and can be seen most clearly in the traces representing whiskers moving freely in air (two of these are shown per panel). The arrow in each panel indicates the time at which a whisker deflects past the vertical bar. A. The whisker starting at an angular position of approximately 65 degrees is initially retarded in the whisk cycle until it flicks past the bar to move at a greater angular velocity than the whisking movement. A small oscillation occurs at the time indicated by the horizontal arrow and represents a half cycle of a damped oscillation. B. Similar to (A), the whisker caught behind the bar starts at approximately 45 degrees and jumps (vertical arrow) past the bar at the 20 ms timepoint causing an oscillation (horizontal arrow). C. Two whiskers (bottom two traces) flick past the bar one immediately after the other causing a single half cycle of damped oscillation in one whisker and three half-cycles in the other. Note the resonances are different frequencies. D. An example where the caudal whisker, starting at approximately 25 degrees, moves in the opposite direction to the other two whiskers during this phase of the whisk cycle. (From Hartmann *et al.* [2003], with kind permission of the authors and the Society for Neuroscience.)

same parameters. In the case of the whisker, the "string" is only held at one end. One other difference from a musical string is that the whisker is tapered, which results in resonant frequencies that are not necessarily harmonics of the first or fundamental resonance. The first resonance of the D-row of whiskers has been measured by driving them at a range of frequencies (Table 8.2).

**Table 8.2**. *Lowest frequency resonance of the D-row whiskers of a rat*

| Whisker | D1 | D2 | D3 | D4 |
|---|---|---|---|---|
| First resonance (Hz) | 50 | 91 | 126 | 85 |

From Hartmann *et al.*, 2003.

In general, the resonant frequency increases as the whiskers become shorter and thinner. The measured resonances range between approximately 27 and 260 Hz for the larger whiskers but can be as high as 750 Hz for the shorter anterior vibrissae.

It is not clear at present whether the resonance information is used by the whisker system in the rodent. However, a number of physical models have been made that demonstrate that resonance can, in principle, be used to solve a number of haptic problems. Using metal whiskers of various lengths, Hipp *et al.* (2006) scanned different textures and found that the textures could be distinguished based on two parameters derived from the movement signal at the whisker base, namely the modulation power (which is related to the modulation amplitude of the signal) and the modulation centroid (which is a measure of the frequency spectrum).

Another mechanical parameter of the whisker that might potentially be used to determine the distance of an object in the rodent's tactile environment is the force created at the base of the whisker when the whisker bends against that object. The whiskers are arranged in a two-dimensional array capable, for any given head position, of decoding vertical position by whisker row and horizontal position by the timing of contact during a whisk cycle. However, the distance of the object from the face is ambiguous, particularly if several whiskers of different lengths make contact at the same time. In theory, the third dimension of distance could be represented by the bending moment in the whisker and the torque it creates at the base of the whisker. In a demonstration of the technique, a sculptured face was scanned with four artificial whiskers and the three-dimensional shape reproduced (Figure 8.4), using timing information and the rate of change of force registered during bending (Solomon and Hartmann, 2006). In principle, a single whisker can be used to the same effect by keeping track of pitch and yaw during the scan (Clements and Rahn, 2006).

These studies provide an rationale for discovering whether the follicle innervation might be able to detect the rate of change of force. Modeling the behavior of receptors at the level of the ring sinus (Gottschaldt *et al.*, 1973), the mechanical properties of the glassy membrane can be shown to create the first-time derivative of the force at whisker base (Mitchinson *et al.*, 2004). The model is able

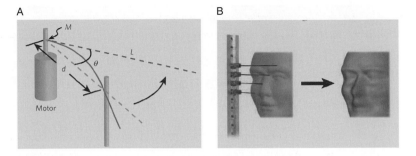

**Figure 8.4.** Determining distance from bending moment in whisker scans of a surface. A. A whisker makes contact with a vertical bar at a distance $d$ from the pivot point. The rotation of the motor through $\theta$ degrees causes the whisker to bend and create a bending moment at the pivot point that can be measured as, $d = C \, \theta/\tau$ where $C$ is $3EI$ (and $E$ is Young's modulus of elasticity and $I$ the second-order cross-sectional moment of the whisker), $\theta$ is the displacement angle and $\tau$ is the torque at the pivot point (Kaneko *et al.*, 1998). B. Four whiskers are used to scan a face and the contact time and bending moments used to calculate the contours of the surface. The four steel spring whiskers scanned the sculpted face at evenly spaced heights and angles and a smooth surface was fitted to the contact points. The face on the right was reconstructed from the data gathered in this way. (Reproduced from Solomon and Hartmann [2006], with kind permission of the V. Jacob, J. LeCam, J-Y. Tiercelin and D. Shulz and the *Nature* Publishing Group.)

to capture the natural responses measured in brainstem neurons for similar contact, pressure and detachment signals using slowly and rapidly adapting receptors. Conversely, it was found that the responses measured during free whisking in air by Szwed *et al.* (2003) could not be seen in this model, suggesting that free air responses may derive from different receptors in a different location within the follicle (Mitchinson *et al.*, 2004).

### 8.2.2    *Studying natural whisking responses*

Studies of barrel cortex function have typically and to some extent purposely used simple single-whisker stimulation to try to understand cortical function. However, having made considerable progress in this direction, there is a trend in the field to understand how more complex natural stimuli are integrated in the barrel system, especially given that the rodent actively moves its whiskers to touch objects in the environment. There are broadly two choices when embarking on such a project; one is to make the stimulus more complex in an attempt to reproduce a more natural stimulus and the other is to record responses during the natural movements the animal makes, preferably during a particular stereotypical whisking task.

Making the stimulus more realistic means making the stimulator more complex (Figure 8.5). Multichannel whisker stimulators have been built that consist

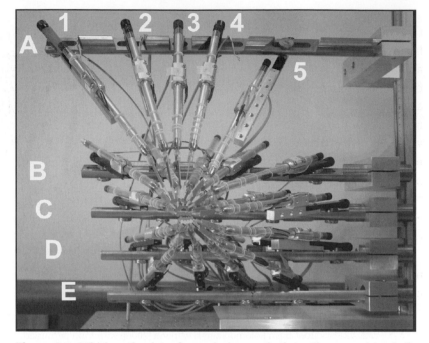

**Figure 8.5.** Whisker stimulator for producing synthetic tactile scenes. A total of 25 piezoelectric stimulators are arranged in a 5 × 5 array to stimulate whiskers 1–5 in rows A–E of the whisker pad. The angle of each stimulator can be adjusted independently so that each whisker starts at its resting position. The stimulator can be used to deliver sparse noise for reverse or forward correlation analysis (10 ms rise time, 10 ms hold time, 20 Hz repetition rate) or complex stimuli such as a bar moving at constant speed (0.125– 1.25 m/s) in a particular orientation. (The figure is reported in Jacob *et al.* [2006] and was kindly supplied by the authors.)

of five (Rodgers *et al.*, 2006) or 16 miniature solonoid actuators (Krupa *et al.*, 2001), or 25 stimulators using piezoelectric wafers (Jacob *et al.*, 2006). Complex stimulators can be used to provide spatial noise inputs to all the whiskers at different times, and a reverse or forward correlation procedure can be used to reconstruct the receptive field. Alternatively, complex stimulators can be used to synthesize tactile scenes, such as horizontal bars that are swept across the whiskers at various orientations (Jacob *et al.*, 2006). Complex stimulators hold the promise of allowing us to understand a greater repertoire of barrel cortex processing than has been possible so far. For example, studies using complex stimuli have shown that coincidence detection between whiskers, such as occurs when a bar is moved across the whisker array, may be signaled by "high gamma" oscillations at around 350 Hz (Rodgers *et al.*, 2006). High gamma-frequency activity has been implicated in cognitive processing in human cortex (Canolty *et al.*, 2006) and may convey saliency in rat cortex.

Allowing the animal to create the sensory response during a discrimination task adds a further dimension to the neuronal firing patterns recorded in the barrel cortex because motor signals, whisk-phase responses (Chapter 5) and anticipatory firing patterns are all possible in addition to the sensory response that arises from contact. Krupa *et al.* (2004) found that layer V/VI cells appear to anticipate the sensory contact during a tactile discrimination task. Aligning the responses of neurons recorded during the task to the moment of contact using video analysis showed that some layer V/VI cells fired for several hundreds of milliseconds before contact but reduced their firing rate directly around the period of contact for up to 200 ms or so. It would be interesting to compare the behavior of these neurons in an animal naive to the task where anticipation was eliminated from the equation. It would also be valuable to track the evolution of the response from first whisk to later whisks in the trial.

Whisk-phase responses can be seen to modulate the membrane potential of neurons in barrel cortex judging by intracellular recordings made in whole-cell mode (Crochet and Petersen, 2006). The depolarizations made during contact have a faster rise time and are larger than those correlated with whisking, but they could potentially have an effect on the probability of firing if the two occurred in phase. The response to passive stimulation during the whisk cycle tended to be quite small and variable in this study, while the individual whisker contacts during intentional contact during the whisk cycle were robust and less variable (Crochet and Petersen, 2006). An extra dimension of neuronal firing that is likely to enhance sensory discrimination is, therefore, present in neuronal recordings made in awake behaving animals when they whisk to detect an object or to investigate an object that they know is present. This is an new area of research that will most probably require multidisciplinary input to elucidate the mechanism.

One further highly innovative method for measuring responses in awake behaving animals comes from adaptation of the intrinsic imaging technique (Grinvald *et al.*, 1986; Masino *et al.*, 1993) and involves using fiber optic wave guides to deliver single wavelength illumination to the cortex and to detect the absorbed or reflected light (Ferezou *et al.*, 2006). The fiber optic wave guides are 8 μm diameter, giving a high level of spatial resolution, and can be arranged into a 3 mm$^2$ array of 9000 fibers, potentially giving complete coverage of the mouse if not the rat posterior medial barrel cortex (Ferezou *et al.*, 2006). Using an optical imaging method has the added advantage of allowing remote whisker stimulation. A ferromagnetic bead can be attached to the whisker and moved by a magnetic field. The electrical field generated by the electromagnet would normally create a large noise signal and disrupt any electrical recordings, but optical recordings are, of course, unaffected. Using these methods, the response of the cortex to stimulation of a single C2 whisker was similar to that predicted by recordings in anesthetized animals; the initial latency of response was approximately 10 ms and the depolarization spread out from the epicenter of the principal barrel to neighboring barrels over a period of 70 ms or so (Figure 5.2). As with the studies described above, the response to passive stimulation was found to be weaker when it occurred during a whisk cycle than when it occurred during a period of quiet waking (Ferezou et al., 2006). Nevertheless, during active whisking, a similar level of response and similar spatiotemporal dynamics were measured to those found during isoflurane anesthesia. These studies both validate the original findings made in anesthetized animals and open up the possibility of understanding far more complex responses made during behavioral whisking tasks.

## 8.3    Studying synaptic physiology

### 8.3.1    The thalamocortical slice preparation

Barrel cortex offers a number of advantages for studying synaptic physiology, chief among which is the ability to identify the pathway being studied within the general framework of the columnar system. Using laser photostimulation and caged glutamate, the individual contributions of septal and barrel-column pathways as well as inhibitory and excitatory pathways have been described (Schubert et al., 2001; Shepherd et al., 2003; Bureau et al., 2006). In addition, the invention of the thalamocortical slice preparation has allowed a clearly defined monosynaptic pathway to be studied in development and later in life. Since the development of the thalamocortical slice from the original anatomy (Bernardo et al., 1986) to the physiological implementation (Agmon and Connors, 1991), this preparation has enabled a number of important discoveries, including the existence of a critical period for LTP (Crair and Malenka, 1995), the presence and developmental elimination of silent synapses (Isaac et al., 1997) and the nature of thalamocortical LTD (Feldman et al., 1998).

Studies in early development have also benefited from the high input resistance of the layer IV neurons at early postnatal ages, allowing very small inputs, including miniature excitatory postsynaptic currents (mEPSCs), to be measured more accurately and the postsynaptic membrane voltage to be controlled reasonably well from the soma. As a consequence, a detailed picture of the nature and plasticity of the thalamocortical synapse has emerged. For example, using extracellular strontium to desynchronize vesicular release, Bannister et al. (2005) have shown that spontaneous or evoked mEPSCs fall into two classes distinguished by their different timecourses. The slower mEPSCs result from kainate-linked conductances and the faster mEPSC from AMPA-linked conductances (Bannister *et al.*, 2005). The fact that kainate can be activated by a single quantum of transmitter suggests that the slow timecourse is not a consequence of glutamate spill overacting on extrasynaptic receptors. Evoked mEPSCs either have both AMPA and kainate currents (i.e. they co exist) or just have kainate-like responses. The high input resistance of these cells (5–600 Mohms) allows a high signal-to-noise ratio to be achieved and allows, for example, quantal analysis of small kainate currents to resolve a peak amplitude of 1.8 pA and non-stationary fluctuation analysis to resolve conductance values of approximately 3 pS.

Similarly, Lu *et al.* (2003) have shown that AC1 is required for AMPA receptor trafficking at the thalamocortical synapse during mouse cortical barrel map development, again using extracellular strontium to look at evoked mEPSCs, this time in *barrelless* animals, which lack functional ACI. The mEPSC amplitudes were found to be 62% of wild-type levels in the *barrelless* animals. Since the level of GluR1 expression on the cell surface is also reduced in these mutants, these results suggests that ACI, and perhaps PKA phosphorylation of the Ser-845 site on GluR1, is necessary for the insertion or removal of AMPA channels in these young animals. The occurrence of LTP at this synapse has also been shown to require PKC and NMDA receptor activation (Scott *et al.*, 2007). Therefore, the picture that emerges is one of PKA and PKC controlling AMPA receptor insertion during kainate receptor elimination during the first postnatal week of development of the thalamocortical synapse.

Interestingly, LTP does not cause a great increase in the amplitude of synaptic potentials following induction, but rather it produces an increase in synaptic current (Daw *et al.*, 2006). Increased synaptic current improves the fidelity of spike timing at the thalamocortical synapse. The functional need for this mechanism may lie in the fact that, in the mature animal, the thalamocortical synapses on to excitatory cells are relatively weak. Convergent weak input is, therefore, required to depolarize the cell, and this only occurs with a high level of thalamic synchrony. High synchrony tends to occur only for the principal whisker, thereby limiting the receptive field and improving the spatial acuity of the mapping from thalamus to cortex (Sections 5.2.1 and 5.3.3). Altering the voltage amplitude of the input by potentiation would disrupt this mechanism by reducing the need for synchrony, while increasing the current would benefit the mechanism by improving the coupling between input spike timing and output spike timing.

### 8.3.2    *Intracortical pathways*

The intrinsic architecture of the barrel cortex has also been exploited recently to understand plasticity at the circuit level. Laser scanning photostimulation has been used to release caged glutamate at known locations while recording intracellularly from a particular cell, allowing the cells excitatory and inhibitory inputs to be mapped. Using this method, Shepherd *et al.* (2003) have described opposite changes in the connectivity of septal and barrel-columns in response to whisker deprivation. While whisker deprivation causes the expected decrease in connectivity between layers IV and layer II/III within a barrel-column, the analogous pathway in the septal locations actually increased in efficacy with the same treatment. A high level of detail is potentially available using this methodology. For example, using thalamocortical slices of mouse barrel cortex, Bureau *et al.* (2006) showed that the VPm and POm pathways from the thalamus activate separate circuits within the cortex. While the VPm route connects to layer III cells via layer IV within the barrel-column, the POm input is preferentially routed to layer II cells via layer Va cells (Bureau *et al.*, 2006). The plasticity of these pathways have yet to be examined, but the technique shows how it can, in principle, be applied to quite complex problems.

Finally on this topic, the ability to use whisker trimming to induce plasticity and then to examine its effect in a cortical slice has recently been applied to studying whether or not AMPA receptor insertion occurs in layer II/III cells during development. The critical period for connecting layer IV to layers II/III occurs between P11 and P14 in the rat barrel cortex (Maravall *et al.*, 2004). Therefore, Takahashi *et al.* (2003) trimmed the whiskers during this period to see whether it prevented insertion of particular AMPA receptor subunits. They found that trimming the whiskers during the critical period prevented the change in rectification properties normally seen with AMPA receptor currents. Rectification properties allow recognition of GluR1 homomeric channels. Increased GluR1 insertion resulted in greater EPSCs at hyperpolarized compared with depolarized potentials. The process of increased rectification was prevented in whisker-trimmed animals, indicating that it reduced the level of GluR1 insertion. The fact that insertion occurred rather than, for example, alteration of the conductance state of the channels was demonstrated by infecting the cortical cells with a virus that coded for the cytoplasmic tail of GluR1 and was known to prevent the insertion process. The expressed construct also contained green fluorescent protein, allowing neurons in which insertion is impaired to be spotted in a slice. Using these techniques, it was found that the rectification properties were decreased in cells expressing the antagonistic cytoplasmic tail, showing that insertion normally occurs during the critical period provided the whiskers are intact. Conversely, insertion of the GluR2 subunit was not experience dependent. A construct that prevented insertion of GluR2 subunits caused a decrease in AMPA-linked currents in infected cells, and the effect occurred independent of whether the whiskers were present or not.

These methods are, therefore, capable of providing detailed understanding of the molecular and neurophysiological development of the thalamocortical synapse and the description will no doubt continue to be embellished in the future. One unexplored but tractable area in this field is the thalamic input on to inhibitory cells within layer IV, where little is known about the development and plasticity at present. Given the varied synaptic physiology of the different inhibitory cell subtypes of layer IV (Section 3.4.4) this is likely to be an interesting and fruitful area of research in the future.

## 8.4    Modeling cortical function

### 8.4.1    Modeling barrels

The cerebral cortex is without argument an extremely complex structure, containing many different types of cell and a high level of synaptic interconnectivity. Traditionally, methods of cortical analysis are aimed at studying a single cell in detail or at most several cells at a time. However, even then, unless the recordings are made as part of a multiple intracellular recording, it is not possible to know the connectivity between the recorded cells. Computer modeling offers a method for bridging the gap between cellular and circuit level analysis by combining the detailed cellular knowledge from single- or paired-cell recording with a broader anatomical knowledge of intracortical pathways gained from pathway tracing and photostimulation experiments.

The basic building block for constructing a model of the cortex is of course the cortical column, as discussed in Chapters 1 and 5. A reasonable first step on a journey to build a model of the cortex is to build a model of a cortical column and then to link several columns together. In principle, the commonality of columnar structure across cortical areas could present an argument for simply choosing any area of cortex for such an endeavor. However, in practice, there are sufficient differences between sensory and association cortex, as well as differences between somatosensory, visual and auditory cortex, to make it necessary to choose a particular cortical area to model. In this respect, the barrel cortex is a good system to choose, not only because there is a large amount of single-cell information available (Chapter 3) but also because the anatomical barrel-columns are easy to identify and the thalamic and intracortical connections are largely known (Chapter 2). One could model visual cortex instead of barrel cortex, but there are two factors that make this a less attractive option at present. The first is that the columnar structure of the visual cortex is far more complex than that of the somatosensory, involving orientation, ocular dominance and retinotopic columns, before even considering spatial frequency maps and color coding. The second is that there are insufficient cellular and synaptic physiological data available for visual cortex at present. Furthermore, obtaining such information is not straightforward in the binocular species one might wish to model, such as cats and primates.

Early modeling studies in barrel cortex focused on the main thalamocortical input layer within the barrel itself. A remarkable degree of progress was possible simply from a knowledge of the receptive field properties of thalamocortical relay neurons and layer IV inhibitory and excitatory receptive fields, which led to insights into the requirement for synchronous thalamic input and the potential for the thalamus to control cortical tonic inhibition (Kyriazi and Simons, 1993; Kyriazi *et al.*, 1996b, Pinto *et al.*, 1996, 2003). The original model of the barrel comprised 70 excitatory and 30 inhibitory cortical cells activated by thalamic inputs from VPm neurons. The proportion of thalamic synapses were set at 18% of the total input to both cell types based on realistic estimates (Section 2.4.1), and the remaining synapses were, therefore, intracortical. The synaptic weights were chosen to account for several different factors including the location of the synapses on the dendritic tree and the greater efficacy of inhibition in the circuit. The fact that the neurons in the model represented a relatively small fraction of the total in the real barrel resulted in EPSPs and IPSPs being much larger than those measured in practice to allow that action potentials could be evoked in the barrel neurons (Kyriazi and Simons, 1993).

The model was able to replicate neuronal responses to a 200 ms "step and hold" stimulus when driven by real spike trains recorded from thalamocortical neurons in vivo, including the differences seen in practice between RS units and FS units (Kyriazi and Simons, 1993). One of the interesting ideas to emerge from this study was the notion of network tension, which was defined as the ratio of intrinsic (intracortical) to extrinsic (thalamic) network drive. Clearly, the cortical barrel is highly interconnected and, therefore, the intrinsic drive within the barrel is a highly significant factor in shaping the response. An analysis of the model showed that if extrinsic drive increases then so too must intrinsic drive, in other words tension must remain constant within bounds. The reason for this behavior is that tonic thalamic input preferentially increases intracortical inhibition more than excitation; therefore, in order for the phasic excitation to overcome inhibition, intracortical excitation must be increased in the model to compensate. The model could be made realistic over a wide range of tensions, but when the input drive was relatively weak the network parameters needed to be tuned more finely to achieve a realistic output (Kyriazi and Simons, 1993).

Many of these attributes can be traced to the behavior of inhibition in the model. This was further explored in a model of the barrel by Pinto *et al.* (1996) in which the three pools of neurons were reduced to three neuron types (thalamocortical, spiny and aspiny). This allowed an analytical approach to the circuit behavior. Phase-plane analysis of the circuit (where excitatory and inhibitory components are plotted orthogonal to one another) allowed the trajectory of the response to stimulation to be plotted over time. Using this method, it becomes clear that if the thalamic drive increases rapidly during a sensory response excitation is able to outrun inhibition and a significant spiking response is evoked in the spiny stellate cell population. Conversely, if the thalamic input is ramped slowly, inhibition dominates the circuit before the maximum thalamic drive occurs, thereby suppressing the excitatory response (Pinto *et al.*, 2003).

### 8.4.2    *Toward simulation of a cortical column*

More recent studies of cortical function have benefited from an increase in computer performance. As computing power increases, it becomes possible to model more neurons and to add more features to each neuron. Consequently, the number of neurons involved in the simulations has increased from 100 (Kyriazi and Simons, 1993) to 1000 cells in a recent model of general cortex (Traub *et al.*, 2005) and 10 000 in the case of the "Blue Brain" project, which aims to model a complete somatosensory column (Markram, 2006). Similarly, the neurons have changed from being nodal summation points with a spike threshold and an S-shaped input–output curve to multicompartmental models with realistic synaptic and active membrane currents. With bigger and faster computers, it becomes possible to model extra features of cellular response such as the short-term dynamics of synaptic currents and spike accommodation as well as to increase the variety of cell types included to take into account, for example, the different synaptic properties of different inhibitory cell subtypes.

Recent studies have used the extra computing capacity to explore oscillatory rhythms in cortical circuits. While not explicitly a model of barrel cortex, the Traub model of a cortical column (Traub *et al.*, 2005) draws on parameters measured in barrel cortex in addition to those from visual cortex and hippocampus. The model includes two types of inhibitory cell (FS and LTS), two types of layer V pyramidal cell (IB bursting and RS), two types of layer II/III pyramidal cell (RS and fast-rhythmic bursting) as well as layer VI pyramidal cells and layer IV spiny stellate cells. The model is able to replicate a number of oscillatory behaviors including sleep spindles (10–15 Hz), gamma oscillations (about 30 Hz) and very fast oscillations (> 70 Hz). Although the model contains a higher proportion of fast-rhythmic bursting neurons than so far encountered in barrel cortex, and a large number of excitatory axo-axonic connections that have not yet been encountered experimentally, the model could in practice be adapted to model a barrel cortex column, and as such throws light on how a barrel-column might operate.

Increasing the timing parameters in the circuit allows cortical rhythms to be modeled more realistically. The field has recently focused on the issue of active touch and the possible role of rhythmic whisking. A natural resonance occurs within the thalamocortical circuit at spindle frequencies of 10–15 Hz, which might be exploited in some beneficial way by whisking at 4–12 Hz. Experimental evidence shows that the longer latency components of the response to whisker deflection ($> 15$ ms) are increased at stimulus frequencies in the range 3–10 Hz, and this has been modeled for a single barrel (Garabedian *et al.*, 2003). The model implies that the combination of slow inhibition and thalamocortical adaptation give rise to the band-pass characteristics of the barrel (Garabedian *et al.*, 2003).

The future is impossible to predict of course; nevertheless, one can imagine that a great deal of progress can be made in modeling barrel cortex in future years by using parallel computing and faster processors. If the right parameters could be determined for the subcomponents of the neuronal circuits, one could also imagine that significant speed improvements could be achieved by producing customized chips containing silicon neurons, rather than purely relying on software to model circuit behavior. The path to a complete model of cortical function could proceed through the single-column stage to the point where several columns are joined in simple arrays before coupling other cortical areas together. One of the requirements for progress is obviously the need for sufficient computing power, but that will no doubt increase substantially with time. Another issue that will need to be solved is the need to build complete databases for the experimental evidence as it becomes available. Ideally, databases would carry information in a standard format so that any modeling group could access the information. Similarly, if models were available in more detail within journals, then the work could be replicated and built on more easily, for example to test a model against recently acquired experimental data. The newly formed International Neuroinformatics Coordination Facility has recently embarked on a course that should, if adopted, lead to standardization and interoperability of models and databases (Eckersley *et al.*, 2003; Bjaalie and Grillner, 2007). In the initial stages of development, it would also makes sense for cortical modelers to standardize on a system and, given the large amount of data available for barrel cortex already, it would seem a good test-bed system for such a task.

## 8.5    Genetic analysis of barrel cortex

Genetic manipulation has been of great benefit in understanding the function of molecules that are not otherwise amenable to manipulation by traditional pharmacological methods. Reverse genetics allows the phenotypic trait(s) caused by a known mutation to be identified, while forward genetics allows the genetic origins of a particular phenotypic trait to be identified. In both cases, the unknown element can take some time to unveil. Reverse genetics suffers from redundancy and compensation in the affected gene and can result in an obscure phenotype that takes careful experimentation to discover. Forward genetics suffers from requiring large numbers of animals and from only arriving at the identity of the particular genes involved relatively slowly (Flint *et al.*, 2005), though development of new bioinformatic tools and methodologies promises to reduce this time in the future (Chesler *et al.*, 2005). Nevertheless, both methods have led to major advances in neuroscience in recent years and both have their advantages.

### 8.5.1    *Forward genetic approaches*

Forward genetics methods are particularly useful where polygenic processes are involved. Common examples of polygenic traits in neuroscience research include a number of neuropsychiatry diseases such as schizophrenia and specification of cortical areas during development of the brain. Presently, there is a great deal of interest in the genes involved in cortical development (Section 4.2.1) and, recently, forward genetic methods have been applied to identifying factors that determine barrel cortex identity. The size, shape, pattern and position of the barrel cortex are readily defined and quantifiable phenotypic traits and, therefore, can potentially be analyzed using forward genetics. In a study of 15 strains of recombinant inbred mice, quantitative trait locus analysis has been used to look at variation in barrel cortex size and shape (Li *et al.*, 2005). DBA/2 J mice were found to have a larger barrel field than C57/Bl6 mice despite having smaller brain sizes than the C57/Bl6 strain, indicating that separate factors control brain size and barrel field size. Furthermore, crosses between the inbred strains showed that the parameter of barrel cortex size varied continuously across the strains, suggesting that the trait is indeed polygenic. In a separate study, again using recombinant inbred strains, the positions of individual barrels in C57/Bl6 and DBA/2J were accurately measured and the barrel cortex shown to vary in shape as well as in size (Airey *et al.*, 2006). The degree of systematic variation was less than that caused by expression of *Emx2* in transgenic *nestin–Emx2* mice, for example (Hamasaki *et al.*, 2004), but the differences were nevertheless measurable and reproducible. The existence of spatial gradients in *Emx2* expression during development of the cortex affects the location of boundaries between cortical areas. Therefore, genetic differences between the recombinant inbred strains that mimic that behavior may lead to identification of further cortical morphogens. The fact that the genomes of the C57/Bl6 and DBA/2J strains are fully sequenced should facilitate this process.

Spontaneous mutations in inbred lines have certainly been of great use in barrel cortex research in the past; example include the *barrelless* mouse, which has a deficiency in ACI (Welker *et al.*, 1996), and the mouse strains originally bred by Van der Loos *et al.* (1986) to show that supernumary whiskers on the snout always resulted in supernumary barrels in the cortex. The *barrelless* mutation has led to insights in thalamocortical development, and the strains with supernumary whiskers provided some of the first evidence that the periphery dictated the central pattern of cortical barrels.

At present it is not clear whether forward genetic methods will blossom in barrel cortex research in the near future or not. Mutagenesis using *N*-ethylnitrosourea can increase the number of mutations available and a screen can be performed to detect particular phenotypes. However, the large number of animals required for this type of work may make progress slower than would be ideal. Yet forward genetics offers a systematic method for discovering new genes involved in barrel cortex specification, which is an important goal not easily achieved by other means. The other major branch of genetic analysis is reverse genetics and this is discussed in the next section.

### 8.5.2    *Reverse genetic approaches*

Serendipity can play its part in reverse genetic approaches as well as in forward genetics. For example, the Tg8 line of transgenic mice were found to have a deficiency in monoamine oxidase type A (MAO-A) owing to insertion of an interferon-$\beta$ transgene by chance at a critical site for the gene coding MAO-A. The mutation led to an increase in serotonin expression during early development. It was found that MAO-A knockouts do not have cortical barrels despite having a normal barrel pattern in the thalamus (Cases *et al.*, 1995; see Section 4.3.2). Subsequent studies using directed knockout of the 5-HT transporter, vesicular monoamine transporter and the 5-HT$_{1B}$ receptor, and combinations of these, have revealed that excess levels of serotonin in either the MAO-A mutant or the 5-HT transporter knockout disrupt thalamocortical axon growth by acting on the presynaptically expressed 5HT$_{1B}$ receptor (Rebsam *et al.*, 2002).

In general, reverse genetic approaches have been more directed than serendipitous and very successful in following up on leads from previous studies. The list is too long to detail even a small percentage of the examples in this area, but typical of the approach are the follow-up studies made on the subunits composing PKA in the light of discovery of the phenotype of the *barrelless* animals. The work originated with the observation that this mutant mouse had a deficiency in ACI. If ACI exerts its effect via PKA, then one might expect the barrelless phenotype to occur in mutants lacking particular subunits of PKA. The PKA holoenzyme is composed of two catalytic subunits and two regulatory subunits and can be assembled from two variants of the catalytic subunit (C1 and C2, [*Prkaca* and *Prkacb*]) and two of four variants of the regulatory subunits (RIα, RIβ, RIIα, RIIβ [*Prkar1a*, *Prkar1b*, *Prkar2a*, and *Prkar2b*]). The RIα subunit knockout is lethal and so cannot be investigated this way, which incidentally is a limitation of the reverse genetic approach. However, analysis of the non-lethal null mutants for each of the other subunits showed a selective effect of RIIβ on barrel formation and a lack of effect of the other subunits (Watson *et al.*, 2006). Because RIIβ is located post-synaptically, the observation implicates a postsynaptic ACI/PKA pathway in barrel development. This interpretation is consistent with three further observations, namely the lower levels of postsynaptic GluR1 insertion found in the *barrelless* animals (Lu *et al.*, 2003), the lower expression of GluR1 in synaptosome preparations (Watson *et al.*, 2006) and the lack of AMPA receptor insertion in developing layer IV thalamocortical synapses in the RIIβ mutants (Inan *et al.*, 2006).

The presence or absence of the barrel field has been a quick and easy phenotype to check in mutations that affect neuronal development. The barrel phenotype has been useful in two areas: first, where the role of a specific developmental factor is the prime subject of the experiment, and, second, where the presence of an intact barrel field indicates normal development in a mutation designed to address a non-developmental question. In the latter case, the gene knockout experiment is aimed at disrupting a protein that produces a phenotype in adult animals, but as the mutation is present from conception and, therefore, could theoretically produce a developmental effect. Some studies have cited normal development of the barrel cortex as evidence that a mutation does not cause a substantial developmental abnormality that could otherwise explain the adult phenotype (Orr-Urtreger *et al.*, 1997; Glazewski *et al.*, 2000; Cybulska-Klosowicz *et al.*, 2004; Harwell *et al.*, 2005). Conversely, in many cases the gene knockout experiment is purposely aimed at disrupting a protein that produces a developmental phenotype. Recent studies that have shed light on the role of various factors in development through the barrel phenotype include Hoxa2, which is necessary for axon targeting between principalis and VPm thalamus (Oury *et al.*, 2006), EMX2, which controls the relative rostrolateral position and size of barrel cortex (Hamasaki *et al.*, 2004), and fibroblast growth factor 8, which creates positional cues for thalamocortical innervation of barrel cortex (Shimogori and Grove, 2005).

At present it is not known whether a specific gene is required to code uniquely for barrel cortex. Certainly, genes influencing position of cortical areas are usually expressed in gradients rather than confined to barrel cortex. However, two publications have reported where a randomly inserted reporter gene has been expressed locally in barrel cortex rather than in gradients across cortical areas. The first report of this kind was made by Cohen-Tannoudji *et al.* (1992), who

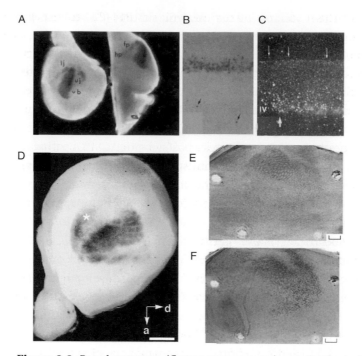

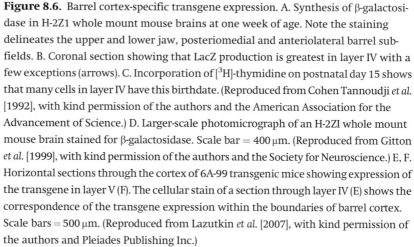

**Figure 8.6.** Barrel cortex-specific transgene expression. A. Synthesis of β-galactosidase in H-2Z1 whole mount mouse brains at one week of age. Note the staining delineates the upper and lower jaw, posteriomedial and anteriolateral barrel subfields. B. Coronal section showing that LacZ production is greatest in layer IV with a few exceptions (arrows). C. Incorporation of [³H]-thymidine on postnatal day 15 shows that many cells in layer IV have this birthdate. (Reproduced from Cohen Tannoudji *et al.* [1992], with kind permission of the authors and the American Association for the Advancement of Science.) D. Larger-scale photomicrograph of an H-2ZI whole mount mouse brain stained for β-galactosidase. Scale bar = 400 μm. (Reproduced from Gitton *et al.* [1999], with kind permission of the authors and the Society for Neuroscience.) E, F. Horizontal sections through the cortex of 6A-99 transgenic mice showing expression of the transgene in layer V (F). The cellular stain of a section through layer IV (E) shows the correspondence of the transgene expression within the boundaries of barrel cortex. Scale bars = 500 μm. (Reproduced from Lazutkin *et al.* [2007], with kind permission of the authors and Pleiades Publishing Inc.)

showed that a subset of layer IV cells located in the barrels of the barrel cortex expressed the *LacZ* reporter gene. The H-2ZI mice are a strain in which a *LacZ* reporter gene is coupled to the class I major histocompatibility complex regulatory sequence (Cohen-Tannoudji et al., 1992). Because of the nature of the transgenic technique employed, the transgene is located in different positions in the genome in different strains made with the same construct. By chance, one strain expressed the reporter gene only in the barrel cortex, as shown in Figure 8.6.

Transplants of the cortex of H-2ZI transgenics at P14–P16 to either cortex or cerebellum of wild-type hosts maintained their expression of the transgene (Cohen-Tannoudji *et al.*, 1994). The timepoint for transplantation occurs at the point just before the layer IV cells are born (Section 4.1.2) which suggests a very early stage of determination for layer and area. The transgene's expression normally occurs coincident with thalamocortical invasion of the cortical plate if left in its natural cortical location (Gitton *et al.*, 1999). However, determination can occur in the absence of thalamocortical afferent ingrowth because transgene expression is present in explants transplanted in the cerebellum (Cohen-Tannoudji *et al.*, 1994). To date, the positional cues surrounding the transgene are not known, so the causative factors for barrel-specific layer IV expression remain to be determined.

The second report of barrel-specific transgene expression was the 6A-99 construct created using the gene-trapping method (Salminen *et al.*, 1998). The *LacZ* reporter gene was randomly inserted in the genome by viral transfer into stem cells, which were then used to create blastocysts and hence the mouse strains (Lazutkin *et al.*, 2007). The reporter was expressed in a deeper layer than layer IV (most probably layer V) of barrel cortex and adjacent SII cortex (Figure 8.6 E, F). The layer specificity of the genes in 6A-99 and H-2ZI constructs are intriguing given that individual progenitor cells give rise to cells in different layers of cortex, albeit at different times in development.

In conclusion, a genetic analysis of the barrel cortex is eminently feasible in the mouse. Forward and reverse genetic studies not only promise to give great insight into the nature of the barrel cortex itself and the developmental processes that shape it, but they also create the tools necessary to make advances in other fields of barrel cortex research. In this respect, the holy grail of barrel cortex genetic analysis would be to discover a promoter that was uniquely active in barrel cortex or several promoters unique to subsets of barrel cortex cells.

## 8.6    Conclusions

Research aimed at understanding barrel cortex and research aimed at understanding neuronal function using barrel cortex as a test system have seen steady and in some cases explosive growth since the discovery of the barrel fields in the early 1970s. One of the strengths of this field is the almost bewildering array of techniques that can be brought to bear. In this chapter, studies using intrinsic optical imaging, MRI, optical in vivo imaging, robotics, behavioral tracking, forward and reverse genetics and computer modeling have all aided progress in understanding barrel cortex function and have built upon the traditional methods of anatomical pathway tracing and electrophysiological recording. The real promise for the future in this area probably lies in using combinations of these methods to tackle questions. For example, one can imagine using a combination of behavioral, transgenic, knockout and cortical blood flow measurement techniques to discover the role of angiogenic factors in recovery from stroke. Similarly, progress in understanding active touch will require not only a knowledge of whisker mechanics and innovative methods of in vivo cortical imaging but also careful design of behavioral paradigms for haptic tasks. Building models to simulate cortical function will require detailed multicellular electrophysiological recordings of cellular properties and synaptic connections, computer modeling and, of course, good communication between the two disciplines. Such work has already started, and these fields have gravitated naturally toward barrel cortex as a tractable system in which to understand this diverse set of inter-related questions. It will be fascinating to see what the next 30 years holds for barrel cortex research.

# References

Abbott, L. F., Regehr, W. G. (2004) Synaptic computation. *Nature* **431**: 796–803.

Abbott, L. F., Varela, J. A., Sen, K., Nelson, S. B. (1997) Synaptic depression and cortical gain control. *Science* **275**: 220–224.

Abdel-Majid, R. M., Leong, W. L., Schalkwyk, L. C., *et al.* (1998) Loss of adenylyl cyclase I activity disrupts patterning of mouse somatosensory cortex. *Nat Genet* **19**: 289–291.

Agmon, A., Connors, B. W. (1991) Thalamocortical responses of mouse somatosensory (barrel) cortex in vitro. *Neuroscience* **41**: 365–379.

Agmon, A., Connors, B. W. (1992) Correlation between intrinsic firing patterns and thalamocortical synaptic responses of neurons in mouse barrel cortex. *J Neurosci* **12**: 319–329.

Agmon, A., Hollrigel, G., O'Dowd, D. K. (1996) Functional GABAergic synaptic connection in neonatal mouse barrel cortex. *J Neurosci* **16**: 4684–4695.

Ahissar, E., Kleinfeld, D. (2003) Closed-loop neuronal computations: focus on vibrissa somatosensation in rat. *Cereb Cortex* **13**: 53–62.

Ahissar, E., Sosnik, R., Haidarliu, S. (2000) Transformation from temporal to rate coding in a somatosensory thalamocortical pathway. *Nature* **406**: 302–306.

Ahissar, E., Sosnik, R., Bagdasarian, K., Haidarliu, S. (2001) Temporal frequency of whisker movement. II. Laminar organization of cortical representations. *J Neurophysiol* **86**: 354–367.

Airey, D. C., Wu, F., Guan, M., Collins, C. E. (2006) Geometric morphometrics defines shape differences in the cortical area map of C57BL/6J and DBA/2J inbred mice. *BMC Neurosci* **7**: 63.

Alberini, C. M., Ghirardi, M., Metz, R., Kandel, E. R. (1994) *C/EBP* is an immediate-early gene required for the consolidation of long-term facilitation in *Aplysia*. *Cell* **76**: 1099–1114.

Allen, C. B., Celikel, T., Feldman, D. E. (2003) Long-term depression induced by sensory deprivation during cortical map plasticity in vivo. *Nat Neurosci* **6**: 291–299.

Alloway, K. D., Zhang, M., Chakrabarti, S. (2004) Septal columns in rodent barrel cortex: functional circuits for modulating whisking behavior. *J Comp Neurol* **480**: 299–309.

Amitai, Y., Gibson, J. R., Beierlein, M., *et al.* (2002) The spatial dimensions of electrically coupled networks of interneurons in the neocortex. *J Neurosci* **22**: 4142–4152.

Andermann, M. L., Moore, C. I. (2006) A somatotopic map of vibrissa motion direction within a barrel column. *Nat Neurosci* **9**: 543–551.

Anderson, P. A., Olavarria, J., Van Sluyters, R. C. (1988) The overall pattern of ocular dominance bands in cat visual cortex. *J Neurosci* **8**: 2183–2200.

Antonini, A., Stryker, M. P. (1993) Rapid remodeling of axonal arbors in the visual cortex. *Science* **260**: 1819–1821.

Armstrong-James, M., Callahan, C. A. (1991) Thalamo-cortical processing of vibrissal information in the rat. II. Spatiotemporal convergence in the thalamic ventroposterior medial nucleus (VPm) and its relevance to generation of receptive fields of S1 cortical "barrel" neurones. *J Comp Neurol* **303**: 211–224.

Armstrong-James, M., Fox, K. (1987) Spatiotemporal convergence and divergence in the rat S1 "barrel" cortex. *J Comp Neurol* **263**: 265–281.

Armstrong-James, M., George, M. J. (1988) Influence of anesthesia on spontaneous activity and receptive field size of single units in rat Sm1 neocortex. *Exp Neurol* **99**: 369–387.

Armstrong-James, M., Callahan, C. A., Friedman, M. A. (1991) Thalamo-cortical processing of vibrissal information in the rat. I. Intracortical origins of surround but not centre-receptive fields of layer IV neurones in the rat S1 barrel field cortex. *J Comp Neurol* **303**: 193–210.

Armstrong-James, M., Fox, K., Das-Gupta, A. (1992) Flow of excitation within rat barrel cortex on striking a single vibrissa. *J Neurophysiol* **68**: 1345–1358.

Armstrong-James, M., Welker, E., Callahan, C. A. (1993) The contribution of NMDA and non-NMDA receptors to fast and slow transmission of sensory information in the rat SI barrel cortex. *J Neurosci* **13**: 2149–2160.

Armstrong-James, M., Diamond, M. E., Ebner, F. F. (1994) An innocuous bias in whisker use in adult rats modifies receptive fields of barrel cortex neurons. *J Neurosci* **14**: 6978–6991.

Arnold, P. B., Li, C. X., Waters, R. S. (2001) Thalamocortical arbors extend beyond single cortical barrels: an in vivo intracellular tracing study in rat. *Exp Brain Res* **136**: 152–168.

Aroniadou-Anderjaska, V., Keller, A. (1995) LTP in the barrel cortex of adult rats. *Neuroreport* **6**: 2297–2300.

Artola, A., Singer, W. (1987) Long-term potentiation and NMDA receptors in rat visual cortex. *Nature* **330**: 649–652.

Artola, A., Brocher, S., Singer, W. (1990) Different voltage-dependent thresholds for inducing long-term depression and long-term potentiation in slices of rat visual cortex. *Nature* **347**: 69–72.

Arvidsson, J., Rice, F. L. (1991) Central projections of primary sensory neurons innervating different parts of the vibrissae follicles and intervibrissal skin on the mystacial pad of the rat. *J Comp Neurol* **309**: 1–16.

Ayata, C., Ma, J., Meng, W., Huang, P., Moskowitz, M. A. (1996) L-NA-sensitive rCBF augmentation during vibrissal stimulation in type III nitric oxide synthase mutant mice. *J Cereb Blood Flow Metab* **16**: 539–541.

Bailey, K. R., Mair, R. G. (2005) Lesions of specific and nonspecific thalamic nuclei affect prefrontal cortex-dependent aspects of spatial working memory. *Behav Neurosci* **119**: 410–419.

Baldi, A., Calia, E., Ciampini, A., *et al.* (2000) Deafferentation-induced apoptosis of neurons in thalamic somatosensory nuclei of the newborn rat: critical period and rescue from cell death by peripherally applied neurotrophins. *Eur J Neurosci* **12**: 2281–2290.

Banke, T. G., Bowie, D., Lee, H., *et al.* (2000) Control of GluR1 AMPA receptor function by cAMP-dependent protein kinase. *J Neurosci* **20**: 89–102.

Bannister, N. J., Benke, T. A., Mellor, J., *et al.* (2005) Developmental changes in AMPA and kainate receptor-mediated quantal transmission at thalamocortical synapses in the barrel cortex. *J Neurosci* **25**: 5259–5271.

Barria, A., Muller, D., Derkach, V., Griffith, L. C., Soderling, T. R. (1997) Regulatory phosphorylation of AMPA-type glutamate receptors by CaM-KII during long-term potentiation. *Science* **276**: 2042–2045.

Barrionuevo, G., Schottler, F., Lynch, G. (1980) The effects of repetitive low frequency stimulation on control and "potentiated" synaptic responses in the hippocampus. *Life Sci* **27**: 2385–2391.

Barth, A. L., McKenna, M., Glazewski, S., *et al.* (2000) Upregulation of cAMP response element-mediated gene expression during experience-dependent plasticity in adult neocortex. *J Neurosci* **20**: 4206–4216.

Baumbach, G. L., Sigmund, C. D., Faraci, F. M. (2004) Structure of cerebral arterioles in mice deficient in expression of the gene for endothelial nitric oxide synthase. *Circ Res* **95**: 822–829.

Beierlein, M., Connors, B. W. (2002) Short-term dynamics of thalamocortical and intracortical synapses onto layer 6 neurons in neocortex. *J Neurophysiol* **88**: 1924–1932.

Beierlein, M., Gibson, J. R., Connors, B. W. (2000) A network of electrically coupled interneurons drives synchronized inhibition in neocortex. *Nat Neurosci* **3**: 904–910.

Beierlein, M., Gibson, J. R., Connors, B. W. (2003) Two dynamically distinct inhibitory networks in layer 4 of the neocortex. *J Neurophysiol* **90**: 2987–3000.

Belford, G. R., Killackey, H. P. (1979) The development of vibrissae representation in subcortical trigeminal centers of the neonatal rat. *J Comp Neurol* **188**: 63–74.

Bellocchio, E. E., Hu, H., Pohorille, A., *et al.* (1998) The localization of the brain-specific inorganic phosphate transporter suggests a specific presynaptic role in glutamatergic transmission. *J Neurosci* **18**: 8648–8659.

Bender, V. A., Bender, K. J., Brasier, D. J., Feldman, D. E. (2006) Two coincidence detectors for spike timing-dependent plasticity in somatosensory cortex. *J Neurosci* **26**: 4166–4177.

Bennett-Clarke, C. A., Leslie, M. J., Chiaia, N. L., Rhoades, R. W. (1993) Serotonin 1B receptors in the developing somatosensory and visual cortices are located on thalamocortical axons. *Proc Natl Acad Sci USA* **90**: 153–157.

Bennett-Clarke, C. A., Leslie, M. J., Lane, R. D., Rhoades, R. W. (1994) Effect of serotonin depletion on vibrissa-related patterns of thalamic afferents in the rat's somatosensory cortex. *J Neurosci* **14**: 7594–7607.

Benshalom, G., White, E. L. (1986) Quantification of thalamocortical synapses with spiny stellate neurons in layer IV of mouse somatosensory cortex. *J Comp Neurol* **253**: 303–314.

Berendse, H. W., Groenewegen, H. J. (1991) Restricted cortical termination fields of the midline and intralaminar thalamic nuclei in the rat. *Neuroscience* **42**: 73–102.

Bernardo, K. L., Woolsey, T. A. (1987) Axonal trajectories between mouse somatosensory thalamus and cortex. *J Comp Neurol* **258**: 542–564.

Bernardo, K. L., Ma, P. M., Woolsey, T. A. (1986) In vitro labeling of axonal projections in the mammalian central nervous system. *J Neurosci Meth* **16**: 89–101.

Bernardo, K. L., McCasland, J. S., Woolsey, T. A., Strominger, R. N. (1990a) Local intra- and interlaminar connections in mouse barrel cortex. *J Comp Neurol* **291**: 231–255.

Bernardo, K. L., McCasland, J. S., Woolsey, T. A. (1990b) Local axonal trajectories in mouse barrel cortex. *Exp Brain Res* **82**: 247–253.

Berwick, J., Martin, C., Martindale, J., *et al.* (2002) Hemodynamic response in the unanesthetized rat: intrinsic optical imaging and spectroscopy of the barrel cortex. *J Cereb Blood Flow Metab* **22**: 670–679.

Bina, K. G., Guzman, P., Broide, R. S., *et al.* (1995) Localization of alpha 7 nicotinic receptor subunit mRNA and alpha-bungarotoxin binding sites in developing mouse somatosensory thalamocortical system. *J Comp Neurol* **363**: 321–332.

Bindman, L. J., Murphy, K. P., Pockett, S. (1988) Postsynaptic control of the induction of long-term changes in efficacy of transmission at neocortical synapses in slices of rat brain. *J Neurophysiol* **60**: 1053–1065.

Binshtok, A. M., Fleidervish, I. A., Sprengel, R., Gutnick, M. J. (2006) NMDA receptors in layer 4 spiny stellate cells of the mouse barrel cortex contain the NR2 C subunit. *J Neurosci* **26**: 708–715.

Bisler, S., Schleicher, A., Gass, P., *et al.* (2002) Expression of c-Fos, ICER, Krox-24 and JunB in the whisker-to-barrel pathway of rats: time course of induction upon whisker stimulation by tactile exploration of an enriched environment. *J Chem Neuroanat* **23**: 187–198.

Bjaalie, J. G., Grillner, S. (2007) Global informatics: the International Neuroinformatics Coordinating Facility. *J Neurosci* **27**: 3613–3615.

Blackstone, C., Sheng, M. (1999) Protein targeting and calcium signaling microdomains in neuronal cells. *Cell Calcium* **26**: 181–192.

Bliss, T. V., Lomo, T. (1970) Plasticity in a monosynaptic cortical pathway. *J Physiol* **207**: 61P.

Bliss, T. V., Lomo, T. (1973) Long-lasting potentiation of synaptic transmission in the dentate area of the anaesthetized rabbit following stimulation of the perforant path. *J Physiol* **232**: 331–356.

Blue, M. E., Martin, L. J., Brennan, E. M., Johnston, M. V. (1997) Ontogeny of non-NMDA glutamate receptors in rat barrel field cortex: I. Metabotropic receptors. *J Comp Neurol* **386**: 16–28.

Bodor, A. L., Katona, I., Nyiri, G., *et al.* (2005) Endocannabinoid signaling in rat somatosensory cortex: laminar differences and involvement of specific interneuron types. *J Neurosci* **25**: 6845–6856.

Boehm, J., Kang, M. G., Johnson, R. C., *et al.* (2006) Synaptic incorporation of AMPA receptors during LTP is controlled by a PKC phosphorylation site on GluR1. *Neuron* **51**: 213–225.

Bourassa, J., Pinault, D., Deschenes, M. (1995) Corticothalamic projections from the cortical barrel field to the somatosensory thalamus in rats: a single-fibre study using biocytin as an anterograde tracer. *Eur J Neurosci* **7**: 19–30.

Bourtchuladze, R., Frenguelli, B., Blendy, J., *et al.* (1994) Deficient long-term memory in mice with a targeted mutation of the cAMP-responsive element-binding protein. *Cell* **79**: 59–68.

Boylan, C. B., Bennett-Clarke, C. A., Crissman, R. S., Mooney, R. D., Rhoades, R. W. (2000) Clorgyline treatment elevates cortical serotonin and temporarily disrupts the vibrissae-related pattern in rat somatosensory cortex. *J Comp Neurol* **427**: 139–149.

Bramham, C. R., Srebro, B. (1987) Induction of long-term depression and potentiation by low- and high-frequency stimulation in the dentate area of the anesthetized rat: magnitude, time course and EEG. *Brain Res* **405**: 100–107.

Brecht, M., Schneider, M., Sakmann, B., Margrie, T. W. (2004) Whisker movements evoked by stimulation of single pyramidal cells in rat motor cortex. *Nature* **427**: 704–710.

Bredt, D. S., Ferris, C. D., Snyder, S. H. (1992) Nitric oxide synthase regulatory sites. Phosphorylation by cyclic AMP-dependent protein kinase, protein kinase C, and calcium/calmodulin protein kinase; identification of flavin and calmodulin binding sites. *J Biol Chem* **267**: 10976–10981.

Brodmann, K. (1909) *Vergleichende Lokalisationlehre der Grosshirnrinde*. Leipzig: Barth.

Broide, R. S., Robertson, R. T., Leslie, F. M. (1996) Regulation of alpha7 nicotinic acetylcholine receptors in the developing rat somatosensory cortex by thalamocortical afferents. *J Neurosci* **16**: 2956–2971.

Brown, C. E., Dyck, R. H. (2003) Experience-dependent regulation of synaptic zinc is impaired in the cortex of aged mice. *Neuroscience* **119**: 795–801.

Brumberg, J. C., Pinto, D. J., Simons, D. J. (1996) Spatial gradients and inhibitory summation in the rat whisker barrel system. *J Neurophysiol* **76**: 130–140.

Bruno, R. M., Sakmann, B. (2006) Cortex is driven by weak but synchronously active thalamocortical synapses. *Science* **312**: 1622–1627.

Bruno, R. M., Simons, D. J. (2002) Feedforward mechanisms of excitatory and inhibitory cortical receptive fields. *J Neurosci* **22**: 10966–10975.

Bruno, R. M., Khatri, V., Land, P. W., Simons, D. J. (2003) Thalamocortical angular tuning domains within individual barrels of rat somatosensory cortex. *J Neurosci* **23**: 9565–9574.

Bugbee, N. M., Goldman-Rakic, P. S. (1983) Columnar organization of corticocortical projections in squirrel and rhesus monkeys: similarity of column width in species differing in cortical volume. *J Comp Neurol* **220**: 355–364.

Buhl, E. H., Tamas, G., Fisahn, A. (1998) Cholinergic activation and tonic excitation induce persistent gamma oscillations in mouse somatosensory cortex in vitro. *J Physiol* **513**: 117–126.

Bureau, I., von Saint Paul, F., Svoboda, K. (2006) Interdigitated paralemniscal and lemniscal pathways in the mouse barrel cortex. *PLoS Biol* **4**: e382.

Calford, M. B., Tweedale, R. (1991a) Immediate expansion of receptive fields of neurons in area 3b of macaque monkeys after digit denervation. *Somatosens Mot Res* **8**: 249–260.

Calford, M. B., Tweedale, R. (1991b) Acute changes in cutaneous receptive fields in primary somatosensory cortex after digit denervation in adult flying fox. *J Neurophysiol* **65**: 178–187.

Calford, M. B., Tweedale, R. (1991c) C-fibres provide a source of masking inhibition to primary somatosensory cortex. *Proc Biol Sci* **243**: 269–275.

Calia, E., Persico, A. M., Baldi, A., Keller, F. (1998) BDNF and NT-3 applied in the whisker pad reverse cortical changes after peripheral deafferentation in neonatal rats. *Eur J Neurosci* **10**: 3194–3200.

Canolty, R. T., Edwards, E., Dalal, S. S., *et al.* (2006) High gamma power is phase-locked to theta oscillations in human neocortex. *Science* **313**: 1626–1628.

Cantallops, I., Haas, K., Cline, H. T. (2000) Postsynaptic CPG15 promotes synaptic maturation and presynaptic axon arbor elaboration in vivo. *Nat Neurosci* **3**: 1004–1011.

Carmichael, S. T., Wei, L., Rovainen, C. M., Woolsey, T. A. (2001) New patterns of intracortical projections after focal cortical stroke. *Neurobiol Dis* **8**: 910–922.

Carpenter, G. A., Milenova, B. L. (2002) Redistribution of synaptic efficacy supports stable pattern learning in neural networks. *Neural Comput* **14**: 873–888.

Carroll, S. B., Gates, J., Keys, D. N., *et al.* (1994) Pattern formation and eyespot determination in butterfly wings. *Science* **265**: 109–114.

Carvell, G. E., Simons, D. J. (1995) Task- and subject-related differences in sensorimotor behavior during active touch. *Somatosens Mot Res* **12**: 1–9.

Carvell, G. E., Simons, D. J. (1996) Abnormal tactile experience early in life disrupts active touch. *J Neurosci* **16**: 2750–2757.

Cases, O., Seif, I., Grimsby, J., *et al.* (1995) Aggressive behavior and altered amounts of brain serotonin and norepinephrine in mice lacking MAOA. *Science* **268**: 1763–1766.

Cases, O., Vitalis, T., Seif, I., *et al.* (1996) Lack of barrels in the somatosensory cortex of monoamine oxidase A-deficient mice: role of a serotonin excess during the critical period. *Neuron* **16**: 297–307.

Castro-Alamancos, M. A., Donoghue, J. P., Connors, B. W. (1995) Different forms of synaptic plasticity in somatosensory and motor areas of the neocortex. *J Neurosci* **15**: 5324–5333.

Catalano, S. M., Robertson, R. T., Killackey, H. P. (1996) Individual axon morphology and thalamocortical topography in developing rat somatosensory cortex. *J Comp Neurol* **367**: 36–53.

Catania, K. C., Kaas, J. H. (1997) Organization of somatosensory cortex and distribution of corticospinal neurons in the eastern mole (*Scalopus aquaticus*). *J Comp Neurol* **378**: 337–353.

Celikel, T., Szostak, V. A., Feldman, D. E. (2004) Modulation of spike timing by sensory deprivation during induction of cortical map plasticity. *Nat Neurosci* **7**: 534–541.

Chagnac-Amitai, Y., Connors, B. W. (1989) Synchronized excitation and inhibition driven by intrinsically bursting neurons in neocortex. *J Neurophysiol* **62**: 1149–1162.

Chagnac-Amitai, Y., Luhmann, H. J., Prince, D. A. (1990) Burst generating and regular spiking layer 5 pyramidal neurons of rat neocortex have different morphological features. *J Comp Neurol* **296**: 598–613.

Chakrabarti, S., Alloway, K. D. (2006) Differential origin of projections from SI barrel cortex to the whisker representations in SII and MI. *J Comp Neurol* **498**: 624–636.

Chapman, P. F., White, G. L., Jones, M. W., *et al.* (1999) Impaired synaptic plasticity and learning in aged amyloid precursor protein transgenic mice. *Nat Neurosci* **2**: 271–276.

Chen, B. E., Lendvai, B., Nimchinsky, E. A., *et al.* (2000) Imaging high-resolution structure of GFP-expressing neurons in neocortex in vivo. *Learn Mem* **7**: 433–441.

Chesler, E. J., Lu, L., Shou, S., *et al.* (2005) Complex trait analysis of gene expression uncovers polygenic and pleiotropic networks that modulate nervous system function. *Nat Genet* **37**: 233–242.

Chiaia, N. L., Rhoades, R. W., Bennett-Clarke, C. A., Fish, S. E., Killackey, H. P. (1991) Thalamic processing of vibrissal information in the rat. I. Afferent input to the medial ventral posterior and posterior nuclei. *J Comp Neurol* **314**: 201–216.

Chiaia, N. L., Fish, S. E., Bauer, W. R., Bennett-Clarke, C. A., Rhoades, R. W. (1992) Postnatal blockade of cortical activity by tetrodotoxin does not disrupt the formation of vibrissa-related patterns in the rat's somatosensory cortex. *Brain Res Dev Brain Res* **66**: 244–250.

Chiaia, N. L., Zhang, S., Crissman, R. S., Rhoades, R. W. (2000) Effects of neonatal axoplasmic transport attenuation on the response properties of vibrissae-sensitive neurons in the trigeminal principal sensory nucleus of the rat. *Somatosens Mot Res* **17**: 273–283.

Cho, K., Aggleton, J. P., Brown, M. W., Bashir, Z. I. (2001) An experimental test of the role of postsynaptic calcium levels in determining synaptic strength using perirhinal cortex of rat. *J Physiol* **532**: 459–466.

Clark, S. A., Allard, T., Jenkins, W. M., Merzenich, M. M. (1988) Receptive fields in the body-surface map in adult cortex defined by temporally correlated inputs. *Nature* **332**: 444–445.

Clem, R. L., Barth, A. (2006) Pathway-specific trafficking of native AMPARs by in vivo experience. *Neuron* **49**: 663–670.

Clements, T. N., Rahn, C. D. (2006) Three-dimensional contact imaging with an actuated whisker. *IEEE Trans Robotics* **22**: 844–848.

Cline, H. T., Debski, E. A., Constantine-Paton, M. (1987) N-Methyl-D-aspartate receptor antagonist desegregates eye-specific stripes. *Proc Natl Acad Sci USA* **84**: 4342–4345.

Cohen-Tannoudji, M., Morello, D., Babinet, C. (1992) Unexpected position-dependent expression of H-2 and beta 2-microglobulin/*lacZ* transgenes. *Mol Reprod Dev* **33**: 149–159.

Cohen-Tannoudji, M., Babinet, C., Wassef, M. (1994) Early determination of a mouse somatosensory cortex marker. *Nature* **368**: 460–463.

Conn, P. J., Pin, J. P. (1997) Pharmacology and functions of metabotropic glutamate receptors. *Annu Rev Pharmacol Toxicol* **37**: 205–237.

Connors, B. W., Kriegstein, A. R. (1986) Cellular physiology of the turtle visual cortex: distinctive properties of pyramidal and stellate neurons. *J Neurosci* **6**: 164–177.

Connors, B. W., Benardo, L. S., Prince, D. A. (1983) Coupling between neurons of the developing rat neocortex. *J Neurosci* **3**: 773–782.

Constantine-Paton, M., Law, M. I. (1978) Eye-specific termination bands in tecta of three-eyed frogs. *Science* **202**: 639–641.

Cooper, N. G., Steindler, D. A. (1986) Lectins demarcate the barrel subfield in the somatosensory cortex of the early postnatal mouse. *J Comp Neurol* **249**: 157–169.

Couve, A., Moss, S. J., Pangalos, M. N. (2000) GABAB receptors: a new paradigm in G protein signaling. *Mol Cell Neurosci* **16**: 296–312.

Cowan, A. I., Stricker, C. (2004) Functional connectivity in layer IV local excitatory circuits of rat somatosensory cortex. *J Neurophysiol* **92**: 2137–2150.

Cox, S. B., Woolsey, T. A., Rovainen, C. M. (1993) Localized dynamic changes in cortical blood flow with whisker stimulation corresponds to matched vascular and neuronal architecture of rat barrels. *J Cereb Blood Flow Metab* **13**: 899–913.

Crabtree, J. W., Collingridge, G. L., Isaac, J. T. (1998) A new intrathalamic pathway linking modality-related nuclei in the dorsal thalamus. *Nat Neurosci* **1**: 389–394.

Crair, M. C., Malenka, R. C. (1995) A critical period for long-term potentiation at thalamocortical synapses. *Nature* **375**: 325–328.

Crochet, S., Petersen, C. C. (2006) Correlating whisker behavior with membrane potential in barrel cortex of awake mice. *Nat Neurosci* **9**: 608–610.

Cruikshank, S., Lewis, T., Connors, B. W. (2007) Synaptic basis for intense thalamocortical activation of feedforward inhibitory cells in neocortex. *Nat Neurosci* **10**: 462–468.

Cunningham, M. O., Whittington, M. A., Bibbig, A., *et al.* (2004) A role for fast rhythmic bursting neurons in cortical gamma oscillations in vitro. *Proc Natl Acad Sci USA* **101**: 7152–7157.

Cybulska-Klosowicz, A., Zakrzewska, R., Pyza, E., Kossut, M., Schachner, M. (2004) Reduced plasticity of cortical whisker representation in adult tenascin-C-deficient mice after vibrissectomy. *Eur J Neurosci* **20**: 1538–1544.

D'Alcantara, P., Schiffmann, S. N., Swillens, S. (2003) Bidirectional synaptic plasticity as a consequence of interdependent Ca$^{2+}$-controlled phosphorylation and dephosphorylation pathways. *Eur J Neurosci* **17**: 2521–2528.

Dagnew, E., Latchamsetty, K., Erinjeri, J. P., *et al.* (2003) Glutamate receptor blockade alters the development of intracortical connections in rat barrel cortex. *Somatosens Mot Res* **20**: 77–84.

Dale, A., Fortin, D. A., Levine, E. S. (2007) Differential effects of endocannabinoids on glutamatergic and GABAergic inputs to layer 5 pyramidal neurons. *Cereb Cortex* **17**: 163–174.

Datwani, A., Iwasato, T., Itohara, S., Erzurumlu, R. S. (2002) Lesion-induced thalamocortical axonal plasticity in the S1 cortex is independent of NMDA receptor function in excitatory cortical neurons. *J Neurosci* **22**: 9171–9175.

Davis, B. M., Fundin, B. T., Albers, K. M., *et al.* (1997) Overexpression of nerve growth factor in skin causes preferential increases among innervation to specific sensory targets. *J Comp Neurol* **387**: 489–506.

Davis, H. P., Squire, L. R. (1984) Protein synthesis and memory: a review. *Psychol Bull* **96**: 518–559.

Davis, T. L., Kwong, K. K., Weisskoff, R. M., Rosen, B. R. (1998) Calibrated functional MRI: mapping the dynamics of oxidative metabolism. *Proc Natl Acad Sci USA* **95**: 1834–1839.

Daw, M. I., Bannister, N. V., Isaac, J. T. (2006) Rapid, activity-dependent plasticity in timing precision in neonatal barrel cortex. *J Neurosci* **26**: 4178–4187.

Daw, N. W., Gordon, B., Fox, K. D., *et al.* (1999) Injection of MK-801 affects ocular dominance shifts more than visual activity. *J Neurophysiol* **81**: 204–215.

De Felipe, J., Marco, P., Fairen, A., Jones, E. G. (1997) Inhibitory synaptogenesis in mouse somatosensory cortex. *Cereb Cortex* **7**: 619–634.

De Paola, V., Holtmaat, A., Knott, G., *et al.* (2006) Cell type-specific structural plasticity of axonal branches and boutons in the adult neocortex. *Neuron* **49**: 861–875.

Deans, M. R., Gibson, J. R., Sellitto, C., Connors, B. W., Paul, D. L. (2001) Synchronous activity of inhibitory networks in neocortex requires electrical synapses containing connexin36. *Neuron* **31**: 477–485.

Dempsey, E., Morison, R. (1943) Electrical activity of the thalamocortical relay system. *Am J Physiol* **138**: 283–296.

Derdikman, D., Yu, C., Haidarliu, S., *et al.* (2006) Layer-specific touch-dependent facilitation and depression in the somatosensory cortex during active whisking. *J Neurosci* **26**: 9538–9547.

Derkach, V., Barria, A., Soderling, T. R. (1999) Ca$^{2+}$/calmodulin-kinase II enhances channel conductance of alpha-amino-3-hydroxy-5-methyl-4-isoxazolepropionate type glutamate receptors. *Proc Natl Acad Sci USA* **96**: 3269–3274.

Descarries, L., Lemay, B., Doucet, G., Berger, B. (1987) Regional and laminar density of the dopamine innervation in adult rat cerebral cortex. *Neuroscience* **21**: 807–824.

Deschenes, M., Bourassa, J., Parent, A. (1995) Two different types of thalamic fibers innervate the rat striatum. *Brain Res* **701**: 288–292.

Deschenes, M., Veinante, P., Zhang, Z. W. (1998) The organization of corticothalamic projections: reciprocity versus parity. *Brain Res Brain Res Rev* **28**: 286–308.

Diamond, M. E. (1995) *Somatosensory Thalamus of the Rat*. London: Plenum.

Diamond, M. E., Armstrong-James, M., Ebner, F. F. (1992a) Somatic sensory responses in the rostral sector of the posterior group (POm) and in the ventral posterior medial nucleus (VPM) of the rat thalamus. *J Comp Neurol* **318**: 462–476.

Diamond, M. E., Armstrong-James, M., Budway, M. J., Ebner, F. F. (1992b) Somatic sensory responses in the rostral sector of the posterior group (POm) and in the ventral posterior medial nucleus (VPM) of the rat thalamus: dependence on the barrel field cortex. *J Comp Neurol* **319**: 66–84.

Diamond, M. E., Armstrong-James, M., Ebner, F. F. (1993) Experience-dependent plasticity in adult rat barrel cortex. *Proc Natl Acad Sci USA* **90**: 2082–2086.

Dirnagl, U., Niwa, K., Lindauer, U., Villringer, A. (1994) Coupling of cerebral blood flow to neuronal activation: role of adenosine and nitric oxide. *Am J Physiol* **267**: H296–301.

Dodt, H. U., Schierloh, A., Eder, M., Zieglgansberger, W. (2003) Circuitry of rat barrel cortex investigated by infrared-guided laser stimulation. *Neuroreport* **14**: 623–627.

Dorfl, J. (1985) The innervation of the mystacial region of the white mouse: A topographical study. *J Anat* **142**: 173–184.

Dudek, S. M., Bear, M. F. (1992) Homosynaptic long-term depression in area CA1 of hippocampus and effects of N-methyl-D-aspartate receptor blockade. *Proc Natl Acad Sci USA* **89**: 4363–4367.

Dunn-Meynell, A. A., Levin, B. E. (1993) Alpha 1-adrenoceptors in the adult rat barrel field: effects of deafferentation and norepinephrine removal. *Brain Res* **623**: 25–32.

Durham, D., Woolsey, T. A. (1984) Effects of neonatal whisker lesions on mouse central trigeminal pathways. *J Comp Neurol* **223**: 424–447.

Eckersley, P., Egan, G. F., Amari, S., *et al.* (2003) Neuroscience data and tool sharing: a legal and policy framework for neuroinformatics. *Neuroinformatics* **1**: 149–165.

Ehrlich, I., Malinow, R. (2004) Postsynaptic density 95 controls AMPA receptor incorporation during long-term potentiation and experience-driven synaptic plasticity. *J Neurosci* **24**: 916–927.

Ekerot, C. F., Kano, M. (1985) Long-term depression of parallel fibre synapses following stimulation of climbing fibres. *Brain Res* **342**: 357–360.

Eliceiri, B. P., Cheresh, D. A. (2001) Adhesion events in angiogenesis. *Curr Opin Cell Biol* **13**: 563–568.

Engert, F., Bonhoeffer, T. (1999) Dendritic spine changes associated with hippocampal long-term synaptic plasticity. *Nature* **399**: 66–70.

Ericson, J., Muhr, J., Placzek, M., *et al.* (1995) Sonic hedgehog induces the differentiation of ventral forebrain neurons: a common signal for ventral patterning within the neural tube. *Cell* **81**: 747–756.

Ericson, J., Morton, S., Kawakami, A., Roelink, H., Jessell, T. M. (1996) Two critical periods of sonic hedgehog signaling required for the specification of motor neuron identity. *Cell* **87**: 661–673.

Erzurumlu, R. S., Jhaveri, S. (1990) Thalamic axons confer a blueprint of the sensory periphery onto the developing rat somatosensory cortex. *Brain Res Dev Brain Res* **56**: 229–234.

Erzurumlu, R. S., Killackey, H. P. (1983) Development of order in the rat trigeminal system. *J Comp Neurol* **213**: 365–380.

Fabri, M., Burton, H. (1991) Ipsilateral cortical connections of primary somatic sensory cortex in rats. *J Comp Neurol* **311**: 405–424.

Fagiolini, M., Pizzorusso, T., Berardi, N., Domenici, L., Maffei, L. (1994) Functional postnatal development of the rat primary visual cortex and the role of visual experience: dark rearing and monocular deprivation. *Vision Res* **34**: 709–720.

Fairen, A., DeFelipe, J., Regidor, J. (1984) *Cellular Components of the Cerebral Cortex.* New York: Plenum.

Favorov, O. V., Diamond, M. E., Whitsel, B. L. (1987) Evidence for a mosaic representation of the body surface in area 3b of the somatic cortex of cat. *Proc Natl Acad Sci USA* **84**: 6606–6610.

Fee, M. S., Mitra, P. P., Kleinfeld, D. (1997) Central versus peripheral determinants of patterned spike activity in rat vibrissa cortex during whisking. *J Neurophysiol* **78**: 1144–1149.

Feldman, D. E. (2000) Timing-based LTP and LTD at vertical inputs to layer II/III pyramidal cells in rat barrel cortex. *Neuron* **27**: 45–56.

Feldman, D. E., Brecht, M. (2005) Map plasticity in somatosensory cortex. *Science* **310**: 810–815.

Feldman, D. E., Nicoll, R. A., Malenka, R. C., Isaac, J. T. (1998) Long-term depression at thalamocortical synapses in developing rat somatosensory cortex. *Neuron* **21**: 347–357.

Feldman, M. L. (1984) *Morphology of the Neocortical Pyramidal Neuron.* New York: Plenum.

Feldmeyer, D., Sakmann, B. (2000) Synaptic efficacy and reliability of excitatory connections between the principal neurones of the input (layer 4) and output layer (layer 5) of the neocortex. *J Physiol* **525**: 31–39.

Feldmeyer, D., Egger, V., Lubke, J., Sakmann, B. (1999) Reliable synaptic connections between pairs of excitatory layer 4 neurones within a single "barrel" of developing rat somatosensory cortex. *J Physiol* **521**: 169–190.

Feldmeyer, D., Lubke, J., Silver, R. A., Sakmann, B. (2002) Synaptic connections between layer 4 spiny neurone-layer 2/3 pyramidal cell pairs in juvenile rat barrel cortex: physiology and anatomy of interlaminar signalling within a cortical column. *J Physiol* **538**: 803–822.

Feldmeyer, D., Roth, A., Sakmann, B. (2005) Monosynaptic connections between pairs of spiny stellate cells in layer 4 and pyramidal cells in layer 5A indicate that lemniscal and paralemniscal afferent pathways converge in the infragranular somatosensory cortex. *J Neurosci* **25**: 3423–3431.

Feldmeyer, D., Lubke, J., Sakmann, B. (2006) Efficacy and connectivity of intracolumnar pairs of layer 2/3 pyramidal cells in the barrel cortex of juvenile rats. *J Physiol* **575**: 583–602.

Ferezou, I., Bolea, S., Petersen, C. C. (2006) Visualizing the cortical representation of whisker touch: voltage-sensitive dye imaging in freely moving mice. *Neuron* **50**: 617–629.

Ferster, D. (1986) Orientation selectivity of synaptic potentials in neurons of cat primary visual cortex. *J Neurosci* **6**: 1284–1301.

Finnerty, G. T., Roberts, L. S., Connors, B. W. (1999) Sensory experience modifies the short-term dynamics of neocortical synapses. *Nature* **400**: 367–371.

Fischer, M., Kaech, S., Knutti, D., Matus, A. (1998) Rapid actin-based plasticity in dendritic spines. *Neuron* **20**: 847–854.

Fischer, M., Kaech, S., Wagner, U., Brinkhaus, H., Matus, A. (2000) Glutamate receptors regulate actin-based plasticity in dendritic spines. *Nat Neurosci* **3**: 887–894.

Fischer, Q. S., Beaver, C. J., Yang, Y., *et al.* (2004) Requirement for the RIIbeta isoform of PKA, but not calcium-stimulated adenylyl cyclase, in visual cortical plasticity. *J Neurosci* **24**: 9049–9058.

Flint, J., Valdar, W., Shifman, S., Mott, R. (2005) Strategies for mapping and cloning quantitative trait genes in rodents. *Nat Rev Genet* **6**: 271–286.

Foehring, R. C., van Brederode, J. F., Kinney, G. A., Spain, W. J. (2002) Serotonergic modulation of supragranular neurons in rat sensorimotor cortex. *J Neurosci* **22**: 8238–8250.

Fox, K. (1992) A critical period for experience-dependent synaptic plasticity in rat barrel cortex. *J Neurosci* **12**: 1826–1838.

Fox, K. (1994) The cortical component of experience-dependent synaptic plasticity in the rat barrel cortex. *J Neurosci* **14**: 7665–7679.

Fox, K. (1995) The critical period for long-term potentiation in primary sensory cortex. *Neuron* **15**: 485–488.

Fox, K. (1996) The role of excitatory amino acid transmission in development and plasticity of SI barrel cortex. *Prog Brain Res* **108**: 219–234.

Fox, K. (2002) Pathways and mechanisms for plasticity in the barrel cortex. *Neuroscience* **111**: 799–84.

Fox, K., Armstrong-James, M. (1986) The role of the anterior intralaminar nuclei and N-methyl-D-aspartate receptors in the generation of spontaneous bursts in rat neocortical neurones. *Exp Brain Res* **63**: 505–518.

Fox, K., Sato, H., Daw, N. (1989) The location and function of NMDA receptors in cat and kitten visual cortex. *J Neurosci* **9**: 2443–2454.

Fox, K., Schlaggar, B. L., Glazewski, S., O'Leary, D. D. (1996a) Glutamate receptor blockade at cortical synapses disrupts development of thalamocortical and columnar organization in somatosensory cortex. *Proc Natl Acad Sci USA* **93**: 5584–5589.

Fox, K., Glazewski, S., Chen, C. M., Silva, A., Li, X. (1996b) Mechanisms underlying experience-dependent potentiation and depression of vibrissae responses in barrel cortex. *J Physiol* (Paris) **90**: 263–269.

Fox, K., Wallace, H., Glazewski, S. (2002) Is there a thalamic component to experience-dependent cortical plasticity? *Philos Trans R Soc Lond B Biol Sci* **357**: 1709–1715.

Fox, K., Wright, N., Wallace, H., Glazewski, S. (2003) The origin of cortical surround receptive fields studied in the barrel cortex. *J Neurosci* **23**: 8380–8391.

Frankland, P. W., Bontempi, B., Talton, L. E., Kaczmarek, L., Silva, A. J. (2004) The involvement of the anterior cingulate cortex in remote contextual fear memory. *Science* **304**: 881–883.

Fremeau, R. T., Jr., Troyer, M. D., Pahner, I., *et al.* (2001) The expression of vesicular glutamate transporters defines two classes of excitatory synapse. *Neuron* **31**: 247–260.

Friedberg, M. H., Lee, S. M., Ebner, F. F. (1999) Modulation of receptive field properties of thalamic somatosensory neurons by the depth of anesthesia. *J Neurophysiol* **81**: 2243–2252.

Friedberg, M. H., Lee, S. M., Ebner, F. F. (2004) The contribution of the principal and spinal trigeminal nuclei to the receptive field properties of thalamic VPM neurons in the rat. *J Neurocytol* **33**: 75–85.

Froc, D. J., Racine, R. J. (2005) Interactions between LTP- and LTD-inducing stimulation in the sensorimotor cortex of the awake freely moving rat. *J Neurophysiol* **93**: 548–556.

Fukuchi-Shimogori, T., Grove, E. A. (2001) Neocortex patterning by the secreted signaling molecule FGF8. *Science* **294**: 1071–1074.

Fundin, B. T., Pfaller, K., Rice, F. L. (1997) Different distributions of the sensory and autonomic innervation among the microvasculature of the rat mystacial pad. *J Comp Neurol* **389**: 545–568.

Gabernet, L., Jadhav, S. P., Feldman, D. E., Carandini, M., Scanziani, M. (2005) Somatosensory integration controlled by dynamic thalamocortical feed-forward inhibition. *Neuron* **48**: 315–327.

Galarreta, M., Hestrin, S. (2001) Electrical synapses between GABA-releasing interneurons. *Nat Rev Neurosci* **2**: 425–433.

Garabedian, C. E., Jones, S. R., Merzenich, M. M., Dale, A., Moore, C. I. (2003) Band-pass response properties of rat SI neurons. *J Neurophysiol* **90**: 1379–1391.

Gehring, W. J. (1987) Homeo boxes in the study of development. *Science* **236**: 1245–1252.

Gehring, W. J. (1993) Exploring the homeobox. *Gene* **135**: 215–221.

Gerrits, R. J., Stein, E. A., Greene, A. S. (1998) Laser-Doppler flowmetry utilizing a thinned skull cranial window preparation and automated stimulation. *Brain Res Brain Res Protoc* **3**: 14–21.

Gerrits, R. J., Stein, E. A., Greene, A. S. (2001) Anesthesia alters NO-mediated functional hyperemia. *Brain Res* **907**: 20–26.

Ghazanfar, A. A., Krupa, D. J., Nicolelis, M. A. (2001) Role of cortical feedback in the receptive field structure and nonlinear response properties of somatosensory thalamic neurons. *Exp Brain Res* **141**: 88–100.

Ghosh, A., Shatz, C. J. (1992) Involvement of subplate neurons in the formation of ocular dominance columns. *Science* **255**: 1441–1443.

Gibson, J. M., Welker, W. I. (1983a) Quantitative studies of stimulus coding in first-order vibrissa afferents of rats. 2. Adaptation and coding of stimulus parameters. *Somatosens Res* **1**: 95–117.

Gibson, J. M., Welker, W. I. (1983b) Quantitative studies of stimulus coding in first-order vibrissa afferents of rats. 1. Receptive field properties and threshold distributions. *Somatosens Res* **1**: 51–67.

Gibson, J. R., Beierlein, M., Connors, B. W. (1999) Two networks of electrically coupled inhibitory neurons in neocortex. *Nature* **402**: 75–79.

Giese, K. P., Fedorov, N. B., Filipkowski, R. K., Silva, A. J. (1998) Autophosphorylation at Thr286 of the alpha calcium-calmodulin kinase II in LTP and learning. *Science* **279**: 870–873.

Gil, Z., Amitai, Y. (1996) Properties of convergent thalamocortical and intracortical synaptic potentials in single neurons of neocortex. *J Neurosci* **16**: 6567–6578.

Gil, Z., Connors, B. W., Amitai, Y. (1997) Differential regulation of neocortical synapses by neuromodulators and activity. *Neuron* **19**: 679–686.

Gilbert, C. D., Kelly, J. P. (1975) The projections of cells in different layers of the cat's visual cortex. *J Comp Neurol* **163**: 81–105.

Ginsberg, M. D., Castella, Y., Dietrich, W. D., Watson, B. D., Busto, R. (1989) Acute thrombotic infarction suppresses metabolic activation of ipsilateral somatosensory cortex: evidence for functional diaschisis. *J Cereb Blood Flow Metab* **9**: 329–341.

Gioanni, Y., Rougeot, C., Clarke, P. B., *et al.* (1999) Nicotinic receptors in the rat prefrontal cortex: increase in glutamate release and facilitation of mediodorsal thalamo-cortical transmission. *Eur J Neurosci* **11**: 18–30.

Girod, R., Barazangi, N., McGehee, D., Role, L. W. (2000) Facilitation of glutamatergic neurotransmission by presynaptic nicotinic acetylcholine receptors. *Neuropharmacology* **39**: 2715–2725.

Gitton, Y., Cohen-Tannoudji, M., Wassef, M. (1999) Specification of somatosensory area identity in cortical explants. *J Neurosci* **19**: 4889–4898.

Glade, N., Demongeot, J., Tabony, J. (2002) Comparison of reaction–diffusion simulations with experiment in self-organised microtubule solutions. *C R Biol* **325**: 283–294.

Glazewski, S., Fox, K. (1996) Time course of experience-dependent synaptic potentiation and depression in barrel cortex of adolescent rats. *J Neurophysiol* **75**: 1714–1729.

Glazewski, S., Chen, C. M., Silva, A., Fox, K. (1996) Requirement for alpha-CaMKII in experience-dependent plasticity of the barrel cortex. *Science* **272**: 421–423.

Glazewski, S., Herman, C., McKenna, M., Chapman, P. F., Fox, K. (1998a) Long-term potentiation in vivo in layers II/III of rat barrel cortex. *Neuropharmacology* **37**: 581–592.

Glazewski, S., McKenna, M., Jacquin, M., Fox, K, (1998b) Experience-dependent depression of vibrissae responses in adolescent rat barrel cortex. *Eur J Neurosci* **10**: 2107–2116.

Glazewski, S., Barth, A. L., Wallace, H., *et al.* (1999) Impaired experience-dependent plasticity in barrel cortex of mice lacking the alpha and delta isoforms of CREB. *Cereb Cortex* **9**: 249–256.

Glazewski, S., Giese, K. P., Silva, A., Fox, K. (2000) The role of alpha-CaMKII autophosphorylation in neocortical experience-dependent plasticity. *Nat Neurosci* **3**: 911–918.

Goldreich, D., Kyriazi, H. T., Simons, D. J. (1999) Functional independence of layer IV barrels in rodent somatosensory cortex. *J Neurophysiol* **82**: 1311–1316.

Gottlieb, J. P., Keller, A. (1997) Intrinsic circuitry and physiological properties of pyramidal neurons in rat barrel cortex. *Exp Brain Res* **115**: 47–60.

Gottschaldt, K. M., Iggo, A., Young, D. W. (1973) Functional characteristics of mechanoreceptors in sinus hair follicles of the cat. *J Physiol* **235**: 287–315.

Grinvald, A., Lieke, E., Frostig, R. D., Gilbert, C. D., Wiesel, T. N. (1986) Functional architecture of cortex revealed by optical imaging of intrinsic signals. *Nature* **324**: 361–364.

Gross, J., Schnitzler, A., Timmermann, L., Ploner, M. (2007) Gamma oscillations in human primary somatosensory cortex reflect pain perception. *PLoS Biol* **5**: e133.

Grosshans, D. R., Clayton, D. A., Coultrap, S. J., Browning, M. D. (2002) LTP leads to rapid surface expression of NMDA but not AMPA receptors in adult rat CA1. *Nat Neurosci* **5**: 27–33.

Haidarliu, S., Ahissar, E. (2001) Size gradients of barreloids in the rat thalamus. *J Comp Neurol* **429**: 372–387.

Haidarliu, S., Sosnik, R., Ahissar, E. (1999) Simultaneous multi-site recordings and iontophoretic drug and dye applications along the trigeminal system of anesthetized rats. *J Neurosci Meth* **94**: 27–40.

Hall, W. C., Ebner, F. F. (1970) Thalamotelencephalic projections in the turtle (*Pseudemys scripta*). *J Comp Neurol* **140**: 101–122.

Hallas, B. H., Jacquin, M. F. (1990) Structure–function relationships in rat brain stem subnucleus interpolaris. IX. Inputs from subnucleus caudalis. *J Neurophysiol* **64**: 28–45.

Hamada, Y., Miyashita, E., Tanaka, H. (1999) Gamma-band oscillations in the "barrel cortex" precede rat's exploratory whisking. *Neuroscience* **88**: 667–671.

Hamasaki, T., Leingartner, A., Ringstedt, T., O'Leary, D. D. (2004) EMX2 regulates sizes and positioning of the primary sensory and motor areas in neocortex by direct specification of cortical progenitors. *Neuron* **43**: 359–372.

Hamori, J., Savy, C., Madarasz, M., *et al.* (1986) Morphological alterations in subcortical vibrissal relays following vibrissal follicle destruction at birth in the mouse. *J Comp Neurol* **254**: 166–183.

Hand, P. J. (1982) *Plasticity of the Rat Barrel System*. New York: Academic Press.

Hannan, A. J., Blakemore, C., Katsnelson, A., *et al.* (2001) PLC-beta1, activated via mGluRs, mediates activity-dependent differentiation in cerebral cortex. *Nat Neurosci* **4**: 282–288.

Hardingham, N., Fox, K. (2006) The role of nitric oxide and GluR1 in presynaptic and postsynaptic components of neocortical potentiation. *J Neurosci* **26**: 7395–7404.

Hardingham, N. R., Fox, K. (2007). A role of PKA in the reversal of depression in layer II/III barrel cortex. *Proceedings of the Annual Meeting of the Society for Neuroscience*, San Diego, CA, abstract 146.12/L22.

Hardingham, N., Glazewski, S., Pakhotin, P., *et al.* (2003) Neocortical long-term potentiation and experience-dependent synaptic plasticity require alpha-calcium/calmodulin-dependent protein kinase II autophosphorylation. *J Neurosci* **23**: 4428–4436.

Hardingham, N. R., Bannister, N. J., Read, J. C., *et al.* (2006) Extracellular calcium regulates postsynaptic efficacy through group 1 metabotropic glutamate receptors. *J Neurosci* **26**: 6337–6345.

Hardingham, N. R., Wright, N. F., Fox, K. (2006) The role of GluR1 and cannabinoid receptors in neocortical LTD and experience-dependent depression. *Proceedings of the Annual Meeting of the Society for Neuroscience*, Atlanta, GA, abstract 732.13/G12.

Harris, J. A., Miniussi, C., Harris, I. M., Diamond, M. E. (2002) Transient storage of a tactile memory trace in primary somatosensory cortex. *J Neurosci* **22**: 8720–8725.

Harris, R. M., Woolsey, T. A. (1979) Morphology of Golgi-impregnated neurons in mouse cortical barrels following vibrissae damage at different post-natal ages. *Brain Res* **161**: 143–149.

Harris, R. M., Woolsey, T. A. (1981) Dendritic plasticity in mouse barrel cortex following postnatal vibrissa follicle damage. *J Comp Neurol* **196**: 357–376.

Harris, R. M., Woolsey, T. A. (1983) Computer-assisted analyses of barrel neuron axons and their putative synaptic contacts. *J Comp Neurol* **220**: 63–79.

Hartings, J. A., Temereanca, S., Simons, D. J. (2000) High responsiveness and direction sensitivity of neurons in the rat thalamic reticular nucleus to vibrissa deflections. *J Neurophysiol* **83**: 2791–2801.

Hartmann, M. J., Johnson, N. J., Towal, R. B., Assad, C. (2003) Mechanical characteristics of rat vibrissae: resonant frequencies and damping in isolated whiskers and in the awake behaving animal. *J Neurosci* **23**: 6510–6519.

Harvey, M. A., Sachdev, R. N., Zeigler, H. P. (2001) Cortical barrel field ablation and unconditioned whisking kinematics. *Somatosens Mot Res* **18**: 223–227.

Harwell, C., Burbach, B., Svoboda, K., Nedivi, E. (2005) Regulation of *cpg15* expression during single whisker experience in the barrel cortex of adult mice. *J Neurobiol* **65**: 85–96.

Hayashi, Y., Shi, S. H., Esteban, J. A., *et al.* (2000) Driving AMPA receptors into synapses by LTP and CaMKII: requirement for GluR1 and PDZ domain interaction. *Science* **287**: 2262–2267.

He, J., Devonshire, I. M., Mayhew, J. E., Papadakis, N. G. (2007) Simultaneous laser Doppler flowmetry and arterial spin labeling MRI for measurement of functional perfusion changes in the cortex. *Neuroimage* **34**: 1391–1404.

Henderson, T. A., Woolsey, T. A., Jacquin, M. F. (1992) Infraorbital nerve blockade from birth does not disrupt central trigeminal pattern formation in the rat. *Brain Res Dev Brain Res* **66**: 146–152.

Henderson, T. A., Rhoades, R. W., Bennett-Clarke, C. A., *et al.* (1993) NGF augmentation rescues trigeminal ganglion and principalis neurons, but not brainstem or cortical whisker patterns, after infraorbital nerve injury at birth. *J Comp Neurol* **336**: 243–260.

Henderson, T. A., Johnson, E. M., Jr., Osborne, P. A., Jacquin, M. F. (1994) Fetal NGF augmentation preserves excess trigeminal ganglion cells and interrupts whisker-related pattern formation. *J Neurosci* **14**: 3389–3403.

Hensch, T. K., Fagiolini, M., Mataga, N., *et al.* (1998a) Local GABA circuit control of experience-dependent plasticity in developing visual cortex. *Science* **282**: 1504–1508.

Hensch, T. K., Gordon, J. A., Brandon, E. P., *et al.* (1998b) Comparison of plasticity in vivo and in vitro in the developing visual cortex of normal and protein kinase A RIbeta-deficient mice. *J Neurosci* **18**: 2108–2117.

Herkenham, M. (1979) The afferent and efferent connections of the ventromedial thalamic nucleus in the rat. *J Comp Neurol* **183**: 487–517.

Herkenham, M. (1980) Laminar organization of thalamic projections to the rat neocortex. *Science* **207**: 532–535.

Heynen, A. J., Yoon, B. J., Liu, C. H., *et al.* (2003) Molecular mechanism for loss of visual cortical responsiveness following brief monocular deprivation. *Nat Neurosci* **6**: 854–862.

Hickmott, P. W., Steen, P. A. (2005) Large-scale changes in dendritic structure during reorganization of adult somatosensory cortex. *Nat Neurosci* **8**: 140–142.

Higley, M. J., Contreras, D. (2003) Nonlinear integration of sensory responses in the rat barrel cortex: an intracellular study in vivo. *J Neurosci* **23**: 10190–10200.

Hipp, J., Arabzadeh, E., Zorzin, E., *et al.* (2006) Texture signals in whisker vibrations. *J Neurophysiol* **95**: 1792–1799.

Hoeflinger, B. F., Bennett-Clarke, C. A., Chiaia, N. L., Killackey, H. P., Rhoades, R. W. (1995) Patterning of local intracortical projections within the vibrissae representation of rat primary somatosensory cortex. *J Comp Neurol* **354**: 551–563.

Hoffer, Z. S., Hoover, J. E., Alloway, K. D. (2003) Sensorimotor corticocortical projections from rat barrel cortex have an anisotropic organization that facilitates integration of inputs from whiskers in the same row. *J Comp Neurol* **466**: 525–544.

Hoffman, D. A., Sprengel, R., Sakmann, B. (2002) Molecular dissection of hippocampal theta-burst pairing potentiation. *Proc Natl Acad Sci USA* **99**: 7740–7745.

Hollmann, M., Heinemann, S. (1994) Cloned glutamate receptors. *Annu Rev Neurosci* **17**: 31–108.

Holtmaat, A. J., Trachtenberg, J. T., Wilbrecht, L., *et al.* (2005) Transient and persistent dendritic spines in the neocortex in vivo. *Neuron* **45**: 279–291.

Hoogland, P. V., Welker, E., van der Loos, H. (1987) Organization of the projections from barrel cortex to thalamus in mice studied with *Phaseolus vulgaris*-leucoagglutinin and HRP. *Exp Brain Res* **68**: 73–87.

Hoogland, P. V., Wouterlood, F. G., Welker, E., Van der Loos, H. (1991) Ultrastructure of giant and small thalamic terminals of cortical origin: a study of the projections from the barrel cortex in mice using *Phaseolus vulgaris* leuco-agglutinin (PHA-L). *Exp Brain Res* **87**: 159–172.

Hubel, D. H., Wiesel, T. N. (1977) Ferrier lecture. Functional architecture of macaque monkey visual cortex. *Proc R Soc Lond B Biol Sci* **198**: 1–59.

Hubel, D. H., Wiesel, T. N., Stryker, M. P. (1978) Anatomical demonstration of orientation columns in macaque monkey. *J Comp Neurol* **177**: 361–380.

Huber, K. M., Roder, J. C., Bear, M. F. (2001) Chemical induction of mGluR5- and protein synthesis-dependent long-term depression in hippocampal area CA1. *J Neurophysiol* **86**: 321–325.

Hurwitz, B. E., Dietrich, W. D., McCabe, P. M., *et al.* (1990) Sensory–motor deficit and recovery from thrombotic infarction of the vibrissal barrel-field cortex. *Brain Res* **512**: 210–220.

Husi, H., Ward, M. A., Choudhary, J. S., Blackstock, W. P., Grant, S. G. (2000) Proteomic analysis of NMDA receptor-adhesion protein signaling complexes. *Nat Neurosci* **3**: 661–669.

Inan, M., Lu, H. C., Albright, M. J., She, W. C., Crair, M. C. (2006) Barrel map development relies on protein kinase A regulatory subunit II beta-mediated cAMP signaling. *J Neurosci* **26**: 4338–4349.

Ince-Dunn, G., Hall, B. J., Hu, S. C., *et al.* (2006) Regulation of thalamocortical patterning and synaptic maturation by NeuroD2. *Neuron* **49**: 683–695.

Irikura, K., Maynard, K. I., Moskowitz, M. A. (1994) Importance of nitric oxide synthase inhibition to the attenuated vascular responses induced by topical L-nitroarginine during vibrissal stimulation. *J Cereb Blood Flow Metab* **14**: 45–48.

Isaac, J. T., Crair, M. C., Nicoll, R. A., Malenka, R. C. (1997) Silent synapses during development of thalamocortical inputs. *Neuron* **18**: 269–280.

Ismailov, I., Kalikulov, D., Inoue, T., Friedlander, M. J. (2004) The kinetic profile of intracellular calcium predicts long-term potentiation and long-term depression. *J Neurosci* **24**: 9847–9861.

Itami, C., Kimura, F., Kohno, T., *et al.* (2003) Brain-derived neurotrophic factor-dependent unmasking of "silent" synapses in the developing mouse barrel cortex. *Proc Natl Acad Sci USA* **100**: 13069–13074.

Ito, M. (1985) Processing of vibrissa sensory information within the rat neocortex. *J Neurophysiol* **54**: 479–490.

Ito, M., Kano, M. (1982) Long-lasting depression of parallel fiber–Purkinje cell transmission induced by conjunctive stimulation of parallel fibers and climbing fibers in the cerebellar cortex. *Neurosci Lett* **33**: 253–258.

Ito, M., Kato, M. (2002) Analysis of variance study of the rat cortical layer 4 barrel and layer 5b neurones. *J Physiol* **539**: 511–522.

Iwasato, T., Datwani, A., Wolf, A. M., *et al.* (2000) Cortex-restricted disruption of NMDAR1 impairs neuronal patterns in the barrel cortex. *Nature* **406**: 726–731.

Jaarsma, D., Sebens, J. B., Korf, J. (1991) Localization of NMDA and AMPA receptors in rat barrel field. *Neurosci Lett* **133**: 233–236.

Jablonka, J., Kossut, M. (2006) Focal stroke in the barrel cortex of rats enhances ipsilateral response to vibrissal input. *Acta Neurobiol Exp* (Wars) **66**: 261–266.

Jablonka, J. A., Witte, O. W., Kossut, M. (2007) Photothrombotic infarct impairs experience-dependent plasticity in neighboring cortex. *Neuroreport* **18**: 165–169.

Jablonska, B., Smith, A. L., Kossut, M., Skangiel-Kramska, J. (1998) Development of laminar distributions of kainate receptors in the somatosensory cortex of mice. *Brain Res* **791**: 325–329.

Jacob, V., Le Cam, J., Shulz, D. E. (2006) Spatiotemporally complex tactile stimuli delivered through a multi-actuator whisker stimulator. In *Proceedings of the Annual Meeting of the Society for Neuroscience*, pp. 145.120. Atlanta, GA: Society for Neuroscience.

Jacquin, M. F., Woerner, D., Szczepanik, A. M., *et al.* (1986) Structure–function relationships in rat brainstem subnucleus interpolaris. I. Vibrissa primary afferents. *J Comp Neurol* **243**: 266–279.

Jacquin, M. F., Stennett, R. A., Renehan, W. E., Rhoades, R. W. (1988a) Structure–function relationships in the rat brainstem subnucleus interpolaris: II. Low and high threshold trigeminal primary afferents. *J Comp Neurol* **267**: 107–130.

Jacquin, M. F., Golden, J., Panneton, W. M. (1988b) Structure and function of barrel "precursor" cells in trigeminal nucleus principalis. *Brain Res* **471**: 309–314.

Jacquin, M. F., Barcia, M., Rhoades, R. W. (1989) Structure–function relationships in rat brainstem subnucleus interpolaris: IV. Projection neurons. *J Comp Neurol* **282**: 45–62.

Jacquin, M. F., Wiegand, M. R., Renehan, W. E. (1990) Structure–function relationships in rat brain stem subnucleus interpolaris. VIII. Cortical inputs. *J Neurophysiol* **64**: 3–27.

Jacquin, M. F., Renehan, W. E., Rhoades, R. W., Panneton, W. M. (1993a) Morphology and topography of identified primary afferents in trigeminal subnuclei principalis and oralis. *J Neurophysiol* **70**: 1911–1936.

Jacquin, M. F., McCasland, J. S., Henderson, T. A., Rhoades, R. W., Woolsey, T. A. (1993b) 2-DG uptake patterns related to single vibrissae during exploratory behaviors in the hamster trigeminal system. *J Comp Neurol* **332**: 38–58.

Jacquin, M. F., Rhoades, R. W., Klein, B. G. (1995) Structure–function relationships in rat brainstem subnucleus interpolaris. XI. Effects of chronic whisker trimming from birth. *J Comp Neurol* **356**: 200–224.

Jeanmonod, D., Rice, F. L., Van der Loos, H. (1981) Mouse somatosensory cortex: alterations in the barrelfield following receptor injury at different early postnatal ages. *Neuroscience* **6**: 1503–1535.

Jensen, K. F., Killackey, H. P. (1987) Terminal arbors of axons projecting to the somatosensory cortex of the adult rat. I. The normal morphology of specific thalamocortical afferents. *J Neurosci* **7**: 3529–3543.

Jones, E. G. (1985) *The Thalamus.* New York: Plenum Press.

Kamal, A., Ramakers, G. M., Urban, I. J., De Graan, P. N., Gispen, W. H. (1999) Chemical LTD in the CA1 field of the hippocampus from young and mature rats. *Eur J Neurosci* **11**: 3512–3516.

Kaneko, M., Kanayama, N., Tsuji, T. (1998) Active antenna for contact sensing. *IEEE Trans Robotics Automation* **14**: 278–291.

Katz, D. B., Simon, S. A., Moody, A., Nicolelis, M. A. (1999) Simultaneous reorganization in thalamocortical ensembles evolves over several hours after perioral capsaicin injections. *J Neurophysiol* **82**: 963–977.

Kawaguchi, Y. (1995) Physiological subgroups of nonpyramidal cells with specific morphological characteristics in layer II/III of rat frontal cortex. *J Neurosci* **15**: 2638–2655.

Kawaguchi, Y., Kubota, Y. (1997) GABAergic cell subtypes and their synaptic connections in rat frontal cortex. *Cereb Cortex* **7**: 476–486.

Keller, A., Carlson, G. C. (1999) Neonatal whisker clipping alters intracortical, but not thalamocortical projections, in rat barrel cortex. *J Comp Neurol* **412**: 83–94.

Keller, A., White, E. L. (1987) Synaptic organization of GABAergic neurons in the mouse SmI cortex. *J Comp Neurol* **262**: 1–12.

Kelly, M. K., Carvell, G. E., Kodger, J. M., Simons, D. J. (1999) Sensory loss by selected whisker removal produces immediate disinhibition in the somatosensory cortex of behaving rats. *J Neurosci* **19**: 9117–9125.

Kennedy, M. B. (2000) Signal-processing machines at the postsynaptic density. *Science* **290**: 750–754.

Kennerley, A. J., Berwick, J., Martindale, J., *et al.* (2005) Concurrent fMRI and optical measures for the investigation of the hemodynamic response function. *Magn Reson Med* **54**: 354–365.

Kharazia, V. N., Weinberg, R. J. (1994) Glutamate in thalamic fibers terminating in layer IV of primary sensory cortex. *J Neurosci* **14**: 6021–6032.

Kidd, F. L., Isaac, J. T. (1999) Developmental and activity-dependent regulation of kainate receptors at thalamocortical synapses. *Nature* **400**: 569–573.

Kidd, F. L., Coumis, U., Collingridge, G. L., Crabtree, J. W., Isaac, J. T. (2002) A presynaptic kainate receptor is involved in regulating the dynamic properties of thalamocortical synapses during development. *Neuron* **34**: 635–646.

Killackey, H. P. (1973) Anatomical evidence for cortical subdivisions based on vertically discrete thalamic projections from the ventral posterior nucleus to cortical barrels in the rat. *Brain Res* **51**: 326–331.

Killackey, H. P., Belford, G. R. (1979) The formation of afferent patterns in the somatosensory cortex of the neonatal rat. *J Comp Neurol* **183**: 285–303.

Killackey, H. P., Belford, G. R. (1980) Central correlates of peripheral pattern alterations in the trigeminal system of the rat. *Brain Res* **183**: 205–210.

Killackey, H. P., Ebner, F. (1973) Convergent projection of three separate thalamic nuclei on to a single cortical area. *Science* **179**: 283–285.

Killackey, H. P., Belford, G., Ryugo, R., Ryugo, D. K. (1976) Anomalous organization of thalamocortical projections consequent to vibrissae removal in the newborn rat and mouse. *Brain Res* **104**: 309–315.

Kim, C. H., Chung, H. J., Lee, H. K., Huganir, R. L. (2001) Interaction of the AMPA receptor subunit GluR2/3 with PDZ domains regulates hippocampal long-term depression. *Proc Natl Acad Sci USA* **98**: 11725–11730.

Kim, H. G., Fox, K., Connors, B. W. (1995) Properties of excitatory synaptic events in neurons of primary somatosensory cortex of neonatal rats. *Cereb Cortex* **5**: 148–157.

Kim, U., Ebner, F. F. (1999) Barrels and septa: separate circuits in rat barrels field cortex. *J Comp Neurol* **408**: 489–505.

Kirkwood, A., Silva, A., Bear, M. F. (1997) Age-dependent decrease of synaptic plasticity in the neocortex of alphaCaMKII mutant mice. *Proc Natl Acad Sci USA* **94**: 3380–3383.

Kleinfeld, D., Berg, R. W., O'Connor, S. M. (1999) Anatomical loops and their electrical dynamics in relation to whisking by rat. *Somatosens Mot Res* **16**: 69–88.

Kleinfeld, D., Ahissar, E., Diamond, M. E. (2006) Active sensation: insights from the rodent vibrissa sensorimotor system. *Curr Opin Neurobiol* **16**: 434–444.

Knott, G. W., Quairiaux, C., Genoud, C., Welker, E. (2002) Formation of dendritic spines with GABAergic synapses induced by whisker stimulation in adult mice. *Neuron* **34**: 265–273.

Knott, G. W., Holtmaat, A., Wilbrecht, L., Welker, E., Svoboda, K. (2006) Spine growth precedes synapse formation in the adult neocortex in vivo. *Nat Neurosci* **9**: 1117–1124.

Knutsen, P. M., Pietr, M., Ahissar, E. (2006) Haptic object localization in the vibrissal system: behavior and performance. *J Neurosci* **26**: 8451–8464.

Koralek, K. A., Jensen, K. F., Killackey, H. P. (1988) Evidence for two complementary patterns of thalamic input to the rat somatosensory cortex. *Brain Res* **463**: 346–351.

Koralek, K. A., Olavarria, J., Killackey, H. P. (1990) Areal and laminar organization of corticocortical projections in the rat somatosensory cortex. *J Comp Neurol* **299**: 133–150.

Kossut, M., Hand, P. (1984) Early development of changes in cortical representation of C3 vibrissa following neonatal denervation of surrounding vibrissa receptors: a 2-deoxyglucose study in the rat. *Neurosci Lett* **46**: 7–12.

Kossut, M., Juliano, S. L. (1999) Anatomical correlates of representational map reorganization induced by partial vibrissectomy in the barrel cortex of adult mice. *Neuroscience* **92**: 807–817.

Kossut, M., Hand, P. J., Greenberg, J., Hand, C. L. (1988) Single vibrissal cortical column in SI cortex of rat and its alterations in neonatal and adult vibrissa-deafferented animals: a quantitative 2DG study. *J Neurophysiol* **60**: 829–852.

Kriegstein, A. R., Connors, B. W. (1986) Cellular physiology of the turtle visual cortex: synaptic properties and intrinsic circuitry. *J Neurosci* **6**: 178–191.

Kristt, D. A., Waldman, J. V. (1982) Developmental reorganization of acetylcholinesterase-rich inputs to somatosensory cortex of the mouse. *Anat Embryol* (Berl) **164**: 331–342.

Krupa, D. J., Ghazanfar, A. A., Nicolelis, M. A. (1999) Immediate thalamic sensory plasticity depends on corticothalamic feedback. *Proc Natl Acad Sci USA* **96**: 8200–8205.

Krupa, D. J., Brisben, A. J., Nicolelis, M. A. (2001) A multi-channel whisker stimulator for producing spatiotemporally complex tactile stimuli. *J Neurosci Meth* **104**: 199–208.

Krupa, D. J., Wiest, M. C., Shuler, M. G., Laubach, M., Nicolelis, M. A. (2004) Layer-specific somatosensory cortical activation during active tactile discrimination. *Science* **304**: 1989–1992.

Kurokawa, J., Motoike, H. K., Rao, J., Kass, R. S. (2004) Regulatory actions of the A-kinase anchoring protein Yotiao on a heart potassium channel downstream of PKA phosphorylation. *Proc Natl Acad Sci USA* **101**: 16374–16378.

Kyriazi, H. T., Simons, D. J. (1993) Thalamocortical response transformations in simulated whisker barrels. *J Neurosci* **13**: 1601–1615.

Kyriazi, H. T., Carvell, G. E., Brumberg, J. C., Simons, D. J. (1996a) Effects of baclofen and phaclofen on receptive field properties of rat whisker barrel neurons. *Brain Res* **712**: 325–328.

Kyriazi, H. T., Carvell, G. E., Brumberg, J. C., Simons, D. J. (1996b) Quantitative effects of GABA and bicuculline methiodide on receptive field properties of neurons in real and simulated whisker barrels. *J Neurophysiol* **75**: 547–560.

Laaris, N., Keller, A. (2002) Functional independence of layer IV barrels. *J Neurophysiol* **87**: 1028–1034.

Land, P. W., Simons, D. J. (1985) Cytochrome oxidase staining in the rat SmI barrel cortex. *J Comp Neurol* **238**: 225–235.

Land, P. W., Buffer, S. A., Jr., Yaskosky, J. D. (1995) Barreloids in adult rat thalamus: three-dimensional architecture and relationship to somatosensory cortical barrels. *J Comp Neurol* **355**: 573–588.

Lanuza, E., Novejarque, A., Moncho-Bogani, J., Hernandez, A., Martinez-Garcia, F. (2002) Understanding the basic circuitry of the cerebral hemispheres: the case of lizards and its implications in the evolution of the telencephalon. *Brain Res Bull* **57**: 471–473.

Lavallee, P., Deschenes, M. (2004) Dendroarchitecture and lateral inhibition in thalamic barreloids. *J Neurosci* **24**: 6098–6105.

Lavdas, A. A., Grigoriou, M., Pachnis, V., Parnavelas, J. G. (1999) The medial ganglionic eminence gives rise to a population of early neurons in the developing cerebral cortex. *J Neurosci* **19**: 7881–7888.

Lavenex, P., Amaral, D. G. (2000) Hippocampal–neocortical interaction: a hierarchy of associativity. *Hippocampus* **10**: 420–430.

Lazutkin, A. A., Meyer, B. I., Anokhin, K. V. (2007) [Transgene *6A-99* is a molecular marker of developing somatosensory cortex in mice.] *Ontogenez* **38**: 21–32.

Lebrand, C., Cases, O., Wehrle, R., *et al.* (1998) Transient developmental expression of monoamine transporters in the rodent forebrain. *J Comp Neurol* **401**: 506–524.

Lee, H. K., Kameyama, K., Huganir, R. L., Bear, M. F. (1998) NMDA induces long-term synaptic depression and dephosphorylation of the GluR1 subunit of AMPA receptors in hippocampus. *Neuron* **21**: 1151–1162.

Lee, K. J., Woolsey, T. A. (1975) A proportional relationship between peripheral innervation density and cortical neuron number in the somatosensory system of the mouse. *Brain Res* **99**: 349–353.

Lee, L. J., Erzurumlu, R. S. (2005) Altered parcellation of neocortical somatosensory maps in *N*-methyl-D-aspartate receptor-deficient mice. *J Comp Neurol* **485**: 57–63.

Lee, L. J., Iwasato, T., Itohara, S., Erzurumlu, R. S. (2005) Exuberant thalamocortical axon arborization in cortex-specific NMDAR1 knockout mice. *J Comp Neurol* **485**: 280–292.

Lee, S. H., Simons, D. J. (2004) Angular tuning and velocity sensitivity in different neuron classes within layer 4 of rat barrel cortex. *J Neurophysiol* **91**: 223–229.

Lee, S. M., Weisskopf, M. G., Ebner, F. F. (1991) Horizontal long-term potentiation of responses in rat somatosensory cortex. *Brain Res* **544**: 303–310.

Leergaard, T. B., Alloway, K. D., Mutic, J. J., Bjaalie, J. G. (2000) Three-dimensional topography of corticopontine projections from rat barrel cortex: correlations with corticostriatal organization. *J Neurosci* **20**: 8474–8484.

Lendvai, B., Stern, E. A., Chen, B., Svoboda, K. (2000) Experience-dependent plasticity of dendritic spines in the developing rat barrel cortex in vivo. *Nature* **404**: 876–881.

LeVay, S., Wiesel, T. N., Hubel, D. H. (1980) The development of ocular dominance columns in normal and visually deprived monkeys. *J Comp Neurol* **191**: 1–51.

Li, C. X., Wei, X., Lu, L., Peirce, J. L., Williams, R. W., Waters, R. S. (2005) Genetic analysis of barrel field size in the first somatosensory area (SI) in inbred and recombinant inbred strains of mice. *Somatosens Mot Res* **22**: 141–150.

Li, X., Glazewski, S., Lin, X., Elde, R., Fox, K. (1995) Effect of vibrissae deprivation on follicle innervation, neuropeptide synthesis in the trigeminal ganglion, and S1 barrel cortex plasticity. *J Comp Neurol* **357**: 465–481.

Lichtenstein, S. H., Carvell, G. E., Simons, D. J. (1990) Responses of rat trigeminal ganglion neurons to movements of vibrissae in different directions. *Somatosens Mot Res* **7**: 47–65.

Lidov, H. G., Grzanna, R., Molliver, M. E. (1980) The serotonin innervation of the cerebral cortex in the rat: an immunohistochemical analysis. *Neuroscience* **5**: 207–227.

Lindvall, O., Bjorklund, A., Moore, R. Y., Stenevi, U. (1974) Mesencephalic dopamine neurons projecting to neocortex. *Brain Res* **81**: 325–331.

Lisman, J. E. (1985) A mechanism for memory storage insensitive to molecular turnover: a bistable autophosphorylating kinase. *Proc Natl Acad Sci USA* **82**: 3055–3057.

Lisman, J. E., Goldring, M. A. (1988) Feasibility of long-term storage of graded information by the $Ca^{2+}$/calmodulin-dependent protein kinase molecules of the postsynaptic density. *Proc Natl Acad Sci USA* **85**: 5320–5324.

Liu, X. B., Jones, E. G. (1996) Localization of alpha type II calcium calmodulin-dependent protein kinase at glutamatergic but not gamma-aminobutyric acid (GABAergic) synapses in thalamus and cerebral cortex. *Proc Natl Acad Sci USA* **93**: 7332–7336.

Liu, X. B., Jones, E. G. (2003) Fine structural localization of connexin-36 immunoreactivity in mouse cerebral cortex and thalamus. *J Comp Neurol* **466**: 457–467.

Lopez-Bendito, G., Cautinat, A., Sanchez, J. A., *et al.* (2006) Tangential neuronal migration controls axon guidance: a role for neuregulin-1 in thalamocortical axon navigation. *Cell* **125**: 127–142.

Lorento de Nó, R. (1922) La corteza cerebral del ratón. *Trab Lab Invest Boil* (Madrid) **20**: 41–78.

Lorente de Nó, R. (1992) The cerebral cortex of the mouse (a first contribution – the "acoustic" cortex). *Somatosens Mot Res* **9**: 3–36.

Lotto, B., Upton, L., Price, D. J., Gaspar, P. (1999) Serotonin receptor activation enhances neurite outgrowth of thalamic neurones in rodents. *Neurosci Lett* **269**: 87–90.

LoTurco, J. J., Blanton, M. G., Kriegstein, A. R. (1991) Initial expression and endogenous activation of NMDA channels in early neocortical development. *J Neurosci* **11**: 792–799.

Louderback, K. M., Glass, C. S., Shamalla-Hannah, L., Erickson, S. L., Land, P. W. (2006) Subbarrel patterns of thalamocortical innervation in rat somatosensory cortical barrels: organization and postnatal development. *J Comp Neurol* **497**: 32–41.

Lu, H. C., She, W. C., Plas, D. T., *et al.* (2003) Adenylyl cyclase I regulates AMPA receptor trafficking during mouse cortical "barrel" map development. *Nat Neurosci* **6**: 939–947.

Lu, S. M., Lin, R. C. (1993) Thalamic afferents of the rat barrel cortex: a light- and electron-microscopic study using *Phaseolus vulgaris* leucoagglutinin as an anterograde tracer. *Somatosens Mot Res* **10**: 1–16.

Lubke, J., Egger, V., Sakmann, B., Feldmeyer, D. (2000) Columnar organization of dendrites and axons of single and synaptically coupled excitatory spiny neurons in layer 4 of the rat barrel cortex. *J Neurosci* **20**: 5300–5311.

Lubke, J., Roth, A., Feldmeyer, D., Sakmann, B. (2003) Morphometric analysis of the columnar innervation domain of neurons connecting layer 4 and layer 2/3 of juvenile rat barrel cortex. *Cereb Cortex* **13**: 1051–1063.

Luis de la Iglesia, J. A., Lopez-Garcia, C. (1997) A Golgi study of the principal projection neurons of the medial cortex of the lizard *Podarcis hispanica*. *J Comp Neurol* **385**: 528–564.

Luo, L. (2002) Actin cytoskeleton regulation in neuronal morphogenesis and structural plasticity. *Annu Rev Cell Dev Biol* **18**: 601–635.

Luskin, M. B., Shatz, C. J. (1985) Studies of the earliest generated cells of the cat's visual cortex: cogeneration of subplate and marginal zones. *J Neurosci* **5**: 1062–1075.

Luskin, M. B., Pearlman, A. L., Sanes, J. R. (1988) Cell lineage in the cerebral cortex of the mouse studied in vivo and in vitro with a recombinant retrovirus. *Neuron* **1**: 635–647.

Ma, J., Ayata, C., Huang, P. L., Fishman, M. C., Moskowitz, M. A. (1996) Regional cerebral blood flow response to vibrissal stimulation in mice lacking type I NOS gene expression. *Am J Physiol* **270**: H1085–H1090.

Ma, P. M. (1991) The barrelettes: architectonic vibrissal representations in the brainstem trigeminal complex of the mouse. I. Normal structural organization. *J Comp Neurol* **309**: 161–199.

Ma, Y., Hu, H., Berrebi, A. S., Mathers, P. H., Agmon, A. (2006) Distinct subtypes of somatostatin-containing neocortical interneurons revealed in transgenic mice. *J Neurosci* **26**: 5069–5082.

Maalouf, M., Miasnikov, A. A., Dykes, R. W. (1998) Blockade of cholinergic receptors in rat barrel cortex prevents long-term changes in the evoked potential during sensory preconditioning. *J Neurophysiol* **80**: 529–545.

Maass, W., Natschlager, T., Markram, H. (2002) Real-time computing without stable states: a new framework for neural computation based on perturbations. *Neural Comput* **14**: 2531–2560.

Maass, W., Natschlager, T., Markram, H. (2004) Fading memory and kernel properties of generic cortical microcircuit models. *J Physiol Paris* **98**: 315–330.

Malenka, R. C., Bear, M. F. (2004) LTP and LTD: an embarrassment of riches. *Neuron* **44**: 5–21.

Maletic-Savatic, M., Malinow, R., Svoboda, K. (1999) Rapid dendritic morphogenesis in CA1 hippocampal dendrites induced by synaptic activity. *Science* **283**: 1923–1927.

Malinow, R. (2003) AMPA receptor trafficking and long-term potentiation. *Philos Trans R Soc Lond B Biol Sci* **358**: 707–714.

Malinow, R., Malenka, R. C. (2002) AMPA receptor trafficking and synaptic plasticity. *Annu Rev Neurosci* **25**: 103–126.

Mansour-Robaey, S., Mechawar, N., Radja, F., Beaulieu, C., Descarries, L. (1998) Quantified distribution of serotonin transporter and receptors during the postnatal development of the rat barrel field cortex. *Brain Res Dev Brain Res* **107**: 159–163.

Maravall, M., Koh, I. Y., Lindquist, W. B., Svoboda, K. (2004) Experience-dependent changes in basal dendritic branching of layer 2/3 pyramidal neurons during a critical period for developmental plasticity in rat barrel cortex. *Cereb Cortex* **14**: 655–664.

Marin-Padilla, M. (1978) Dual origin of the mammalian neocortex and evolution of the cortical plate. *Anat Embryol* (Berl) **152**: 109–126.

Marin-Padilla, M., Marin-Padilla, T. M. (1982) Origin, prenatal development and structural organization of layer I of the human cerebral (motor) cortex. A Golgi study. *Anat Embryol* (Berl) **164**: 161–206.

Markram, H. (2006) The blue brain project. *Nat Rev Neurosci* **7**: 153–160.

Markram, H., Tsodyks, M. (1996) Redistribution of synaptic efficacy between neocortical pyramidal neurons. *Nature* **382**: 807–810.

Markram, H., Lubke, J., Frotscher, M., Sakmann, B. (1997) Regulation of synaptic efficacy by coincidence of postsynaptic APs and EPSPs. *Science* **275**: 213–215.

Markram, H., Toledo-Rodriguez, M., Wang, Y., Gupta, A., Silberberg, G., Wu, C. (2004) Interneurons of the neocortical inhibitory system. *Nat Rev Neurosci* **5**: 793–807.

Marsicano, G., Lutz, B. (1999) Expression of the cannabinoid receptor CB1 in distinct neuronal subpopulations in the adult mouse forebrain. *Eur J Neurosci* **11**: 4213–4225.

Martin, C., Martindale, J., Berwick, J., Mayhew, J. (2006) Investigating neural–hemodynamic coupling and the hemodynamic response function in the awake rat. *Neuroimage* **32**: 33–48.

Martinotti, C. (1889) Contributo allo studio della corteccia cerebrale, ed all'origine central dei nervi. *Ann Freniatr Sci Affini* **1**: 314–381.

Martinotti, C. (1890) Beitrag zum Studium der Hirnrinde und dem Centralursprung der Nerven. *Int Monatschr Anat Physiol* **7**: 69–90.

Masino, S. A., Kwon, M. C., Dory, Y., Frostig, R. D. (1993) Characterization of functional organization within rat barrel cortex using intrinsic signal optical imaging through a thinned skull. *Proc Natl Acad Sci USA* **90**: 9998–10002.

Maunsell, J. H., Van Essen, D. C. (1983) The connections of the middle temporal visual area (MT) and their relationship to a cortical hierarchy in the macaque monkey. *J Neurosci* **3**: 2563–2586.

Mayer, M. L., Westbrook, G. L., Guthrie, P. B. (1984) Voltage-dependent block by $Mg^{2+}$ of NMDA responses in spinal cord neurones. *Nature* **309**: 261–263.

McCasland, J. S., Hibbard, L. S. (1997) GABAergic neurons in barrel cortex show strong, whisker-dependent metabolic activation during normal behavior. *J Neurosci* **17**: 5509–5527.

McCasland, J. S., Bernardo, K. L., Probst, K. L., Woolsey, T. A. (1992) Cortical local circuit axons do not mature after early deafferentation. *Proc Natl Acad Sci USA* **89**: 1832–1836.

McCasland, J. S., Hibbard, L. S., Rhoades, R. W., Woolsey, T. A. (1997) Activation of a wide-spread network of inhibitory neurons in barrel cortex. *Somatosens Mot Res* **14**: 138–147.

McCormick, D. A., Bal, T. (1997) Sleep and arousal: thalamocortical mechanisms. *Annu Rev Neurosci* **20**: 185–215.

McKinney, R. A., Capogna, M., Durr, R., Gahwiler, B. H., Thompson, S. M. (1999) Miniature synaptic events maintain dendritic spines via AMPA receptor activation. *Nat Neurosci* **2**: 44–49.

Melzer, P., Smith, C. B. (1998) Plasticity of cerebral metabolic whisker maps in adult mice after whisker follicle removal: I. Modifications in barrel cortex coincide with reorganization of follicular innervation. *Neuroscience* **83**: 27–41.

Mercier, B. E., Legg, C. R., Glickstein, M. (1990) Basal ganglia and cerebellum receive different somatosensory information in rats. *Proc Natl Acad Sci USA* **87**: 4388–4392.

Merzenich, M. M., Kaas, J. H., Wall, J. T., *et al.* (1983a) Progression of change following median nerve section in the cortical representation of the hand in areas 3b and 1 in adult owl and squirrel monkeys. *Neuroscience* **10**: 639–665.

Merzenich, M. M., Kaas, J. H., Wall, J., *et al.* (1983b) Topographic reorganization of somatosensory cortical areas 3b and 1 in adult monkeys following restricted deafferentation. *Neuroscience* **8**: 33–55.

Mesulam, M. M., Mufson, E. J., Levey, A. I., Wainer, B. H. (1983) Cholinergic innervation of cortex by the basal forebrain: cytochemistry and cortical connections of the septal area, diagonal band nuclei, nucleus basalis (substantia innominata), and hypothalamus in the rhesus monkey. *J Comp Neurol* **214**: 170–197.

Metin, C., Frost, D. O. (1989) Visual responses of neurons in somatosensory cortex of hamsters with experimentally induced retinal projections to somatosensory thalamus. *Proc Natl Acad Sci USA* **86**: 357–361.

Micheva, K. D., Beaulieu, C. (1995a) An anatomical substrate for experience-dependent plasticity of the rat barrel field cortex. *Proc Natl Acad Sci USA* **92**: 11834–11838.

Micheva, K. D., Beaulieu, C. (1995b) Postnatal development of GABA neurons in the rat somatosensory barrel cortex: a quantitative study. *Eur J Neurosci* **7**: 419–430.

Micheva, K. D., Beaulieu, C. (1995c) Neonatal sensory deprivation induces selective changes in the quantitative distribution of GABA-immunoreactive neurons in the rat barrel field cortex. *J Comp Neurol* **361**: 574–584.

Micheva, K. D., Beaulieu, C. (1996) Quantitative aspects of synaptogenesis in the rat barrel field cortex with special reference to GABA circuitry. *J Comp Neurol* **373**: 340–354.

Miller, B., Blake, N. M., Erinjeri, J. P., *et al.* (2001) Postnatal growth of intrinsic connections in mouse barrel cortex. *J Comp Neurol* **436**: 17–31.

Miller, M. W. (1985) Cogeneration of retrogradely labeled corticocortical projection and GABA-immunoreactive local circuit neurons in cerebral cortex. *Brain Res* **355**: 187–192.

Miller, M. W. (1995) Relationship of the time of origin and death of neurons in rat somatosensory cortex: barrel versus septal cortex and projection versus local circuit neurons. *J Comp Neurol* **355**: 6–14.

Miller, S. G., Kennedy, M. B. (1985) Distinct forebrain and cerebellar isozymes of type II $Ca^{2+}$/calmodulin-dependent protein kinase associate differently with the postsynaptic density fraction. *J Biol Chem* **260**: 9039–9046.

Miller, S. G., Kennedy, M. B. (1986) Regulation of brain type II $Ca^{2+}$/calmodulin-dependent protein kinase by autophosphorylation: a $Ca^{2+}$-triggered molecular switch. *Cell* **44**: 861–870.

Minnery, B. S., Simons, D. J. (2003) Response properties of whisker-associated trigeminothalamic neurons in rat nucleus principalis. *J Neurophysiol* **89**: 40–56.

Minnery, B. S., Bruno, R. M., Simons, D. J. (2003) Response transformation and receptive field synthesis in the lemniscal trigeminothalamic circuit. *J Neurophysiol* **90**: 1379–1391.

Mitchinson, B., Gurney, K. N., Redgrave, P., *et al.* (2004) Empirically inspired simulated electro-mechanical model of the rat mystacial follicle-sinus complex. *Proc Biol Sci* **271**: 2509–2516.

Molnar, Z., Adams, R., Blakemore, C. (1998) Mechanisms underlying the early establishment of thalamocortical connections in the rat. *J Neurosci* **18**: 5723–5745.

Monaghan, D. T., Cotman, C. W. (1985) Distribution of N-methyl-D-aspartate-sensitive L-[$^3$H]glutamate-binding sites in rat brain. *J Neurosci* **5**: 2909–2919.

Monaghan, D. T., Olverman, H. J., Nguyen, L., *et al.* (1988) Two classes of N-methyl-D-aspartate recognition sites: differential distribution and differential regulation by glycine. *Proc Natl Acad Sci USA* **85**: 9836–9840.

Monconduit, L., Bourgeais, L., Bernard, J. F., Le Bars, D., Villanueva, L. (1999) Ventromedial thalamic neurons convey nociceptive signals from the whole body surface to the dorsolateral neocortex. *J Neurosci* **19**: 9063–9072.

Monteiro, A., French, V., Smit, G., Brakefield, P. M., Metz, J. A. (2001) Butterfly eyespot patterns: evidence for specification by a morphogen diffusion gradient. *Acta Biotheor* **49**: 77–88.

Mosconi, T. M., Rice, F. L. (1991) Sensory innervation of the mystacial pad fur of the ferret. *Neurosci Lett* **121**: 199–202.

Mountcastle, V. B. (1957) Modality and topographic properties of single neurons of cat's somatic sensory cortex. *J Neurophysiol* **20**: 408–434.

Mountcastle, V. B., Powell, T. P. (1959) Neural mechanisms subserving cutaneous sensibility, with special reference to the role of afferent inhibition in sensory perception and discrimination. *Bull Johns Hopkins Hosp* **105**: 201–232.

Mountcastle, V. B., Davies, P. W., Berman, A. L. (1957) Response properties of neurons of cat's somatic sensory cortex to peripheral stimuli. *J Neurophysiol* **20**: 374–407.

Muly, E. C., Maddox, M., Smith, Y. (2003) Distribution of mGluR1alpha and mGluR5 immunolabeling in primate prefrontal cortex. *J Comp Neurol* **467**: 521–535.

Munoz, A., Liu, X. B., Jones, E. G. (1999) Development of metabotropic glutamate receptors from trigeminal nuclei to barrel cortex in postnatal mouse. *J Comp Neurol* **409**: 549–566.

Nadarajah, B., Parnavelas, J. G. (2002) Modes of neuronal migration in the developing cerebral cortex. *Nat Rev Neurosci* **3**: 423–432.

Nagerl, U. V., Eberhorn, N., Cambridge, S. B., Bonhoeffer, T. (2004) Bidirectional activity-dependent morphological plasticity in hippocampal neurons. *Neuron* **44**: 759–767.

Nakao, Y., Itoh, Y., Kuang, T. Y., *et al.* (2001) Effects of anesthesia on functional activation of cerebral blood flow and metabolism. *Proc Natl Acad Sci USA* **98**: 7593–7598.

Nedivi, E., Wu, G. Y., Cline, H. T. (1998) Promotion of dendritic growth by CPG15, an activity-induced signaling molecule. *Science* **281**: 1863–1866.

Neimark, M. A., Andermann, M. L., Hopfield, J. J., Moore, C. I. (2003) Vibrissa resonance as a transduction mechanism for tactile encoding. *J Neurosci* **23**: 6499–6509.

Nicolelis, M. A., Chapin, J. K. (1994) Spatiotemporal structure of somatosensory responses of many-neuron ensembles in the rat ventral posterior medial nucleus of the thalamus. *J Neurosci* **14**: 3511–3532.

Nicolelis, M. A., Chapin, J. K., Lin, R. C. (1991) Thalamic plasticity induced by early whisker removal in rats. *Brain Res* **561**: 344–349.

Nicolelis, M. A., Baccala, L. A., Lin, R. C., Chapin, J. K. (1995) Sensorimotor encoding by synchronous neural ensemble activity at multiple levels of the somatosensory system. *Science* **268**: 1353–1358.

Nicolelis, M. A., Lin, R. C., Chapin, J. K. (1997) Neonatal whisker removal reduces the discrimination of tactile stimuli by thalamic ensembles in adult rats. *J Neurophysiol* **78**: 1691–1706.

Noctor, S. C., Martinez-Cerdeno, V., Ivic, L., Kriegstein, A. R. (2004) Cortical neurons arise in symmetric and asymmetric division zones and migrate through specific phases. *Nat Neurosci* **7**: 136–144.

Nomura, S., Itoh, K., Sugimoto, T., *et al.* (1986) Mystacial vibrissae representation within the trigeminal sensory nuclei of the cat. *J Comp Neurol* **253**:121–133.

North, S., Moenner, M., Bikfalvi, A. (2005) Recent developments in the regulation of the angiogenic switch by cellular stress factors in tumors. *Cancer Lett* **218**: 1–14.

Olausson, B., Shyu, B. C., Rydenhag, B. (1989) Projection from the thalamic intralaminar nuclei on the isocortex of the rat: a surface potential study. *Exp Brain Res* **75**: 543–554.

Olavarria, J., Van Sluyters, R. C., Killackey, H. P. (1984) Evidence for the complementary organization of callosal and thalamic connections within rat somatosensory cortex. *Brain Res* **291**: 364–368.

Oliva, A. A., Jr., Jiang, M., Lam, T., Smith, K. L., Swann, J. W. (2000) Novel hippocampal interneuronal subtypes identified using transgenic mice that express green fluorescent protein in GABAergic interneurons. *J Neurosci* **20**: 3354–3368.

Orr-Urtreger, A., Goldner, F. M., Saeki, M., *et al.* (1997) Mice deficient in the alpha7 neuronal nicotinic acetylcholine receptor lack alpha-bungarotoxin binding sites and hippocampal fast nicotinic currents. *J Neurosci* **17**: 9165–9171.

Oury, F., Murakami, Y., Renaud, J. S., *et al.* (2006) Hoxa2- and rhombomere-dependent development of the mouse facial somatosensory map. *Science* **313**: 1408–1413.

Pasternak, J. R., Woolsey, T. A. (1975) The number, size and spatial distribution of neurons in lamina IV of the mouse SmI neocortex. *J Comp Neurol* **160**: 291–306.

Paxinos, G., Watson, C. (1986) *The Rat Brain in Sterotaxic Coordinates*, 2nd edn. San Diego, CA: Academic Press.

Perez-Garci, E., Gassmann, M., Bettler, B., Larkum, M. E. (2006) The GABAB1b isoform mediates long-lasting inhibition of dendritic Ca2+ spikes in layer 5 somatosensory pyramidal neurons. *Neuron* **50**: 603–616.

Persico, A. M., Mengual, E., Moessner, R., *et al.* (2001) Barrel pattern formation requires serotonin uptake by thalamocortical afferents, and not vesicular monoamine release. *J Neurosci* **21**: 6862–6873.

Peters, A., Harriman, K. M. (1988) Enigmatic bipolar cell of rat visual cortex. *J Comp Neurol* **267**: 409–432.

Peters, A., Jones, E. G. (1984) *Cellular Components of the Cerebral Cortex*. New York: Plenum.

Peters, A., Kimerer, L. M. (1981) Bipolar neurons in rat visual cortex: a combined Golgi–electron microscope study. *J Neurocytol* **10**: 921–946.

Petersen, C. C. (2002) Short-term dynamics of synaptic transmission within the excitatory neuronal network of rat layer 4 barrel cortex. *J Neurophysiol* **87**: 2904–2914.

Petersen, C. C., Grinvald, A., Sakmann, B. (2003) Spatiotemporal dynamics of sensory responses in layer 2/3 of rat barrel cortex measured in vivo by voltage-sensitive dye imaging combined with whole-cell voltage recordings and neuron reconstructions. *J Neurosci* **23**: 1298–1309.

Petersen, R. S., Diamond, M. E. (2000) Spatial-temporal distribution of whisker-evoked activity in rat somatosensory cortex and the coding of stimulus location. *J Neurosci* **20**: 6135–6143.

Petralia, R. S., Wang, Y. X., Singh, S., *et al.* (1997) A monoclonal antibody shows discrete cellular and subcellular localizations of mGluR1 alpha metabotropic glutamate receptors. *J Chem Neuroanat* **13**: 77–93.

Petreanu, L. T., Shepherd, G. M. G., Svoboda, K. (2005) Laser-scanning photostimulation reveals that two classes of layer 5B neurons mediate distinct aspects of experience-dependent plasticity. *Proceedings of the Annual Meeting of the Society for Neuroscience*, Washington, DC, abstract 985.2.

Pierret, T., Lavallee, P., Deschenes, M. (2000) Parallel streams for the relay of vibrissal information through thalamic barreloids. *J Neurosci* **20**: 7455–7462.

Pinto, D. J., Brumberg, J. C., Simons, D. J., Ermentrout, G. B. (1996) A quantitative population model of whisker barrels: re-examining the Wilson–Cowan equations. *J Comput Neurosci* **3**: 247–264.

Pinto, D. J., Brumberg, J. C., Simons, D. J. (2000) Circuit dynamics and coding strategies in rodent somatosensory cortex. *J Neurophysiol* **83**: 1158–1166.

Pinto, D. J., Hartings, J. A., Brumberg, J. C., Simons, D. J. (2003) Cortical damping: analysis of thalamocortical response transformations in rodent barrel cortex. *Cereb Cortex* **13**: 33–44.

Porter, J. T., Johnson, C. K., Agmon, A. (2001) Diverse types of interneurons generate thalamus-evoked feedforward inhibition in the mouse barrel cortex. *J Neurosci* **21**: 2699–2710.

Priest, C. A., Thompson, A. J., Keller, A. (2001) Gap junction proteins in inhibitory neurons of the adult barrel neocortex. *Somatosens Mot Res* **18**: 245–252.

Rabow, L. E., Russek, S. J., Farb, D. H. (1995) From ion currents to genomic analysis: recent advances in GABA$_A$ receptor research. *Synapse* **21**: 189–274.

Radnikow, G., Feldmeyer, D., Lubke, J. (2002) Axonal projection, input and output synapses, and synaptic physiology of Cajal–Retzius cells in the developing rat neocortex. *J Neurosci* **22**: 6908–6919.

Rakic, P. (1971) Guidance of neurones migrating to the fetal monkey neocortex. *Brain Research* **33**: 471–476.

Ramon y Cajal, S. (1911) *Histologie due Systeme Nerveux de l'Homme et des Vertebres.* Paris: Maloine.

Ramon y Cajal, S. (1922) Studien uber die Sehrinde der Katze. *J Psychol Neurol* **29**: 161–181.

Rao, Y., Fischer, Q. S., Yang, Y., *et al.* (2004) Reduced ocular dominance plasticity and long-term potentiation in the developing visual cortex of protein kinase A RII alpha mutant mice. *Eur J Neurosci* **20**: 837–842.

Rebsam, A., Seif, I., Gaspar, P. (2002) Refinement of thalamocortical arbors and emergence of barrel domains in the primary somatosensory cortex: a study of normal and monoamine oxidase a knock-out mice. *J Neurosci* **22**: 8541–8552.

Rema, V., Armstrong-James, M., Ebner, F. F. (1998) Experience-dependent plasticity of adult rat S1 cortex requires local NMDA receptor activation. *J Neurosci* **18**: 10196–10206.

Rema, V., Armstrong-James, M., Jenkinson, N., Ebner, F. F. (2006) Short exposure to an enriched environment accelerates plasticity in the barrel cortex of adult rats. *Neuroscience* **140**: 659–672.

Ren, J. Q. (1991) [Stereological analysis of GABAergic neurons and calcium binding protein parvalbumin-containing neurons in the rat somatosensory cortex.] *Fukuoka Igaku Zasshi* **82**: 659–670.

Ren, J. Q., Aika, Y., Heizmann, C. W., Kosaka, T. (1992) Quantitative analysis of neurons and glial cells in the rat somatosensory cortex, with special reference to GABAergic neurons and parvalbumin-containing neurons. *Exp Brain Res* **92**: 1–14.

Reyes, A., Sakmann, B. (1999) Developmental switch in the short-term modification of unitary EPSPs evoked in layer 2/3 and layer 5 pyramidal neurons of rat neocortex. *J Neurosci* **19**: 3827–3835.

Reyes, A., Lujan, R., Rozov, A., Burnashev, N., Somogyi, P., Sakmann, B. (1998) Target-cell-specific facilitation and depression in neocortical circuits. *Nat Neurosci* **1**: 279–285.

Rhoades, R. W., Strang, V., Bennett-Clarke, C. A., Killackey, H. P., Chiaia, N. L. (1997) Sensitive period for lesion-induced reorganization of intracortical projections within the vibrissae representation of rat's primary somatosensory cortex. *J Comp Neurol* **389**: 185–192.

Rice, D. S., Curran, T. (2001) Role of the reelin signaling pathway in central nervous system development. *Annu Rev Neurosci* **24**: 1005–1039.

Rice, F. L., Van der Loos, H. (1977) Development of the barrels and barrel field in the somatosensory cortex of the mouse. *J Comp Neurol* **171**: 545–560.

Rice, F. L., Gomez, C., Barstow, C., Burnet, A., Sands, P. (1985) A comparative analysis of the development of the primary somatosensory cortex: interspecies similarities during barrel and laminar development. *J Comp Neurol* **236**: 477–495.

Rice, F. L., Mance, A., Munger, B. L. (1986) A comparative light microscopic analysis of the sensory innervation of the mystacial pad. I. Innervation of vibrissal follicle-sinus complexes. *J Comp Neurol* **252**: 154–174.

Rice, F. L., Kinnman, E., Aldskogius, H., Johansson, O., Arvidsson, J. (1993) The innervation of the mystacial pad of the rat as revealed by PGP 9.5 immunofluorescence. *J Comp Neurol* **337**: 366–385.

Riddle, D. R., Purves, D. (1995) Individual variation and lateral asymmetry of the rat primary somatosensory cortex. *J Neurosci* **15**: 4184–4195.

Riva, C., Ross, B., Benedek, G. B. (1972) Laser Doppler measurements of blood flow in capillary tubes and retinal arteries. *Invest Ophthalmol* **11**: 936–944.

Rocamora, N., Welker, E., Pascual, M., Soriano, E. (1996) Upregulation of BDNF mRNA expression in the barrel cortex of adult mice after sensory stimulation. *J Neurosci* **16**: 4411–4419.

Rodgers, K. M., Benison, A. M., Barth, D. S. (2006) Two-dimensional coincidence detection in the vibrissa/barrel field. *J Neurophysiol* **96**: 1981–1990.

Roger, M., Cadusseau, J. (1984) Afferent connections of the nucleus posterior thalami in the rat, with some evolutionary and functional considerations. *J Hirnforsch* **25**: 473–485.

Rovainen, C. M., Woolsey, T. A., Blocher, N. C., Wang, D. B., Robinson, O. F. (1993) Blood flow in single surface arterioles and venules on the mouse somatosensory cortex measured with videomicroscopy, fluorescent dextrans, nonoccluding fluorescent beads, and computer-assisted image analysis. *J Cereb Blood Flow Metab* **13**: 359–371.

Rozas, C., Frank, H., Heynen, A. J., *et al.* (2001) Developmental inhibitory gate controls the relay of activity to the superficial layers of the visual cortex. *J Neurosci* **21**: 6791–6801.

Rumpel, S., Kattenstroth, G., Gottmann, K. (2004) Silent synapses in the immature visual cortex: layer-specific developmental regulation. *J Neurophysiol* **91**: 1097–1101.

Sakurada, O., Sokoloff, L., Jacquet, Y. F. (1978) Local cerebral glucose utilization following injection of beta-endorphin into periaqueductal gray matter in the rat. *Brain Res* **153**: 403–407.

Salin, P. A., Prince, D. A. (1996) Electrophysiological mapping of GABA$_A$ receptor-mediated inhibition in adult rat somatosensory cortex. *J Neurophysiol* **75**: 1589–1600.

Salminen, M., Meyer, B. I., Gruss, P. (1998) Efficient poly A trap approach allows the capture of genes specifically active in differentiated embryonic stem cells and in mouse embryos. *Dev Dyn* **212**: 326–333.

Sawtell, N. B., Frenkel, M. Y., Philpot, B. D., *et al.* (2003) NMDA receptor-dependent ocular dominance plasticity in adult visual cortex. *Neuron* **38**: 977–985.

Scheibel, M. E., Scheibel, A. B. (1967) Structural organization of nonspecific thalamic nuclei and their projection toward cortex. *Brain Res* **6**: 60–94.

Schlaggar, B. L., O'Leary, D. D. (1991) Potential of visual cortex to develop an array of functional units unique to somatosensory cortex. *Science* **252**: 1556–1560.

Schlaggar, B. L., O'Leary, D. D. (1994) Early development of the somatotopic map and barrel patterning in rat somatosensory cortex. *J Comp Neurol* **346**: 80–96.

Schlaggar, B. L., Fox, K., O'Leary, D. D. (1993) Postsynaptic control of plasticity in developing somatosensory cortex. *Nature* **364**: 623–626.

Schliebs, R., Walch, C., Stewart, M. G. (1989) Laminar pattern of cholinergic and adrenergic receptors in rat visual cortex using quantitative receptor autoradiography. *J Hirnforsch* **30**: 303–311.

Schubert, D., Staiger, J. F., Cho, N., *et al.* (2001) Layer-specific intracolumnar and transcolumnar functional connectivity of layer V pyramidal cells in rat barrel cortex. *J Neurosci* **21**: 3580–3592.

Schubert, D., Kotter, R., Zilles, K., Luhmann, H. J., Staiger, J. F. (2003) Cell type-specific circuits of cortical layer IV spiny neurons. *J Neurosci* **23**: 2961–2970.

Schubert, D., Kotter, R., Luhmann, H. J., Staiger, J. F. (2006b) Morphology, electrophysiology and functional input connectivity of pyramidal neurons characterizes a genuine layer Va in the primary somatosensory cortex. *Cereb Cortex* **16**: 223–236.

Schubert, V., Da Silva, J. S., Dotti, C. G. (2006a) Localized recruitment and activation of RhoA underlies dendritic spine morphology in a glutamate receptor-dependent manner. *J Cell Biol* **172**: 453–467.

Scott, B. B., Zaratin, P. F., Gilmartin, A. G., *et al.* (2005) TNF-alpha modulates angiopoietin-1 expression in rheumatoid synovial fibroblasts via the NF-kappa B signalling pathway. *Biochem Biophys Res Commun* **328**: 409–414.

Scott, H. L., Braud, S., Bannister, N. J., Isaac, J. T. (2007) Synaptic strength at the thalamocortical input to layer IV neonatal barrel cortex is regulated by protein kinase C. *Neuropharmacology* **52**: 185–192.

Seidenman, K. J., Steinberg, J. P., Huganir, R., Malinow, R. (2003) Glutamate receptor subunit 2 serine 880 phosphorylation modulates synaptic transmission and mediates plasticity in CA1 pyramidal cells. *J Neurosci* **23**: 9220–9228.

Senft, S. L., Woolsey, T. A. (1991) Growth of thalamic afferents into mouse barrel cortex. *Cereb Cortex* **1**: 308–335.

Shatz, C. J., Stryker, M. P. (1978) Ocular dominance in layer IV of the cat's visual cortex and the effects of monocular deprivation. *J Physiol* **281**: 267–283.

Shepherd, G. M., Pologruto, T. A., Svoboda, K. (2003) Circuit analysis of experience-dependent plasticity in the developing rat barrel cortex. *Neuron* **38**: 277–289.

Shepherd, G. M., Stepanyants, A., Bureau, I., Chklovskii, D., Svoboda, K. (2005) Geometric and functional organization of cortical circuits. *Nat Neurosci* **8**: 782–790.

Sherman, S. M., Guillery, R. W. (2002) The role of the thalamus in the flow of information to the cortex. *Philos Trans R Soc Lond B Biol Sci* **357**: 1695–1708.

Sheth, S. A., Nemoto, M., Guiou, M., *et al.* (2004) Columnar specificity of microvascular oxygenation and volume responses: implications for functional brain mapping. *J Neurosci* **24**: 634–641.

Shi, Y., Ethell, I. M. (2006) Integrins control dendritic spine plasticity in hippocampal neurons through NMDA receptor and $Ca^{2+}$/calmodulin-dependent protein kinase II-mediated actin reorganization. *J Neurosci* **26**: 1813–1822.

Shimegi, S., Ichikawa, T., Akasaki, T., Sato, H. (1999) Temporal characteristics of response integration evoked by multiple whisker stimulations in the barrel cortex of rats. *J Neurosci* **19**: 10164–10175.

Shimegi, S., Akasaki, T., Ichikawa, T., Sato, H. (2000) Physiological and anatomical organization of multiwhisker response interactions in the barrel cortex of rats. *J Neurosci* **20**: 6241–6248.

Shimogori, T., Grove, E. A. (2005) Fibroblast growth factor 8 regulates neocortical guidance of area-specific thalamic innervation. *J Neurosci* **25**: 6550–6560.

Shipley, M. T. (1974) Response characteristics of single units in the rat's trigeminal nuclei to vibrissa displacements. *J Neurophysiol* **37**: 73–90.

Shoykhet, M., Doherty, D., Simons, D. J. (2000) Coding of deflection velocity and amplitude by whisker primary afferent neurons: implications for higher level processing. *Somatosens Mot Res* **17**: 171–180.

Sieghart, W. (2000) Unraveling the function of GABA(A) receptor subtypes. *Trends Pharmacol Sci* **21**: 411–413.

Sik, A., Penttonen, M., Ylinen, A., Buzsaki, G. (1995) Hippocampal CA1 interneurons: an in vivo intracellular labeling study. *J Neurosci* **15**: 6651–6665.

Silva, A. C., Zhang, W., Williams, D. S., Koretsky, A. P. (1995) Multi-slice MRI of rat brain perfusion during amphetamine stimulation using arterial spin labeling. *Magn Reson Med* **33**: 209–214.

Silva, A. J., Stevens, C. F., Tonegawa, S., Wang, Y. (1992) Deficient hippocampal long-term potentiation in alpha-calcium-calmodulin kinase II mutant mice. *Science* **257**: 201–206.

Silver, R. A., Lubke, J., Sakmann, B., Feldmeyer, D. (2003) High-probability uniquantal transmission at excitatory synapses in barrel cortex. *Science* **302**: 1981–1984.

Simons, D. J. (1978) Response properties of vibrissa units in rat SI somatosensory neocortex. *J Neurophysiol* **41**: 798–820.

Simons, D. J. (1985) Temporal and spatial integration in the rat SI vibrissa cortex. *J Neurophysiol* **54**: 615–635.

Simons, D. J., Carvell, G. E. (1989) Thalamocortical response transformation in the rat vibrissa/barrel system. *J Neurophysiol* **61**: 311–330.

Simons, D. J., Land, P. W. (1987) Early experience of tactile stimulation influences organization of somatic sensory cortex. *Nature* **326**: 694–697.

Simons, D. J., Land, P. W. (1994) Neonatal whisker trimming produces greater effects in nondeprived than deprived thalamic barreloids. *J Neurophysiol* **72**: 1434–1437.

Simons, D. J., Woolsey, T. A. (1984) Morphology of Golgi–Cox-impregnated barrel neurons in rat SmI cortex. *J Comp Neurol* **230**: 119–132.

Simpson, K. L., Waterhouse, B. D., Lin, R. C. (2006) Characterization of neurochemically specific projections from the locus coeruleus with respect to somatosensory-related barrels. *Anat Rec A Discov Mol Cell Evol Biol* **288**: 166–173.

Sinclair, R. J., Burton, H. (1991) Tactile discrimination of gratings: psychophysical and neural correlates in human and monkey. *Somatosens Mot Res* **8**: 241–248.

Siucinska, E., Kossut, M. (2006) Short-term sensory learning does not alter parvalbumin neurons in the barrel cortex of adult mice: a double-labeling study. *Neuroscience* **138**: 715–724.

Sjostrom, P. J., Turrigiano, G. G., Nelson, S. B. (2003) Neocortical LTD via coincident activation of presynaptic NMDA and cannabinoid receptors. *Neuron* **39**: 641–654.

Sjostrom, P. J., Turrigiano, G. G., Nelson, S. B. (2004) Endocannabinoid-dependent neocortical layer-5 LTD in the absence of postsynaptic spiking. *J Neurophysiol* **92**: 3338–3343.

Skangiel-Kramska, J., Rajkowska, G., Kosmal, A., Kossut, M. (1992) The distribution of cholinergic muscarinic receptors in the dog frontal lobe. *J Chem Neuroanat* **5**: 391–398.

Sloper, J. J. (1972) Gap junctions between dendrites in the primate neocortex. *Brain Res* **44**: 641–646.

Solomon, J. H., Hartmann, M. J. (2006) Biomechanics: robotic whiskers used to sense features. *Nature* **443**: 525.

Somogyi, P., Tamas, G., Lujan, R., Buhl, E. H. (1998) Salient features of synaptic organisation in the cerebral cortex. *Brain Res Brain Res Rev* **26**: 113–135.

Son, H., Hawkins, R. D., Martin, K., *et al.* (1996) Long-term potentiation is reduced in mice that are doubly mutant in endothelial and neuronal nitric oxide synthase. *Cell* **87**: 1015–1023.

Staiger, J. F., Zilles, K., Freund, T. F. (1996) Distribution of GABAergic elements postsynaptic to ventroposteromedial thalamic projections in layer IV of rat barrel cortex. *Eur J Neurosci* **8**: 2273–2285.

Staiger, J. F., Kotter, R., Zilles, K., Luhmann, H. J. (2000) Laminar characteristics of functional connectivity in rat barrel cortex revealed by stimulation with caged-glutamate. *Neurosci Res* **37**: 49–58.

Staiger, J. F., Flagmeyer, I., Schubert, D., *et al.* (2004) Functional diversity of layer IV spiny neurons in rat somatosensory cortex: quantitative morphology of electrophysiologically characterized and biocytin labeled cells. *Cereb Cortex* **14**: 690–701.

Stanton, P. K., Sejnowski, T. J. (1989) Associative long-term depression in the hippocampus induced by hebbian covariance. *Nature* **339**: 215–218.

Steriade, M., Ropert, N., Kitsikis, A., Oaksen, G. (1981) *Ascending Activating Neuronal Networks in Midbrain Reticular Core and Related Rostral Systems*. New York: Raven Press.

Steriade, M., Deschenes, M., Domich, L., Mulle, C. (1985) Abolition of spindle oscillations in thalamic neurons disconnected from nucleus reticularis thalami. *J Neurophysiol* **54**: 1473–1497.

Stern, E. A., Maravall, M., Svoboda, K. (2001) Rapid development and plasticity of layer 2/3 maps in rat barrel cortex in vivo. *Neuron* **31**: 305–315.

Stern, M. D., Lappe, D. L., Bowen, P. D., *et al.* (1977) Continuous measurement of tissue blood flow by laser-Doppler spectroscopy. *Am J Physiol* **232**: H441–H448.

Stettler, D. D., Yamahachi, H., Li, W., Denk, W., Gilbert, C. D. (2006) Axons and synaptic boutons are highly dynamic in adult visual cortex. *Neuron* **49**: 877–887.

Storm-Mathisen, J., Leknes, A. K., Bore, A. T., *et al.* (1983) First visualization of glutamate and GABA in neurones by immunocytochemistry. *Nature* **301**: 517–520.

Stryker, M. P., Harris, W. A. (1986) Binocular impulse blockade prevents the formation of ocular dominance columns in cat visual cortex. *J Neurosci* **6**: 2117–2133.

Sugino, K., Hempel, C. M., Miller, M. N., *et al.* (2006) Molecular taxonomy of major neuronal classes in the adult mouse forebrain. *Nat Neurosci* **9**: 99–107.

Swadlow, H. A. (2003) Fast-spike interneurons and feedforward inhibition in awake sensory neocortex. *Cereb Cortex* **13**: 25–32.

Swadlow, H. A., Gusev, A. G. (2002) Receptive-field construction in cortical inhibitory interneurons. *Nat Neurosci* **5**: 403–404.

Szwed, M., Bagdasarian, K., Ahissar, E. (2003) Encoding of vibrissal active touch. *Neuron* **40**: 621–630.

Tabony, J. (1994) Morphological bifurcations involving reaction–diffusion processes during microtubule formation. *Science* **264**: 245–248.

Tailby, C., Wright, L. L., Metha, A. B., Calford, M. B. (2005) Activity-dependent maintenance and growth of dendrites in adult cortex. *Proc Natl Acad Sci USA* **102**: 4631–4636.

Takahashi, T., Svoboda, K., Malinow, R. (2003) Experience strengthening transmission by driving AMPA receptors into synapses. *Science* **299**: 1585–1588.

Tamas, G., Buhl, E. H., Lorincz, A., Somogyi, P. (2000) Proximally targeted GABAergic synapses and gap junctions synchronize cortical interneurons. *Nat Neurosci* **3**: 366–371.

Thomson, A. M., Bannister, A. P. (1999) Release-independent depression at pyramidal inputs onto specific cell targets: dual recordings in slices of rat cortex. *J Physiol* **519**(Pt 1): 57–70.

Thomson, A. M., Deuchars, J., West, D. C. (1993) Large, deep layer pyramid-pyramid single axon EPSPs in slices of rat motor cortex display paired pulse and frequency-dependent depression, mediated presynaptically and self-facilitation, mediated postsynaptically. *J Neurophysiol* **70**: 2354–2369.

Timofeeva, E., Merette, C., Emond, C., Lavallee, P., Deschenes, M. (2003) A map of angular tuning preference in thalamic barreloids. *J Neurosci* **23**: 10717–10723.

Timofeeva, E., Lavallee, P., Arsenault, D., Deschenes, M. (2004) Synthesis of multiwhisker-receptive fields in subcortical stations of the vibrissa system. *J Neurophysiol* **91**: 1510–1515.

Toledo-Rodriguez, M., Goodman, P., Illic, M., Wu, C., Markram, H. (2005) Neuropeptide and calcium-binding protein gene expression profiles predict neuronal anatomical type in the juvenile rat. *J Physiol* **567**: 401–413.

Trachtenberg, J. T., Chen, B. E., Knott, G. W., *et al.* (2002) Long-term in vivo imaging of experience-dependent synaptic plasticity in adult cortex. *Nature* **420**: 788–794.

Trageser, J. C., Keller, A. (2004) Reducing the uncertainty: gating of peripheral inputs by zona incerta. *J Neurosci* **24**: 8911–8915.

Traub, R. D., Contreras, D., Cunningham, M. O., *et al.* (2005) Single-column thalamocortical network model exhibiting gamma oscillations, sleep spindles, and epileptogenic bursts. *J Neurophysiol* **93**: 2194–2232.

Trettel, J., Levine, E. S. (2002) Cannabinoids depress inhibitory synaptic inputs received by layer 2/3 pyramidal neurons of the neocortex. *J Neurophysiol* **88**: 534–539.

Trettel, J., Fortin, D. A., Levine, E. S. (2004) Endocannabinoid signalling selectively targets perisomatic inhibitory inputs to pyramidal neurones in juvenile mouse neocortex. *J Physiol* **556**: 95–107.

Tsodyks, M. V., Markram, H. (1997) The neural code between neocortical pyramidal neurons depends on neurotransmitter release probability. *Proc Natl Acad Sci USA* **94**: 719–723.

Turing, A. M. (1990) The chemical basis of morphogenesis, 1953. *Bull Math Biol* **52**: 153–197; discussion 119–152. [Republication of the 1953 paper.]

Tyszkiewicz, J. P., Gu, Z., Wang, X., Cai, X., Yan, Z. (2004) Group II metabotropic glutamate receptors enhance NMDA receptor currents via a protein kinase C-dependent mechanism in pyramidal neurones of rat prefrontal cortex. *J Physiol* **554**: 765–777.

Ungerstedt, U. (1971) Stereotaxic mapping of the monoamine pathways in the rat brain. *Acta Physiol Scand Suppl* **367**: 1–48.

Urban, J., Kossut, M., Hess, G. (2002) Long-term depression and long-term potentiation in horizontal connections of the barrel cortex. *Eur J Neurosci* **16**: 1772–1776.

Valcanis, H., Tan, S. S. (2003) Layer specification of transplanted interneurons in developing mouse neocortex. *J Neurosci* **23**: 5113–5122.

Valverde, F. (1967) Apical dendritic spines of the visual cortex and light deprivation in the mouse. *Exp Brain Res* **3**: 337–352.

Valverde, F. (1971) Rate and extent of recovery from dark rearing in the visual cortex of the mouse. *Brain Res* **33**: 1–11.

Van der Loos, H. (1976) Neuronal circuitry and its development. *Prog Brain Res* **45**: 259–278.

Van der Loos, H., Woolsey, T. A. (1973) Somatosensory cortex: structural alterations following early injury to sense organs. *Science* **179**: 395–398.

Van der Loos, H., Welker, E., Dorfl, J., Rumo, G. (1986) Selective breeding for variations in patterns of mystacial vibrissae of mice. Bilaterally symmetrical strains derived from ICR stock. *J Hered* **77**: 66–82.

Veinante, P., Deschenes, M. (1999) Single- and multi-whisker channels in the ascending projections from the principal trigeminal nucleus in the rat. *J Neurosci* **19**: 5085–5095.

Veinante, P., Jacquin, M. F., Deschenes, M. (2000) Thalamic projections from the whisker-sensitive regions of the spinal trigeminal complex in the rat. *J Comp Neurol* **420**: 233–243.

Venance, L., Rozov, A., Blatow, M., *et al.* (2000) Connexin expression in electrically coupled postnatal rat brain neurons. *Proc Natl Acad Sci USA* **97**: 10260–10265.

Waite, P. M., Cragg, B. G. (1979) The effect of destroying the whisker follicles in mice on the sensory nerve, the thalamocortical radiation and cortical barrel development. *Proc R Soc Lond B Biol Sci* **204**: 41–55.

Waite, P. M., Cragg, B. G. (1982) The peripheral and central changes resulting from cutting or crushing the afferent nerve supply to the whiskers. *Proc R Soc Lond B Biol Sci* **214**: 191–211.

Waite, P. M., Jacquin, M. F. (1992) Dual innervation of the rat vibrissa: responses of trigeminal ganglion cells projecting through deep or superficial nerves. *J Comp Neurol* **322**: 233–245.

Waite, P. M., Taylor, P. K. (1978) Removal of whiskers in young rats causes functional changes in cerebral cortex. *Nature* **274**: 600–602.

Waite, P. M., Marotte, L. R., Mark, R. F. (1991) Development of whisker representation in the cortex of the tammar wallaby *Macropus eugenii*. *Brain Res Dev Brain Res* **58**: 35–41.

Waite, P. M., Li, L., Ashwell, K. W. (1992) Developmental and lesion induced cell death in the rat ventrobasal complex. *Neuroreport* **3**: 485–488.

Wall, P. D., Fitzgerald, M., Nussbaumer, J. C., Van der Loos, H., Devor, M. (1982) Somatotopic maps are disorganized in adult rodents treated neonatally with capsaicin. *Nature* **295**: 691–693.

Wallace, H., Fox, K. (1999a) The effect of vibrissa deprivation pattern on the form of plasticity induced in rat barrel cortex. *Somatosens Mot Res* **16**: 122–138.

Wallace, H., Fox, K. (1999b) Local cortical interactions determine the form of cortical plasticity. *J Neurobiol* **41**: 58–63.

Wallace, H., Glazewski, S., Liming, K., Fox, K. (2001) The role of cortical activity in experience-dependent potentiation and depression of sensory responses in rat barrel cortex. *J Neurosci* **21**: 3881–3894.

Walsh, C., Cepko, C. L. (1988) Clonally related cortical cells show several migration patterns. *Science* **241**: 1342–1345.

Wang, Y., Gupta, A., Toledo-Rodriguez, M., Wu, C. Z., Markram, H. (2002) Anatomical, physiological, molecular and circuit properties of nest basket cells in the developing somatosensory cortex. *Cereb Cortex* **12**: 395–410.

Wang, Y., Toledo-Rodriguez, M., Gupta, A., *et al.* (2004) Anatomical, physiological and molecular properties of Martinotti cells in the somatosensory cortex of the juvenile rat. *J Physiol* **561**: 65–90.

Watanabe, Y., Song, T., Sugimoto, K., *et al.* (2003) Post-synaptic density-95 promotes calcium/calmodulin-dependent protein kinase II-mediated Ser847 phosphorylation of neuronal nitric oxide synthase. *Biochem J* **372**: 465–471.

Watson, R. F., Abdel-Majid, R. M., Barnett, M. W., *et al.* (2006) Involvement of protein kinase A in patterning of the mouse somatosensory cortex. *J Neurosci* **26**: 5393–5401.

Wei, L., Rovainen, C. M., Woolsey, T. A. (1995) Ministrokes in rat barrel cortex. *Stroke* **26**: 1459–1462.

Wei, L., Erinjeri, J. P., Rovainen, C. M., Woolsey, T. A. (2001) Collateral growth and angiogenesis around cortical stroke. *Stroke* **32**: 2179–2184.

Welker, C. (1976) Receptive fields of barrels in the somatosensory neocortex of the rat. *J Comp Neurol* **166**: 173–189.

Welker, C., Woolsey, T. A. (1974) Structure of layer IV in the somatosensory neocortex of the rat: description and comparison with the mouse. *J Comp Neurol* **158**: 437–453.

Welker, E., Van der Loos, H. (1986) Quantitative correlation between barrel-field size and the sensory innervation of the whiskerpad: a comparative study in six strains of mice bred for different patterns of mystacial vibrissae. *J Neurosci* **6**: 3355–3373.

Welker, E., Hoogland, P. V., Van der Loos, H. (1988) Organization of feedback and feedforward projections of the barrel cortex: a PHA-L study in the mouse. *Exp Brain Res* **73**: 411–435.

Welker, E., Armstrong-James, M., Bronchti, G., *et al.* (1996) Altered sensory processing in the somatosensory cortex of the mouse mutant barrelless. *Science* **271**: 1864–1867.

Welker, W. I. (1964) Analysis of sniffing of the the albino rat. *Behaviour* **12**: 223–244.

Weller, W. L. (1972) Barrels in somatic sensory neocortex of the marsupial *Trichosurus vulpecula* (brush-tailed possum). *Brain Res* **43**: 11–24.

Whitaker, V. R., Cui, L., Miller, S., Yu, S. P., Wei, L. (2007) Whisker stimulation enhances angiogenesis in the barrel cortex following focal ischemia in mice. *J Cereb Blood Flow Metab* **27**: 57–68.

White, E. L. (1978) Identified neurons in mouse Sml cortex which are postsynaptic to thalamocortical axon terminals: a combined Golgi–electron microscopic and degeneration study. *J Comp Neurol* **181**: 627–661.

White, E. L., DeAmicis, R. A. (1977) Afferent and efferent projections of the region in mouse SmL cortex which contains the posteromedial barrel subfield. *J Comp Neurol* **175**: 455–482.

White, E. L., Hersch, S. M. (1982) A quantitative study of thalamocortical and other synapses involving the apical dendrites of corticothalamic projection cells in mouse SmI cortex. *J Neurocytol* **11**: 137–157.

White, E. L., Keller, A. (1987) Intrinsic circuitry involving the local axon collaterals of corticothalamic projection cells in mouse SmI cortex. *J Comp Neurol* **262**: 13–26.

White, E. L., Weinfeld, L., Lev, D. L. (1997) A survey of morphogenesis during the early postnatal period in PMBSF barrels of mouse SmI cortex with emphasis on barrel D4. *Somatosens Mot Res* **14**: 34–55.

Whitford, K. L., Dijkhuizen, P., Polleux, F., Ghosh, A. (2002) Molecular control of cortical dendrite development. *Annu Rev Neurosci* **25**: 127–149.

Wiesel, T. N., Hubel, D. H. (1965) Comparison of the effects of unilateral and bilateral eye closure on cortical unit responses in kittens. *J Neurophysiol* **28**: 1029–1040.

Wilent, W. B., Contreras, D. (2004) Synaptic responses to whisker deflections in rat barrel cortex as a function of cortical layer and stimulus intensity. *J Neurosci* **24**: 3985–3998.

Wilent, W. B., Contreras, D. (2005) Dynamics of excitation and inhibition underlying stimulus selectivity in rat somatosensory cortex. *Nat Neurosci* **8**: 1364–1370.

Wilson, R. I., Nicoll, R. A. (2002) Endocannabinoid signaling in the brain. *Science* **296**: 678–682.

Woolsey, T. A. (1990) *Peripheral Alteration and Somatosensory Development.* New York: John Wiley.

Woolsey, T. A., Van der Loos, H. (1970) The structural organization of layer IV in the somatosensory region (SI) of mouse cerebral cortex. The description of a cortical field composed of discrete cytoarchitectonic units. *Brain Res* **17**: 205–242.

Woolsey, T. A., Wann, J. R. (1976) Areal changes in mouse cortical barrels following vibrissal damage at different postnatal ages. *J Comp Neurol* **170**: 53–66.

Woolsey, T. A., Welker, C., Schwartz, R. H. (1975a) Comparative anatomical studies of the SmL face cortex with special reference to the occurrence of "barrels" in layer IV. *J Comp Neurol* **164**: 79–94.

Woolsey, T. A., Dierker, M. L., Wann, D. F. (1975b) Mouse SmI cortex: qualitative and quantitative classification of Golgi-impregnated barrel neurons. *Proc Natl Acad Sci USA* **72**: 2165–2169.

Woolsey, T. A., Rovainen, C. M., Cox, S. B., *et al.* (1996) Neuronal units linked to microvascular modules in cerebral cortex: response elements for imaging the brain. *Cereb Cortex* **6**: 647–660.

Woolston, D. C., La Londe, J. R., Gibson, J. M. (1982) Comparison of response properties of cerebellar- and thalamic-projecting interpolaris neurons. *J Neurophysiol* **48**: 160–173.

Wright, A. K., Norrie, L., Ingham, C. A., Hutton, E. A., Arbuthnott, G. W. (1999) Double anterograde tracing of outputs from adjacent "barrel columns" of rat somatosensory cortex. Neostriatal projection patterns and terminal ultrastructure. *Neuroscience* **88**: 119–133.

Wright, A. K., Norrie, L., Arbuthnott, G. W. (2000) Corticofugal axons from adjacent "barrel" columns of rat somatosensory cortex: cortical and thalamic terminal patterns. *J Anat* **196** (Pt 3): 379–390.

Xiang, Z., Huguenard, J. R., Prince, D. A. (1998) Cholinergic switching within neocortical inhibitory networks. *Science* **281**: 985–988.

Yamada, J., Furukawa, T., Ueno, S., Yamamoto, S., Fukuda, A. (2006) Molecular basis for the GABA$_A$ receptor-mediated tonic inhibition in rat somatosensory cortex. *Cereb Cortex* bhl087 (e-publication).

Yamakado, M. (1995) Remodelling in the array of cell aggregates in somatotopic representation of the facial vibrissae through the trigeminal sensory system of the mouse. *Neurosci Res* **23**: 399–413.

Yang, Y., Fischer, Q. S., Zhang, Y., *et al.* (2005) Reversible blockade of experience-dependent plasticity by calcineurin in mouse visual cortex. *Nat Neurosci* **8**: 791–796.

Yasuda, H., Barth, A. L., Stellwagen, D., Malenka, R. C. (2003) A developmental switch in the signaling cascades for LTP induction. *Nat Neurosci* **6**: 15–16.

Yin, J. C., Wallach, J. S., Del Vecchio, M., *et al.* (1994) Induction of a dominant negative *CREB* transgene specifically blocks long-term memory in *Drosophila. Cell* **79**: 49–58.

Young-Davies, C. L., Bennett-Clarke, C. A., Lane, R. D., Rhoades, R. W. (2000) Selective facilitation of the serotonin(1B) receptor causes disorganization of thalamic afferents and barrels in somatosensory cortex of rat. *J Comp Neurol* **425**: 130–138.

Yuste, R., Peinado, A., Katz, L. C. (1992) Neuronal domains in developing neocortex. *Science* **257**: 665–669.

Zhang, Z., Chopp, M. (2002) Vascular endothelial growth factor and angiopoietins in focal cerebral ischemia. *Trends Cardiovasc Med* **12**: 62–66.

Zhang, Z. W., Deschenes, M. (1997) Intracortical axonal projections of lamina VI cells of the primary somatosensory cortex in the rat: a single-cell labeling study. *J Neurosci* **17**: 6365–6379.

Zhu, J. J., Connors, B. W. (1999) Intrinsic firing patterns and whisker-evoked synaptic responses of neurons in the rat barrel cortex. *J Neurophysiol* **81**: 1171–1183.

Zhu, Y., Stornetta, R. L., Zhu, J. J. (2004) Chandelier cells control excessive cortical excitation: characteristics of whisker-evoked synaptic responses of layer 2/3 nonpyramidal and pyramidal neurons. *J Neurosci* **24**: 5101–5108.

Zucker, E., Welker, W. I. (1969) Coding of somatic sensory input by vibrissae neurons in the rat's trigeminal ganglion. *Brain Res* **12**: 138–156.

Zuo, Y., Yang, G., Kwon, E., Gan, W. B. (2005a) Long-term sensory deprivation prevents dendritic spine loss in primary somatosensory cortex. *Nature* **436**: 261–265.

Zuo, Y., Lin, A., Chang, P., Gan, W. B. (2005b) Development of long-term dendritic spine stability in diverse regions of cerebral cortex. *Neuron* **46**: 181–189.

# Index